Obsessive-Compulsive Disorder in Children and Adolescents

Obsessive-Compulsive Disorder in Children and Adolescents

Edited by

Judith L. Rapoport, M.D.

*Chief, Child Psychiatry Branch,
National Institute of Mental Health,
Bethesda, Maryland*

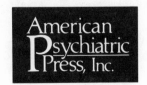

American
Psychiatric
Press, Inc.

1400 K Street, N.W.
Washington, DC 20005

Note: The authors have worked to ensure that all information in this book concerning drug dosages, schedules, and routes of administration is accurate as of the time of publication and consistent with standards set by the U.S. Food and Drug Administration and the general medical community. As medical research and practice advance, however, therapeutic standards may change. For this reason and because human and mechanical errors sometimes occur, we recommend that readers follow the advice of a physician who is directly involved in their care or the care of a members of their family.

Books published by the American Psychiatric Press, Inc., represent the views and opinions of the individual authors and do not necessarily represent the policies and opinions of the Press or the American Psychiatric Association.

Notice: Portions of this book were prepared by employees of the U.S. Government in their official capacity and, as such, are part of the public domain.

Library of Congress Cataloging-in-Publication Data
Obsessive-compulsive disorder in children and adolescents/edited by
   Judith L. Rapoport.—1st ed.
      p. cm.
   Includes bibliographies.
   ISBN 0-88048-282-6
   1. Obsessive-compulsive neurosis in children. 2. Obsessive-
compulsive neurosis in adolescence. I. Rapoport, Judith L.,
1933-   .

   [DNLM: 1. Obsessive-Compulsive Disorder—in adolescence.
2. Obsessive-Compulsive Disorder—in infancy & childhood. WM 176
01455]
RJ506.025027 1988
618.92′85′227—dc19
DNLM/DLC
for Library of Congress   88-24262
                                                       CIP

Contents

III. Associated Measures

IV. The Patients Speak

V. Treatment

VI. Theory and Research

VII. Summary

Contributors

Celia J. Bassaich, M.A.
Speech Pathology Unit, NINCDS

Carol Zaremba Berg, M.A.
Psychologist, Child Psychiatry Branch, NIMH

Nadine P. Connor, M.A.
Speech Pathology Unit, NINCDS

Christiane S. Cox, M.S.
Neuropsychology Section, NINCDS

Mark Davies, M.P.H.
New York State Psychiatric Institute, Columbia
    University, New York, New York

Martha B. Denckla, M.D.
Professor of Neurology and Pediatrics, Johns Hopkins
    University School of Medicine, Baltimore, Maryland

Paul Fedio, Ph.D.
Neuropsychology Section, NINCDS

Martine Flament, M.D.
Child Psychiatry Branch, NIMH

Martin S. Halpern
Rabbi, Shaare Tefila Synagogue, Silver Spring, Maryland

Barbara B. Keller, Ph.D.
Consultant, Child Psychiatry Branch, NIMH

Marge Lenane, M.S.W.
Child Psychiatry Branch, NIMH

Henrietta L. Leonard, M.D.
Clinical Research Fellow, Child Psychiatry Branch, NIMH

Christy L. Ludlow, Ph.D.
Speech Pathology Unit, NINCDS

Charles S. Mansueto, Ph.D.
Professor of Psychology, Bowie State University,
    Bowie, Maryland

Judith L. Rapoport, M.D.
Chief, Child Psychiatry Branch, NIMH

David Shaffer, M.D.
New York State Psychiatric Institute, Columbia
    University, New York, New York

Larry Suess, D.O.
Psychiatry Resident, Texas Technical University,
    El Paso, Texas

Susan E. Swedo, M.D.
Medical Staff Fellow, Child Psychiatry Branch, NIMH

Agnes Whitaker, M.D.
New York State Psychiatric Institute, Columbia
    University, New York, New York

Steven P. Wise, Ph.D.
Chief, Laboratory of Neurophysiology, NIMH

Richard P. Wolff, Ph.D.
Department of Psychiatry, Children's Hospital National
    Medical Center, Washington, D.C.

Section I

Introduction

Chapter 1

Introduction

Judith L. Rapoport, M.D.

Obsessive-compulsive disorder (OCD) is a strange sickness of ritual and doubt run wild. It can begin suddenly and is usually seen as a problem as soon as it begins. *Obsession* derives from the Latin *obsidere*, meaning to besiege; at its worst, this illness is truly a siege. When the thoughts and rituals are intense, one's work and home life disintegrate. This is a serious disease, very much more common than we ever thought. Astonishing as it seems, there may be more than 4 million people in the United States with this disorder. Perhaps one-third of these are children or adolescents. Obsessive-compulsive patients could be reading the same weird script. Senseless thoughts go over and over in their minds, appearing "out of the blue." Certain acts are repeated over and over again. For some, the thoughts are meaningless (just numbers, or a phrase); for others, they are highly charged ideas (e.g., "I have just killed someone"). Some patients are "checkers"; they check lights, doors, appliances, jobs completed 10, 20, or 100 times or repeat peculiar acts over and over again. Others spend hours producing unimportant symmetry. Shoelaces must be exactly even, eyebrows the same to a hair. Most commonly, patients are "washers"; they feel a need to wash over and over again. These problems have similar themes: you can't trust your ordinary good judgment or your

I thank Eleanor Finver for graciously typing and retyping this book, and Deborah Cheslow, M.A., for skilled assistance in the preparation of numerous tables and references.

own senses (which see no dirt, or know the door is locked). Although you "know" you have done nothing harmful, you must go on checking and counting. You can't dismiss the idea of washing; it keeps coming back, and you doubt yourself "Do I really know? I feel something is wrong." Underlying all manifestations of the disorder is the incredible intensity of the urge to wash or to check, or the salience of the thought. As one man told me, "When the thought comes, everything and anything else in my life takes second place!"

The disorder is not new. The first clear accounts go back more than 400 years and are found in the theological literature on scrupulosity (Chapter 18).

My own interest in OCD began during my initial training in general psychiatry. As is true with many psychiatrists, the first patient I saw in my first year of residency is still "with me." Salvatore was a 60-year-old laborer of Italian descent, a valued foreman, a good family man, and a churchgoer who had developed a compulsion to pick up small pieces of trash in his home and on the street. His house was crowded with bags full of trash from the street, which were stored in the halls and on the furniture. His wife's tears and threats to leave were without effect. Over a few months his habit became stronger. He was so unable to resist picking up trash that he could never make it to work. Hospitalization during the 1940s had led to psychosurgery. Prefrontal lobotomy "succeeded" dramatically in decreasing Salvatore's compulsive symptoms; unfortunately, as often happened with those early operations, he suffered disinhibiting personality changes from the surgery itself. Although Sal's disorder had been "cured," he remained disabled from this early and unsatisfactory treatment. His lucid account of the senselessness of his symptoms, whose severity had destroyed his normal life, and their sudden and complete relief with surgery haunted me. This disorder did not seem like other psychiatric disorders. It appeared more separated from the fabric of people's lives, as if some outside agent could suddenly appear and provoke the illness, and could just as suddenly disappear.

In 1974, while visiting colleagues in Stockholm, I learned of a new treatment for obsessions and compulsions: the drug clomipramine. Clomipramine had just been reported by Dr. Lopez-Ibor, a Spanish psychiatrist, to be helpful for obsessive-compulsive adult patients, and was now being tested systematically at the Karolinska Hospital. When I spoke with the patients on the ward, many of them reported that they had been ill since childhood. I saw that the Swedish group had no shortage of patients for their study and reasoned that if this group was so ill in childhood, then children with OCD must be worse all around.

At the National Institute of Mental Health (NIMH), the Child Psychiatry Branch has been studying OCD in children for more than 12 years. Much of the data in this book comes from our ongoing research project on childhood OCD, which is the largest prospective study of children and adolescents with this disorder to date.

At the NIMH, we have used our unique research setting to recruit and study adolescents with OCD. We could recruit patients from all over the country. Because clomipramine is not available in the United States (although it is available in more than 70 other countries), it was a timely research question to see whether clomipramine would help adolescents as it did adults. This would be important to know because treatment might be more effective early on in the disorder than after the disease had progressed for years. It was conceivable, although far from proven, that the prognosis might be altered with long-term care and early detection. Early treatment might also be able to stop the terrible immediate effect of the disorder on children's lives, and prevent the feelings of isolation, depression, and fear that fills each child's day.

There were a number of other compelling reasons to study OCD in childhood. The disorder occurs relatively frequently in children compared with other major psychiatric disorders such as depression, schizophrenia, or other anxiety disorders, which are far more frequent in adults. In contrast, from one-half to one-third of cases of OCD have their onset in childhood or adolescence. Despite this, there is surprisingly little known by most child psychiatrists, psychologists, or pediatricians about this disorder.

Developmentally, it is a commonplace speculation that OCD is an exaggeration of "normal" ritualistic behaviors, such as superstitions or normal developmental childhood rituals. In fact, when examined systematically, the pattern of childhood rituals and common superstitions differs radically from obsessive-compulsive symptomatology. Furthermore, our pediatric obsessive patients are *not* particularly superstitious and do *not* have exaggerated developmental patterns of ritualistic behaviors (Chapter 17).

Although it had been speculated that special timing and style of parenting early in childhood might induce a child to develop OCD, we have not detected any such pattern in how these children were raised, nor idiosyncrasies in toilet training or in other routines, that would account for their obsessional illness. On the other hand, it is clear that special problems are *created* by a child's having OCD. This book shares some experiences of parents who not only had this disorder themselves, but also had to deal with a child with the same problem (Chapters 8 and 9). Their firsthand stories are included to give a clinical richness that most accounts by child psychiatrists lack. Despite the frequency of OCD, many child psychiatrists have not seen, let alone treated, a case.

Since most child psychiatrists lack clinical experience with OCD, one section of this book deals with firsthand accounts of these children at follow-up. Included in these accounts are their ways of coming to terms with the disorder and learning to live with parts that treatment couldn't help (Chapter 10). A great deal of what we know about the disorder is based on accounts like these from children and their parents. For the most part, these are likable "normal" kids. The uniquely alien quality of these compulsions and obsessions contrasts with the "voluntary" nature of the symptoms—supporting the complexity of the concept of "will." Obsessive-compulsive patients frequently describe an inability to "know" the door is locked, even though they remember checking it 50 times. This suggests a psychological score of "knowing," perhaps biologically determined, that is disturbed in OCD (see Chapter 19).

Because the NIMH study comprises the largest systematically examined group of children with OCD to date, we have included descriptive accounts of psychological, neuropsychological, and neurological examination of these patients. It appears that subtle neuropsychological dysfunction is more easily observed in a pediatric population (Chapters 5, 6, and 7).

After just a year into our research, we were getting calls every week from families of children, and from adults with OCD. We had previously had more calls about valid pediatric cases than we had expected could be found in the entire Washington, DC, area. In collaboration with colleagues from Columbia (the New York State Psychiatric Institute), we then surveyed more than 5,000 students in high schools in a county school system. All of the children in school on a particular day filled out a questionnaire about disturbing habits or thoughts. The results were startling. In these "ordinary" schoolchildren, our first impression was confirmed. There were at least 20 cases of OCD. The rate of 1 in 250 in the population means that perhaps 1 million children or adolescents in this country have this problem. Very few have ever asked for help, or have known that it was available; secretiveness appears intrinsic to the disorder (see Chapters 2 and 15).

We do not yet know the boundaries of this problem. We have seen people with odd "habits" who do not have the disorder. One girl, for example, would get up at 6 a.m. every Sunday to spend 3 hours washing the walls of her room. She certainly knew this was odd, but just felt that she "had to do it" and didn't really know why. She said the washing had started quite suddenly about a year before. We could not give her any psychiatric diagnosis because she did not seem very sick and was, for the most part, quite happy. We are puzzled by obsessional features and do not know if they are part of a disease or if they are quirks without clinical significance.

It is too simple to frame this question as just that of the relationship between OCD and compulsive personality. When we examine developmental patterns we are impressed by how a mild circumscribed disorder will, at a later time, reemerge in the form of compulsive personality. Although some of our patients have a compulsive personality as well as OCD, it is clear that most do not. We believe that the strong association seen in adult samples is more probably the influence of the chronic disease.

We also wonder about a group of patients with a great many habits whom we got to know as our "super normals." These children had every minute of their day scheduled. They were on every team and in every club, volunteer, or community group; they also took exercise and music classes. They were good students with very high ambitions, driven, and concerned about the enormous responsibilities they had set for themselves. Extremely organized, neat, and careful, they had answered yes to an unusually high number of questions in our obsessional questionnaire. Yet they felt that their habits were useful, and in no way interfered with their lives. If they had a complaint, it was that they might not meet all their obligations every week of the year. We have no idea if these are simply outstandingly ambitious young people who grow up to achieve a great deal. On the other hand, they might eventually be seen as having obsessional personalities. We are following their lives to find out (Chapter 15).

Despite the interest that individual cases with the disorder have generated over the years, less attention has been paid to treatment. Until about 15 years ago, the recommended treatment was psychotherapy or psychoanalysis. It is ironic that the disorder that best illustrates many key analytic principles should, in its severest form, fail to respond to analytic treatment. Until recently, there were few alternatives, even though follow-up studies with adults did not even hint at advantage for this treatment. At this time, systematic study has shown two newer treatments to be effective: behavior modification and drug treatment with clomipramine.

Behavior therapists have carried out the most extensive treatment research of anyone interested in this disorder. They have paid particular attention to how long their treatments last, and whether regular meetings with the behavior therapist are necessary. They have compared behavioral techniques to see just which are the most useful. Some are much better than others. For example, relaxation alone does not seem to help very much, whereas exposure with response prevention seems the optimal behavior treatment. This technique involves deliberately being in contact with the provoking stimulus, for example dirt or an unlocked door, while deliberately not washing or not checking despite heightened anxiety. Although the technique is initially stressful, follow-up studies have shown that improvement may last for years, or require only minimal "booster" treatments (Chapter 11). The response to behavioral treatment and the biological models of central nervous system dysfunction in OCD have yet to be reconciled.

Behavioral treatment of OCD was pioneered with adult patients during the 1970s (Chapters 11 and 12). Although there is almost no information on treatment of children with this disorder, the marked similarity of presentation in childhood would suggest that behavior therapy should be equally effective with pediatric populations.

Because there is little information on behavioral treatment with younger subjects, we have included a detailed case report to give more depth and "flavor" of work in this area than otherwise would be given. It is likely that exposure with response prevention is the treatment of choice in childhood OCD. It is also likely that individual modification of "technique" will be needed, as occurred with Daniel's treatment (Chapter 12).

Clomipramine is an antidepressant manufactured by CIBA-Geigy Pharmaceuticals that has been used for years to treat depression. Only in the past 15 years has it been recognized as also helpful for OCD (Chapter 13). Controlled trials have shown that the drug is superior to placebo and, most recently, superior to other antidepressants. There is now evidence that at least two other drugs—fluvoxamine and fluoxetine—are also effective in OCD. Clomipramine has excited a great deal of clinical and public interest. This drug does not exert its antiobsessional effect via its antidepressant action, even though it is an excellent antidepressant. Existing data support down-regulation of the serotonin system, although evidence is far from conclusive. An understanding of how clomipramine works will be a major clue to understanding the pathophysiology of OCD, of how the brain provides (releases) rituals of this complex and fascinating disorder. Demonstration of a chemical basis for the complex patterns of guilt, will, danger, cleanliness, and self-control in OCD could provide a biological model for behavior at a level of complexity we never dreamed possible.

A 2- to 5-year follow-up of our patients has shown the chronicity of the disorder for adolescents. For those who remain ill, depression is a major risk. A minority of our teenage patients seem to have "just gotten over it." Anecdotally, some report that they created a "do-it-yourself" behavioral treatment program (Chapter 11). That is, they had forced themselves to endure partly closed doors, dirt, thoughts, or whatever triggered their doubting, checking, or avoidance behavior and had not let themselves behave abnormally. Although they described this as "just getting over it," their stories sound more like a systematic behavioral treatment without a behavior therapist. This has not worked for everyone, but it strengthens the claim of behavioral psychologists that this should be tried. Follow-up studies in adults suggest that half of the obsessional patients continue to have problems. Most patients with OCD had no treatment and all of these studies were done before the newer treatments—behavior modification or clomipramine—were used. Despite new optimism, however, our own follow-up data are disappointing: few of our patients recovered (Chapter 2). The long-term efficacy of clomipramine has yet to be demonstrated.

Patients and their parents have found meeting others with the same problems to be extremely helpful. The patient group movement is not new in psychiatry. Because OCD is often "hidden," both because of the nature of the symptoms and the secretiveness of many patients, obsessive patients are not naturally drawn to patient support groups. The disorder has not been recognized frequently enough in most communities for such groups to be practicable. This will probably change. Clinicians should put patients with OCD in touch with one another. As clinicians develop greater sensitivity to the diagnosis and as greater awareness is acquired on the part of the patients that they can benefit from treatment, support groups for OCD will become more common.

This book was inspired by the recognition that OCD is more common in childhood than had been thought, by the availability of new treatments, and by new biological findings. The relative lack of complicating factors; the ability to obtain more firsthand observational data on the families, environments, and premorbid functioning; and the opportunities for early treatment are compelling reasons for further research with pediatric populations.

Researchers can learn about a biology of ritual, of will, and possibly a biology of knowledge. We hope this book will lead clinicians to recognize, study, and treat children with this disorder. As Aubrey Lewis observed in 1936, the problems of obsessional illness "cover so wide a field, that it is difficult to examine them without also examining the nature of man" (p. 325).

Reference

Lewis A: Problems of obsessional illness. Proceedings of the Royal Society of Medicine 29:325–336, 1936

Section II

Diagnosis

Chapter 2

Phenomenology and Differential Diagnosis of Obsessive-Compulsive Disorder in Children and Adolescents

Susan E. Swedo, M.D.
Judith L. Rapoport, M.D.

Obsessive-compulsive disorder (OCD) is not familiar to most child psychiatrists, even though classic descriptions of the disorder often featured cases with childhood presentation. This review of the diagnosis, phenomenology, and clinical course of the disorder in childhood covers the relevant literature, and then summarizes data from the National Institute of Mental Health (NIMH) cohort.

Pierre Janet (1859–1947) is often cited as developing our modern description of OCD. Although primarily concerned with adults, Janet (1903) described a 5-year-old with typical symptoms. Janet's descriptions seem particularly valid for pediatric subjects. Unlike hysterics, who do not know what troubles them, Janet stressed that obsessional patients may be too embarrassed or constrained to report their feelings, but know exactly what is wrong. "It is fancied crimes, sacrilegious thoughts, sexual perversities which the patient fears are about to be acted upon. The attacks are typically filled with events of the common life" (p. 17). "No reassuring satisfies: the patient must be forever verifying his honesty, cleanliness, sanity, perceptions, and what he did last." Janet was struck by the abnormality of thinking, a "heightening" of reasoning, comparing, correcting, and remembering.

He noted a "mania for interrogation, research, rumination, recall." Observing that these mental operations take on an almost independent life, without practical end or closure, he described them as an "arduous rethinking of the obvious."

Janet (1903) felt that a failure of cognitive abilities, a paralysis of certain functions, produced these symptoms. The functional disturbance in "psychasthenia" (a concept that combined anxiety and obsessive-compulsive symptoms) affected one of the highest and most complex of human functions: the ability to grasp and work with current reality. However, Janet could not reconcile Sherington, Head, and Jackson's notions that whenever there is disturbance of higher functions, simpler responses and lower levels of functioning are released. In OCD he observed a serious disturbance of high-level function with no apparent "low-level" function released. Janet likened obsessional thoughts to "mental tics." The patient was conscious of their existence, but had lost voluntary control over these thoughts. Only minor additions were necessary to capture the clinical characteristics of pediatric obsessive-compulsive populations.

Returning to the child psychiatric literature, Leo Kanner's classic textbook (1935) reviewed the older, primarily German reports on childhood OCD and stressed the social isolation of these children and their "constricted" premorbid personalities, making the important observation that the families became overinvolved with the rituals of the child. This overinvolvement of the parents is a salient difference between the pediatric and adult cases.

Favoring a psychological interpretation, Kanner (1962) stated that the children have been reared with an "overdose of parental perfectionism." The children are taught what is "right" and to strictly avoid "wrong." Kanner also recorded the children's heroic efforts to "reason things out" and to "think of something else" in order to deal with their illness. He too noted the resemblance of some of the "compulsive" movements to tics, and probably was describing mixed cases of Tourette's syndrome and OCD, whose eye blinking and head shaking were hard to distinguish from compulsive rituals.

Berman (1942) described four cases of childhood OCD having symptoms identical to the profiles found in adults (sexual thoughts, counting, fear parent might be killed, and doubts).

Louise Despert's (1955) superb paper, "Differential diagnosis between obsessive-compulsive neurosis and schizophrenia in children," has been largely overlooked, probably due to its publication as a book chapter. Despert presented 401 consecutive cases "from the author's files." Of these, no fewer than 68 cases, all examined personally by Despert, received the diagnosis of obsessive-compulsive neurosis with varying degrees of severity. Males outnumbered females by more than

3:1. Case vignettes illustrated two key points: (a) the child's acute awareness of the abnormality and the undesirability of the symptoms, and (b) the fact that the treating psychotherapist may not be told of the disorder while other (often secondary) symptoms, such as anxiety or depression, are brought forward for treatment.

Freud never described childhood causes of obsessional neurosis per se, but stressed retrospective recall of obsessional behavior in childhood (Freud 1958/1955, 1909/1955, 1913/1950). Freud's theories of pregenital sexual organization as etiological in the "choice" of obsessional neurosis have been particularly stressed, but his formulations are interspersed with speculation about the strong "constitutional" influence (heredity was stressed) on the choice of these symptoms. Freud considered several alternate etiologic formulations and noted the particular difficulty of analyzing obsessive subjects (1913/1950).

Anna Freud (1965) pointed out a crucial difference in the clinical picture of childhood cases:

> While in adults, the individual neurotic symptom usually forms part of a genetically related personality structure, this is not so with children. In children, symptoms occur just as often in isolation, or are coupled with other symptoms and personality traits of a different nature and unrelated origin. Even well defined obsessional symptoms such as bedtime ceremonials or counting compulsions are found in children with otherwise uncontrolled, restless impulsive personalities. . . . (p. 151)

Similarly, Sandler and Joffe (1965) stressed the *variety* of clinical settings in which obsessive-compulsive symptoms appear in childhood.

Judd's (1965) descriptive report of 5 obsessive children, the total population from an inpatient chart survey of 425 childhood psychiatric cases, found premorbid normality and no striking stressful or stringent parental practices.

In his book *Obsessive Children*, Adams (1973) reported a series of 49 cases (39 boys), all 15 years of age or younger. He found punitive bowel training and precipitating events relatively uncommon. Interestingly, aggression toward parents was common in his sample. Adams' informative book is limited, as he himself noted, by its retrospective nature, somewhat unique categorization, and collection from various sites. Nevertheless, the general agreement between his, Judd's (1965), and the prospective NIMH study is striking. Males outnumber females and, in some cases, very early onset (by age 3) is documented.

More recently, Hollingsworth et al. (1980) reported 17 cases (13 male) in a retrospective examination of more than 8,000 clinical records, inpatients and outpatients combined. In addition to male preponderance, there were frequently associated medical disturbances, and poor outcome. Ten cases subsequently were contacted; of these, 7 still suffered from obsessive-compulsive symptoms. Hollingsworth et al. felt the obsessive symptoms were probably defenses against stressful life circumstances.

The NIMH Sample

The NIMH sample of more than 70 children with severe primary OCD is the largest systematically studied group of cases to date. Many earlier clinical observations have been replicated. For example, very early onset in a few cases (before age 3) has been validated by family informants. Symptom pattern (see case illustrations) are strikingly similar to those in adults, with the major difference being sex distribution; in childhood, males outnumber females by more than 2:1.

The early age of onset and prospective nature of the study offers several advantages. Data on early functioning are simpler to collect; early records, developmental history, and interviews with family members are relatively easy to obtain; and fewer complicating disorders and learned behavior patterns confound observations. Despite these advantages, the diagnosis of OCD can be difficult due to the patients' secrecy and the clinicians' lack of familiarity with the disorder.

Presenting Symptoms

Children initially hide their rituals, often disguising hand washing as more frequent voiding, or "scheduling" ritualization for private time. On the average, children have been performing rituals for 4 to 6 months before their parents became aware of the problem. Teachers and peers (like the adult obsessive's employer and co-workers) are unaware of the problem because of the child's partial control.

Parents are baffled by the seemingly willful control, seeing their child suppress rituals at school or with friends, but "having" to do them at home. The children maintain that they expend enormous amounts of effort "controlling" their behaviors in public and have to "let go" when at home. As the illness progresses in severity, the patient is no longer able to resist ritualizing in public.

Parents report daily 3-hour showers, 2 hours checking the door locks, waking them several times each night to recheck, and so on, while the child may deny that a problem exists. Despite this, if OCD is suspected, it is usually easy to ascertain—through family informants combined with interviews with the child—the nature of the compulsive rituals, the degree of interference in the patient's life, and the degrees to which resistance is utilized and is effective.

Interviewers who indicate both an understanding of the child's inability to control his or her "habits" and that they know the child isn't "crazy" will usually find a bright, curious child ready to form an initially rather intellectual alliance. Helping older children become shrewd observers and reporters of their symptoms and getting them curious about the nature of their mysterious disorder can prove supportive in itself. Young children respond to the analogy between obsessive thoughts and "hiccups of the brain."

Diagnostic Criteria

The *Diagnostic and Statistical Manual of Mental Disorders* (DSM-III) (American Psychiatric Association 1980) criteria for the diagnosis of OCD were used for inclusion in the sample. They are: (a) the obsessions or compulsions are present, (b) the obsessions or compulsions are a significant source of distress to the individual or interfere with social or role functioning, and (c) the obsessions or compulsions are not due to another mental disorder, such as Tourette's disorder, schizophrenia, major depression, or organic mental disorder.

With DSM-III-R (American Psychiatric Association 1987), the diagnosis of OCD can now be made in the presence of other Axis I diagnoses, such as schizophrenia, anorexia, and major depression. The NIMH sample, however, excluded subjects with the other Axis I disorders listed above.

DSM-III-R also defines the extent of the impairment necessary for diagnosis. The obsessions or compulsions "cause marked distress, are time-consuming (take more than an hour a day), or interfere with occupational functioning or with usual social activities or relationships with others" (p. 247). All of our cases would meet these levels of impairment.

In the NIMH patient sample, the mean age at onset was 10.2 years, with 7 of the patients having onset at less than 7 years of age.

As shown in Figure 1, males typically begin earlier than females, with mean age of onset for males 9.8 years and for females 11.0 years. The male:female ratio in the NIMH study sample changes with age, as the earlier the age of onset, the more striking is male predominance. Because the disparity in sex distribution is so striking, early onset patients may present a different disease.

A positive family history of OCD is relatively common, occurring in about 20 percent of our series. Father/son pairs predominate ($N = 10$), but two mother/son pairs, two mother/daughter pairs, and

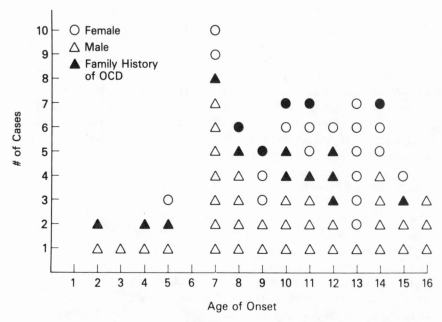

Figure 1. Sex, age of onset, and family history of OCD in NIMH childhood/adolescent OCD sample ($N = 70$).

three father/daughter pairs have also been seen. Three of the 7 "early onset" group have an affected parent.

Differential Diagnosis

The differential diagnosis includes psychotic depression, anorexia/bulimia, autism, Tourette's syndrome, schizophrenia, and phobias, which are each considered briefly.

Psychotic Depression.   Psychotic depression is very rare in childhood. When present, depression is not described as egodystonic and thereby distinguishable from OCD (although young children have trouble identifying thoughts and behaviors as egodystonic). Temporal relationships may also provide a clue; the compulsive behaviors would follow the onset of depression in psychotic depression but precede (secondary) depression in OCD.

Anorexia and Bulimia.   Adult women with OCD have an increased incidence (15 percent) of prior anorexia (Kasvikis et al., in press). The anorexic patient's consuming concern with caloric intake, exercise, and food bears some resemblance to an obsession; washing, checking, and counting rituals are reported. There has been no systematic study of obsessive-compulsive features and bulimia, but such an association is probable (Whitaker, personal communication, August 1988).

The recent report of clomipramine's efficacy in anorexia nervosa (Crisp et al. 1987) and the increased incidence of a history of anorexia in obsessive-compulsive patients makes this relationship intriguing.

Two male patients with OCD presented to the NIMH study with significant weight loss and histories of ritualistic exercising. This weight loss was greater than 25 percent of expected body weight and was secondary to excessive caloric expenditure. The patients had normal body images, however, and easily regained the lost weight. They engaged in hours of highly ritualized exercise daily. One boy spent most of each day lifting weights and doing sit-ups and push-ups. He felt compelled to exercise, repeating exercises until he could do them "perfectly." His exercise routine was time-consuming, leaving little time to eat. He was able to describe his rituals as irrational and undesirable and recognized he was too thin, but was unable to resist the compulsion to exercise.

Patients with OCD obsessed with contamination fears may be unable to eat; in severe cases, almost all food is "contaminated."

Autism. Obsessive-compulsive rituals may superficially resemble the stereotypies seen in autism, but stereotypies of autism are simpler in form than OCD rituals, which are frequently well organized and complex. Ego-dystonicity is a major distinguishing feature as the obsessive patient feels compelled to perform these rituals despite knowing that the ritual is useless and time consuming. In autism, the rituals seem reassuring and lack ego-dystonicity. Other features of autism, such as peculiar speech patterns and severely impaired interpersonal relationships, are not seen in OCD.

Tourette's syndrome. Patients with Tourette's syndrome (TS) frequently have obsessive-compulsive features (Frankel et al. 1986) and obsessive-compulsive patients have an increased incidence of simple motor tics (Adams 1973). The differential diagnosis depends on the predominating symptoms (Green and Pitman 1986). In general, obsessive-compulsive patients have more complex ritualistic compulsions. Both OCD and Tourette's syndrome have a fluctuating course and include partial voluntary control of symptoms. We have seen a number of atypical cases that defy classification, for whom neither diagnosis was quite appropriate because the cases were "transitional" between the two conditions. In the authors' experience, Tourette's patients are more likely to have isolated obsessive-compulsive symptoms rather than the full disorder. Washing is relatively infrequent while touching rituals are relatively common.

Schizophrenia. Insel and Akiskal (1986) suggested that OCD and schizophrenia may coexist. In addition, they speculate that obsessive-compulsive patients exhibit a transient, reactive, affective or paranoid psychosis. Because patients may fall anywhere along a hypothetical insight continuum, some patients would best fit a diagnosis of obsessive-compulsive psychosis.

DSM-III-R allows the concomitant diagnosis of OCD and psychosis. In the NIMH follow-up study (described in the last section of this chapter), 1 patient out of 27 for whom follow-up information was available was subsequently diagnosed as psychotic. In retrospect, it is unclear whether the initial presentation represented pure OCD or whether there were psychotic features at that time.

To obtain a pure culture of obsessive-compulsive patients for study at the NIMH, it has been necessary to exclude those patients with obsessive thoughts or compulsive rituals who evidence psychotic processes. Differentiation has relied on careful history, including insight of the source of the obsessive thoughts (Is it a thought inside your head or a voice? Is someone telling you to do these things?).

Phobias. Phobias are particularly difficult to differentiate; anxiety tension and anxiety generated by obsessions and by phobics' feared objects can be indistinguishable. The content of the obsessions and the phobias may differ, however. Phobias involve fears such as of closed spaces, flying, and heights, whereas obsessions more often center around fears of contamination or of harm coming to oneself or others. Most important, phobics are usually symptom free when not in confrontation with the feared object, whereas distance does not afford the obsessive-compulsive patient any relief.

Representative Cases

Obsessions

Most obsessive thoughts focus on fears: fear of harm, illness, or death; fear of contamination; fear of doing wrong or having done wrong.

The content of the obsessions in our pediatric series closely parallels that found for adults, as shown in Table 1. Some defy categorization, such as a morbid preoccupation with "dumb people," "bad numbers," or a fear of vomiting. Obsessions about numbers are par-

Table 1. Major presenting symptoms for 70 consecutive child and adolescent cases with primary obsessive-compulsive disorder

Symptom	Reported Symptom at Initial Interview	
	N	%
Obsessions		
Concern with dirt, germs, or environmental toxins	28	40
Something terrible happening (fire, death/illness of self or loved one, etc.)	17	24
Symmetry, order, or exactness	12	17
Scrupulosity (religious obsessions)	9	13
Concern or disgust with bodily wastes or secretions (urine, stool, saliva)	6	8
Lucky/unlucky numbers	6	8
Forbidden, aggressive, or perverse sexual thoughts, images, or impulses	3	4
Fear might harm others/self	3	4
Concern with household items	2	3
Intrusive nonsense sounds, words, or music	1	1
Compulsions		
Excessive or ritualized hand washing, showering, bathing, toothbrushing, or grooming	60	85
Repeating rituals (going in/out door, up/down from chair, etc.)	36	51
Checking (doors, locks, stove, appliances, emergency brake on car, paper route, homework, etc.)	32	46
Rituals to remove contact with contaminants	16	23
Touching	14	20
Measures to prevent harm to self or others	11	16
Ordering/arranging	12	17
Counting	13	18
Hoarding/collecting rituals	8	11
Rituals of cleaning household or inanimate objects	4	6
Miscellaneous rituals (e.g., writing, moving, speaking)	18	26

Note. Obsessions or compulsions are totaled; total exceeds 56.

ticularly common among young boys. They describe "safe" numbers, "bad" numbers, having to count, and having to repeat things a certain number of times—significantly interfering with school functioning as the child gets "stuck." The content of obsessions are frequently kept secret.

Fear of harm, illness, or death. For young children and early adolescents, fear of harm is by far the most frequent obsession, usually manifest as concern over their own safety or their parents' safety. Obsessions about death by poisoning, sharp objects, or germs are common. They may fear catastrophic events. Several young boys have become obsessed with tornadoes and developed exhaustive weather checking rituals.

> **Case 1.** A 14-year-old boy, since age 6, had a series of obsessive thoughts concerning harm to self or others. Initially, he was obsessed with thoughts of destructive tornadoes. He had seen a TV documentary on tornadoes in which an entire town had been destroyed, and several people were killed. Around that time, he had also watched the beginning of *The Wizard of Oz* and had seen Dorothy swept from her family by the twister. (He can't remember their reunion at the end of the film and is uncertain whether he ever saw the ending.) His concern about tornadoes was manifested in checking rituals. He would go to the window and check that the sky was clear, or repeatedly ask his mother if there were any tornado warnings. He struggled to master this obsession through an interest in meteorology. At age 6½, he could identify clouds as cirrus or cumulus, and could read the radar weather maps on TV.
>
> Over the next few years, his obsession shifted to concern about power lines and electrocution. In place of the weather, he became expert at currents, resistance, electrical accidents, and safety. His checking rituals now revolved around electrical outlets and light switches, electrical parts of the car and batteries, and power lines. Initially, he would spend hours riding his bike along the base of a high-tension power line near his home to "check that the posts were strong enough." Later, he began to avoid all power lines and developed a lengthy, circuitous route to school that detoured all above-ground power lines and transformers.
>
> Concomitant with these obsessions, the patient suffered from a generalized fear of harm coming to himself or his family. This required extensive "protective" ritualization to keep his mother and father safe, to protect himself and his brother. Particularly at times of separation, such as bedtime, leaving for school, or his parents' departure for work, he would be compelled to repeat actions *perfectly* or to check repetitively. When asked how many times he would have to repeat an action, the patient replied, "It depends. The number isn't always the same. I just have to do it right." When asked how he knew when it was right, he replied, "I don't know. It just *feels* right."
>
> As he entered puberty, his obsessional content shifted from fear of harm to his family, to exclusive concern for harm to himself. He was obsessively concerned about dying, and felt that he was dying or was about to die. He feared poisoning from germs and chemicals. In response to the concern about germs, he began to wash his hands compulsively,

refused to eat any chips if someone else had had their hand in the bag first, and drank lots of water to flush out the poisons from his body. He felt compelled to check the house for dangerous chemicals, as well as to vacuum the house daily to remove toxic dust.

He also began to have obsessive thoughts about intentionally hurting himself. He was clearly able to separate the thoughts from suicidal ideation, but was concerned that he could sit on his shirttail and strangle himself or take too big a bite of food and choke. The patient found these obsessions especially distressing and became quite depressed in response. Suppose he weren't careful enough and he actually did kill himself? Killing himself would be wrong and he would go to hell. On the other hand, he occasionally had volitional thoughts of suicide, particularly as his secondary depression deepened, and that proved he was evil. At this point, his "fear of harming himself" continued, and was joined by obsessive guilt over "evil actions."

Fear of contamination. Contamination fears typically consist of concern with germs, dirt, ink or paint, and excrements. Recently, AIDS obsessions have become quite common, and for several patients, overriding.

> **Case 2.** A 15-year-old boy, after hearing of Rock Hudson's death, began having obsessive fears that his homosexual thoughts would cause him to die of AIDS. He accepted this as irrational, but began spitting in an effort to cleanse his mouth. He had the recurrent obsessive images of a penis injecting the AIDS virus into his mouth and would spit 50 or more times per hour.

> **Case 3.** A 16-year-old girl developed an AIDS obsession after picking up a wrapped, sterile hypodermic needle from the ground behind a doctor's office. Later that day, she became obsessed with the thought that the needle had been used by a drug addict and was contaminated with AIDS. She washed her hands repeatedly to clean them of the virus. Her contamination obsession later shifted from AIDS to rabies (after seeing a frothing dog) and eventually to less specific germ and dirt contamination fears. In response to these obsessions, she had washed so excessively that her arms were permanently scarred.

While usually contamination fears lead to excessive washing, some patients avoid washing and become slovenly. Even those who do wash are often sloppy in other areas of grooming. Red, chapped hands from excessive hand washing are accompanied by untied shoes (as their shoes are contaminated), messy clothes (they were unable to change), greasy hair, or a dirty face.

The baffling inconsistencies raise fundamental questions about the conceptual framework behind obsessions, and suggest discontinuity between state and trait.

Compulsions

As shown in Table 1, the children's rituals are strikingly similar to the adults. Washing/cleaning rituals are by far the most common, but repeating, ordering, and counting are often seen. Other compulsive behaviors that are not performed as rituals include obsessive slowness and hoarding.

Washing/cleaning rituals.   Most of the NIMH patients either presented with washing rituals or had evolved to washing or cleaning rituals at some point in their illness, most commonly hand washing. Patients feel compelled to wash extensively and precisely for minutes to hours each time, or to wash less exhaustively, but more frequently, up to 150 times per day. The washing interferes significantly with getting to school or to bed on time because it is so time consuming.

In two cases, parents had to shut off the water to the house to get the child to leave the shower stall. In another, the patient punched a hole in the glass shower door as his father struggled to pull him out.

> **Case 4.**   An 8-year-old white male (A) was brought in by his mother after 2 years of excessive hand washing. He had, in retrospect, probably started having obsessive thoughts at age 5, when he had refused to sit on the right side of the car where battery acid had been spilled a few weeks earlier. At the time of the spill, his mother had warned him to be careful, as battery acid could burn his skin if splashed onto it. His concern over the battery acid's effects increased and months after all traces of the acid were gone, he was unable to step near the carpet burn, wouldn't pick up anything dropped on that side of the car, and didn't want his younger brother to enter through that car door.
>
> As A's condition worsened, his concern for family safety increased to where he was concerned about fires, accidents, and illness as well. He developed extensive "protective" rituals, which if he were able to perform "perfectly," would keep his family safe. This included checking electric outlets and light switches, rituals at bedtime and on leaving the house, as well as washing rituals. At the time we saw him, he was spending 6 to 8 hours each day checking, washing, or repeating actions until they were "just right."

There may be more *ordering* than cleaning with lining up of stuffed animals or books, sequencing records or tapes, or having precise arrangements of clothes and toys.

Checking.   The obsessive child's checking rituals resemble those of adults, with repetitive checking of doors, windows, light switches, electric sockets, appliances, water faucets, and so on. Sometimes patients report specific thoughts compelling this action, but usually "they can't remember," or aren't aware of such thoughts.

Case 5. A 14-year-old girl spent 3 hours each morning, before leaving for school, checking that the doors were locked, the windows shut, the coffee pot unplugged, and the dog shut up in the garage. When she was finally able to leave the house and go to school, she would often return home midmorning to recheck, starting the ritual all over again. Her tardiness resulted in failing school performance. To get her to school, her parents began to help with her checking rituals. Her mother made up a list that both parents signed and dated each morning. The list included all the patient's checked items, and she was able to take it to school with her each morning. She said that when she felt compelled to leave school to go home and check, she was able to look at the checklist instead and feel reassured.

In response to obsessive thoughts that her carelessness with a curling iron could cause the house to burn down while her parents were sleeping, this patient spent several more hours in the evening checking that the curling iron was unplugged and cool. She would run her fingers over the empty electric outlet 100 to 200 times until she finally could believe that there wasn't a plug in it. Then she would pick up the curling iron, switch it on and off 50 times or more, look for the nonglowing red light (which meant it was off), and feel the coolness of the iron shaft. If something interfered with this ritual, or if it wasn't "just right," she was compelled to start all over.

Repeating. The common ritual of repeating may consist of tapping doorjambs a fixed number of times, walking forward and backward in a circumscribed manner, getting up and down from a chair several times, or other repetitive acts. Sometimes intentionally disguised, passing for impatience or forgetfulness or boredom, repeating rituals less frequently cause significant interference in the patient's life. In our series, locker locks seem to be a particular stumbling block. Patients must repeat the combination a certain number of times until it "feels right." Good-naturedly, one patient joked: "If you only have to repeat three or four times it's okay, but the double digit numbers are killers." One young boy carried all his books with him in a box from class to class. Classmates teased him about this odd behavior but he was compelled to repeat his locker combination so many times that he was constantly late for class. A friend suggested he carry his books in a knapsack, but he replied: "Great idea, guys, only I have to zip and unzip the knapsack 32 times. If anyone talks, sneezes, or coughs while I'm doing it, I have to start over. The box is easier!"

Symmetry. Ritualized symmetry may be limited to a single place or may be more extensive. An 8-year-old boy was compelled to have the right and left sides of his body exactly symmetrical, spending an hour tying and retying his shoelaces to even the two halves of each bow. He also plucked the hairs on his arms and face because they grew to be different lengths. If he plucked 12 on the left, he would pluck 12 on the right. Other children's symmetry routines have included making each

stride length exactly even, or speaking with even stress on all syllables.

Evolution of Symptom Patterns

Typically pediatric patients are seen clinically several years 'after the
onset of OCD. Because prospective follow-up information is also available for a subset of the sample over a 2- to 5-year period, considerable
data are available about change in symptoms over time. Most children
experience a single obsession or compulsion at onset, continue with
this for months to several years, and then gradually shift to a new one.
Over time, at least three-fourths of patients go through a period of
excessive washing. Sexual thoughts or rituals are common in adolescence but usually dissipate by age 18.

The disease has a fluctuating course. The patient may be severely
incapacitated and then, gradually, function more effectively and be
plagued by obsessive thoughts less frequently. Although the transition
from severe to less severe interference is almost always gradual, the
transition from less to more severe severity can be either gradual or
acute.

Associated Disorders

Disorders most commonly associated with childhood OCD follow similar patterns to those reported for adults, with affective and anxiety
disorder most common.

Table 2 gives associated disorders for the first 69 children seen at
the NIMH. The associated disorders are similar to those identified in
our epidemiological study of OCD (see Chapter 15), and therefore are
not an artifact of referral bias.

Depression is frequently associated, with secondary depression
developing in response to the distress or interference from OCD. In
isolated cases, depression predates the OCD. In a follow-up study of
the first 27 subjects, 3 had made life-threatening suicide attempts
(Flament et al., in preparation). The secondary depression may be
quite severe and is typical in its features of other primary depressive
states (Insel 1982).

Phobias and anxiety disorders may occur concurrently with OCD.
Almost one-third of our series also suffered from an anxiety disorder,
and there is an apparent increase in frequency over time. In our pilot
follow-up study, 11 of 25 patients had some form of anxiety disorder,
including social phobia, generalized anxiety, panic disorder, and separation anxiety (see Table 3). It is possible, that these patients experi-

Table 2. NIMH Study of Adolescents with obsessive-compulsive-disorder–associated psychopathology at first admission

	Males (N = 46)	Females (N = 23)	Total (N = 69)	
Associated Diagnosis	N	N	N	%
No other diagnosis	12	6	18	26
Major depression				
Current	11	6	17	23
Lifetime	4	2	6	9
Adjustment disorder with depressed mood	6	3	9	13
Separation anxiety disorder	1	4	5	7
Overanxious disorder	4	7	11	16
Simple phobia	8	4	12	17
Alcohol abuse	2	1	3	4
Substance abuse	1	0	1	1
Conduct disorder	3	2	5	7
Attention deficit disorder	7	0	7	10
Oppositional disorder	5	2	7	10
Enuresis	2	1	3	4
Encopresis	1	1	2	3

Note. Multiple diagnoses given; total exceeds 69.

enced anxiety directly related to their obsessions and this, in turn, generalized over time.

DSM-III-R allows dual diagnosis of OCD and schizophrenia. However, careful differentiation of OCD alone from schizophrenia with OCD is important for prognostication and treatment. In our limited experience, 3 patients with schizophreniform illness and obsessive-compulsive symptoms or disorder received significant benefit from drug treatment of the obsessive-compulsive features.

Tourette's syndrome is conspicuously absent from Table 2. There are a number of reports of obsessions and compulsions in Tourette's patients (Frankel et al. 1986; Greene and Pitman 1986; Pitman et al. 1987), but the incidence of patients with primary OCD who subsequently develop Tourette's is low. Of the 70 childhood patients with OCD treated to date by the NIMH, none have subsequently developed Tourette's syndrome. (Note that any patients who initially manifested both disorders would have been excluded from the NIMH study.)

Motor tics were found in 20 percent of the NIMH study patients, occurring more often in acute cases, in males, and in younger patients. In some cases, touching rituals were utilized to disguise an involuntary tic. It is unknown how the pattern and severity of obsessive-compulsive symptoms differ between Tourette's and primary cases. Prelimi-

Table 3. Diagnosis at 2- to 5-year follow-up

Diagnosis	Obsessive-Compulsive Subjects (N = 25)		Controls (N = 23)	
	N*	%	N	%
Diagnosis of OCD (current)				
No diagnosis	7	28	15	65
OCD only	5	20	0	
OCD plus another disorder	12	48	0	
No OCD, another disorder	1†	4	8	35
OCD plus compulsive personality disorder	5	20	0	
Associated psychopathology at follow-up (lifetime diagnosis)				
Major affective disorder	13	52	1‡	4
Anxiety disorder	11	44	2	9
Psychotic disorder	2	8	0	
Conduct disorder	2	8	3	13
Oppositional disorder	0		1	4
Antisocial personality disorder	1	4	1	4
Immature personality disorder	1	4	1	4
Alcohol abuse	1	4	5	22
Drug abuse	0		5	22
Borderline intellectual functioning	1	4	0	
Suicide attempts	5	20	1	4

* Multiple diagnoses given; total exceeds 25.
† Atypical psychosis.
‡ One manic episode.

nary impressions are that compulsions associated with Tourette's are less likely to involve washing and are usually less severe than in primary OCD.

Probably fewer children than adults with OCD have associated compulsive personality disorder. The lack of standardized instruments for diagnosis of compulsive personality disorder limits work in this area. In both the epidemiological sample and our clinical sample, less than 20 percent of obsessive-compulsive children were judged to have compulsive personality disorder. Nevertheless, our data suggest a complex and important relationship between the two.

Black (1974) summarized the available literature for *adults* with OCD and found moderate to marked obsessional traits reported in 71 percent of 383 patients and no premorbid traits in 29 percent of 451 patients, noting that criteria for evaluating obsessional traits varied widely. In various reports, between 16 and 36 percent of patients with OCD had no obsessional traits before onset of their OCD. Black also noted that 55 percent of *control* patients demonstrated obsessional traits. More recently, Rasmussen et al. (1986) found that the same percentage (55 percent) of his 44 adult patients with OCD had compulsive personality traits before developing OCD.

The relationship between anakastic personality (F60.5), a diagnosis found in ICD-9 (International Classification of Diseases) that is somewhat different from DSM-III compulsive personality disorder, is also unclear. Lewis (1965b) wrote:

> Anakastic personality is a subthreshhold form of OCD in which an isolated symptom is ego dystonic but does not significantly interfere with functioning. In no psychiatric condition is there a more obvious and specific association between *illness* and preceding personality than here, yet we meet people with *severe* obsessional symptoms whose previous personality revealed *no hint of predisposition*; and we meet people with pronounced *unmistakable* anakastic personality who never become mentally ill, in that way or any other. (p. 300)

Systematic data are being collected on the development of both compulsive personality disorder and anakastic personality disorder (see Chapter 17). Both seem to occur in adolescents in about equal frequency. Some children with early onset OCD appear to "form" compulsive personality traits as part of an adaptive coping pattern. If, for example, a child feels compelled to write the number 7 perfectly, he may "deliberately" become slow, careful, and rigid in an effort to "get it right the first time" and "beat the compulsion!" It is not clear what mediates the development of ego dystonicity, and this may be central to understanding the relationship between OCD and compulsive personality.

Prognosis

Follow-up studies of adult obsessive-compulsive patients have stressed the relative "purity" of outcome of uncomplicated cases, with depression being the most common complicating factor (Goodwin et al. 1969; Lo 1967; Welner et al. 1976). Most studies find the disorder to be chronic, with at least half the patients remaining unchanged; moderate disability, social isolation, and celibacy are common. Several studies have reported that symptomatology in childhood predicts poor outcome, but prospective data from juvenile populations are meager.

Berman (1942) reported on 6 child cases from two different institutions, finding good prognosis for a single episode. Long-term follow-up, however, was less favorable. Warren (1965), following 15 previously hospitalized adolescents who were reevaluated 6 to 10 years later, found 50 percent doing poorly and only 2 completely recovered. Hollingsworth et al. (1980) interviewed 10 of 17 cases 6 months to 14 years later, 7 of which still had significant obsessive-compulsive psychopathology.

The first 27 patients in the NIMH study were contacted 2 to 5 years after initial participation in a treatment trial. Twenty-five patients agreed to some form of follow-up contact, a completion rate of 93 percent. The follow-up diagnoses are given in Table 3.

The most striking findings are the continued psychopathology for the patient sample and the mixed diagnostic picture. Only 7 (28 percent) patients received no psychiatric diagnosis and were considered symptom free. Of the 17 (68 percent) patients who still qualified for the diagnosis of OCD, only 5 (20 percent) had OCD as their only diagnosis. The remaining 12 had one or more additional diagnoses, most commonly depressive disorder (recurrent, unipolar depression) and/or an anxiety disorder, including generalized anxiety, social phobia, and separation anxiety.

While 8 patients no longer met criteria for OCD, only 3 of these were considered well. The other 5 all suffered from some disorder: 1 had separation anxiety, 1 unipolar depression, 1 atypical psychosis, and 2 had both depression and an anxiety disorder (phobic and panic disorder, respectively). Thus, regardless of presence of OCD, 13 patients (48 percent) had current or past depressive episodes, and 11 (40 percent) had an anxiety disorder.

Outcome was surprisingly poor for all the patients, and there were virtually *no* significant predictors of outcome. Initial response to clomipramine did not predict outcome, although there had been little active maintenance therapy of any sort in the follow-up interval. Because the follow-up term ranged from 2 to 7 years, the study must be viewed as an intermediate step in the patients' development and disease progression. Future follow-up studies will be of greater interest if related to active treatment programs.

In summary, OCD is a major disturbance of childhood worthy of child psychiatry's greater attention. Because the rational irrationality of children suffering from this disorder causes them to underreport their symptoms, clinicians must be particularly sensitive to this diagnosis. With recognition of OCD's relative frequency and of the availability of effective treatments, it is vital that clinicians be trained to recognize this handicapping condition.

References

Adams PL: Obsessive Children. New York, Penguin Books, 1973

American Psychiatric Association: Diagnostic and Statistical Manual of Mental Disorders, 3rd ed (DSM-III). Washington, DC, American Psychiatric Association, 1980

American Psychiatric Association: Diagnostic and Statistical Manual of Mental Disorders, 3rd ed, revised (DSM-III-R). Washington, DC, American Psychiatric Association, 1987

Berman L: Obsessive-compulsive neurosis in children. J Nerv Ment Dis 95:26–39, 1942

Black A: The natural history of obsessional neurosis, in Obsessional States. Edited by Beech HR. London, Methuen, 1974

Crisp AH, Lacey JH, Crutchfield M: Clomipramine and 'drive' in people with anorexia nervosa: an in-patient study. Br J Psychiatry 150:355–358, 1987

Despert L: Differential diagnosis between obsessive-compulsive neurosis and schizophrenia in children, in Psychopathology of Childhood. Edited by Hoch PH, Zubin J. New York, Grune & Stratton, 1955

Frankel M, Cummings JL, Robertson MM, et al: Obsessions and compulsions in Gilles de la Tourette's syndrome. Neurology 36:378–382, 1986

Freud A: Normality and pathology in childhood. New York, International University Press, 1965

Freud S: Obsessions and phobias: their physical mechanisms and their etiology (1895), in Collected Papers. Vol. 1. Edited by Strachey J. London, Hogarth Press, 1955

Freud S: In notes on a case of obsessional neurosis (1909), in Collected Papers. Vol. 3. Edited by Strachey J. London, Hogarth Press, 1955

Freud S: The predisposition to obsessional neurosis (1913), in Collected Papers. Vol. 2. Edited by Strachey J. London, Hogarth Press, 1950

Goodwin DW, Guze S, Robins E: Follow-up studies in obsessional neurosis. Arch Gen Psychiatry 20:182–187, 1969

Green RC, Pitman RK: Tourette syndrome and obsessive-compulsive disorder, in Obsessive Compulsive Disorders: Theory and Management. Edited by Jenike MA, Baer L, Minichiello WE. Littleton, MA, PSG Publishing Co, 1986

Hollingsworth C, Tanguey P, Grossman L, et al: Longterm outcome of obsessive compulsive disorder in children. J Am Acad Child Psychiatry 19:134–144, 1980

Insel TR: Obsessive compulsive disorder: five clinical questions and a suggested approach. Compr Psychiatry 23:241–251, 1982

Insel TR, Akiskal HS: Obsessive compulsive disorder with psychotic features: a phenomenologic analysis. Am J Psychiatry 143:1527–1533, 1986

Janet P: Les Obsessions et la Psychiasthenie. Vol. 1. Paris, Félix Alan, 1903

Judd L: Obsessive compulsive neurosis in children. Arch Gen Psychiatry 12:136–143, 1965

Kanner L: Child Psychiatry (3rd ed). Springfield, IL, Charles C. Thomas, 1962

Kasvikis YG, Tsakiris F, Marks IM, et al: Women with obsessive compulsive disorder frequently report a past history of anorexia nervosa. (in press)

Lewis A: Obsessional illness, in Patterns of Meaning in Psychiatric Patients. Edited by Marks IM. London, Oxford University Press, 1965a

Lewis A: A note on personality and obsessional neurosis. Psychiatria et Neurologia 150:299–305, 1965b

Lo W: A follow-up study of obsessional neurosis in Hong Kong Chinese. Br J Psychiatry 113:823–832, 1967

Pitman RK, Green RC, Jenike MA, et al: Clinical comparison of Tourette's disorder and obsessive compulsive disorder. Am J Psychiatry 144:1166–1171, 1987

Rasmussen S, Tsuang M: Clinical characteristics and family history in DSM-III OCD. Am J Psychiatry 143:317–322,1986

Sandler M, Joffe W: Notes on obsessional manifestations in children. Psychoanal Study Child 20:425–438, 1965

Warren W: A study of adolescent psychiatric in-patients and the outcome six or more years later. J Child Psychol Psychiatry 6:141–160, 1965

Welner A, Reich T, Robins L: Obsessive compulsive neurosis: record follow-up and family studies, I: inpatient record study. Compr Psychiatry 17:527–539, 1976

Chapter 3

Cognitive Assessment of Obsessive-Compulsive Children

Barbara B. Keller, Ph.D.

Children with obsessive-compulsive disorder (OCD) present with symptoms of excessive checking, repetitive thoughts, and motor rituals that interfere with their daily activities (Flament and Rapoport 1984) and that can interfere with test performance at several levels. These behaviors are likely to complicate cognitive evaluation of these children since their mental efficiency may be at least temporarily compromised by their obsessive-compulsive symptoms. It is important to recognize the subtle, and not so subtle, cognitive complications of this disorder. Obsessive-compulsive children need help coping with school. In addition, psychological test patterns may suggest new research directions.

The Wechsler Intelligence Scale for Children-Revised (WISC-R) (Wechsler 1974) consists of five subtests that require verbal responses to verbal questions (yielding a Verbal IQ) and five subtests that require mostly nonverbal manipulation of materials (yielding a Performance IQ). All of the Performance subtests are timed, and a child who arrives at a correct answer after the time limit earns no points for his or her effort. In contrast, only one of the five verbal subtests has time limits.

Compulsive children may exceed time limits on the WISC-R Performance scale subtests by continuing to align the Block Design cubes and the Object Assembly pieces until they fit perfectly together (Kaufman 1979). Extra time spent on these tasks would generally result in a lowered Performance IQ for the children.

Another pitfall for OCD centers on the preoccupation with detail, which impairs some cases. Adult obsessive-compulsive patients have been observed to be more attentive to unusual details in the Thematic Apperception Test and Rorschach pictures than normal controls (Coursey 1984). If obsessive-compulsive children have difficulty differentiating important from unimportant details, again Performance IQs are likely to be lowered.

Adverse influences on the cognitive test performance of obsessive-compulsive children may also be related to associated psychopathology, such as depression or anxiety (Flament et al. 1987). Memory processes seem to be adversely affected by depression in both encoding and storage processes (Hart et al. 1987; Johnson and Magaro 1987). Anxiety may also interfere with an obsessive-compulsive child's concentration and may result in lowered scores (Sattler 1982). Finally, cognitive rigidity or "field dependence" may negatively influence a child's scores. Kaufman (1979) suggested that children who are somewhat rigid in their thinking or who have difficulty "breaking set" (field dependent) will not do as well on Block Design or Object Assembly tasks as someone who is more field independent and can see things apart from their initial context.

The present report summarizes experience with cognitive testing of 23 obsessive-compulsive children and adolescents with age- and sex-matched controls, the only systematic report of cognitive testing to date in a homogenous prospectively followed sample.

Description of Sample and Measures

Sixteen male and 7 female children and adolescents diagnosed as severe primary OCD were compared with 23 normal controls matched for age, sex, and Full Scale IQ. The WISC-R or the Wechsler Adult Intelligence Scale-Revised (WAIS-R) was administered to everyone. The children and youth were also given the Peabody Individual Achievement Test (PIAT) for academic screening (Dunn and Markwardt 1970) and were rated on test behavior using the Hillside Behavior Rating Scale (Gittelman and Klein 1985). The latter scale was initially developed to rate behavior of attention-deficit disorder in children but was found useful in rating obsessive-compulsive behavior as well. It includes categories of activity level, frustration tolerance, cooperativeness, interest in tasks, impulsivity, and distractibility. The Bender Gestalt Test, other fine-motor tasks, and personality projective tests were administered when clinically needed in diagnosis.

Behavioral Observations

The obsessive-compulsive adolescents appeared anxious and asked more questions for clarification of test procedures. They were more often distracted by external or internal stimuli; a significant difference between obsessive-compulsive children and controls was found on the Hillside scale for the distractibility rating ($p < .009$). The obsessive-compulsive children's response latencies to questions and perceptual tasks were either very short or very long; this style may have adversely affected their performance on timed perceptual tasks where both speed and accuracy were important. In general, testing took longer than expected with the obsessive-compulsive subjects, except for a small subgroup that performed quite impulsively (see below). Normal controls were much more relaxed in approaching the tasks and their response style did not generally adversely affect their performance.

Cognitive Performance

Most patients were in the average to high average Full Scale IQ range. Three obsessive-compulsive subjects scored in the low average range and 2 performed in the superior range. These results are similar to those reported previously (Flament et al. 1985). It is important to note that at the time of testing the obsessive-compulsive children were at least moderately impaired in routine functioning skills (such as decision making); as a result, these ability quotients may be underestimations.

Only one obsessive-compulsive subject has been retested after successful treatment. Initially this 15-year-old boy was unable to complete all of the standardized tests. His response latency was extremely long (about 5 minutes for even simple math questions), and he was unable to copy simple geometric designs on paper. His overall functioning ability, based on a limited sample of questions, was in the borderline category of mental functioning. On retesting, his Full Scale IQ was squarely in the average range, and he no longer showed evidence of the internal distraction that had previously contributed to the impairment of his performance.

Although the obsessive-compulsive subjects had Full Scale and Verbal IQs similar to the controls (see Table 1), they had lower Performance IQs than the controls ($p < .04$). Scores on Block Design were particularly poor.

No sex differences were found on Verbal, Performance, or Full Scale IQs for either the OCD or control groups. There were some differ-

Table 1. Wechsler IQs for obsessive-compulsive and control subjects

	Verbal	Performance	Full scale
OCD	112	109	112
Control	115	114	116
Mean difference	2.48	5.17*	4.30**

*$p < .04$.
**$p < .005$.

ing patterns of subtest results for males and females, however. Male obsessive-compulsive subjects generally scored higher (11.9 ± 3.6) than female obsessive-compulsive subjects (9.8 ± 0.9) on the Picture Completion task of the Performance scale. Perhaps more striking than the mean differences ($p < .05$) are the differences in variabilities of these scores ($p < .003$). While approximately 68 percent of females scored between 9 and 11 (in middle of average range), less than half the males scored in this range. Additional differences in variability of scores did not occur for other perceptual performance tasks, suggesting that it may only be for the skill of "differentiating important from unimportant details" and not a larger perceptual area that this relationship holds. Although no mean verbal subtest differences between obsessive-compulsive males and females were found, males showed greater variability on knowledge of social conventions (Comprehension subscale, $p < .02$) and in immediate recall of spoken numbers (Digit Span, $p < .02$). These variability results must be cautiously interpreted because of the unequal number of obsessive-compulsive males and females included in the comparison. However, among the controls there were no subtests on which there was unequal variability despite the same unequal male/female proportions.

Variation Within the OCD Group

Although as a group, obsessive-compulsive subjects differed from controls, they also differed considerably among themselves. Six (26 percent) had the "organic" indicators of fine-motor and memory deficits. Evaluation of their fine-motor skills was done using the Bender Gestalt with those children who showed awkwardness in copying small geometric forms on the Wechsler scale. Memory was evaluated clinically by test behavior and informal WISC-R subtest pattern analysis. Half of this "organic" group (13 percent of total OCDs) had Verbal–Performance Wechsler discrepancies of 35 or greater, with stronger verbal than perceptual performance scores, a difference typically found in less than 1 percent of children (Sattler 1982).

Obsessive patients, as mentioned, also included a highly impulsive subgroup. About one-third (9) of patients were rated as extremely impulsive in their test behavior. The clearly impulsive patients with OCD may have used this response style as a way to break out of obsessive ruminations and complete tasks in a timely manner; several indicated that this was the case. Those not at all impulsive consisted of the most ruminative, detail-oriented patients as well as some who processed information very slowly. Although it seemed reasonable to expect that the middle one-third in impulsivity would have the most adaptive (and thus optimal) response style, actually there was no significant difference in the Verbal or Performance IQs of these groups.

Discussion

There are several possible explanations for the differences between OCD and control subjects. The obsessive-compulsive subjects may have relatively poor holistic perceptual integration skills and thus "can't see the forest for the trees." Some support for this is provided by Kaufman's (1979) description of the probable impact of cognitive rigidity or field dependence on children's WISC-R subtest scores. He suggested that children who are somewhat rigid in their thinking and who have difficulty "breaking set" will not do as well on Block Design or Object Assembly as field independent children will.

Another explanation is that relatively poor scores on Performance IQ subtests result from anxiety or depression, which differentially affect time-limited tasks. However, quantitative support for this was not found; correlations between Performance IQ and ratings of global anxiety or global depression for the children were not significant.

Although some compulsive children spend extra time aligning the Block Design cubes and Object Assembly pieces so that they "fit" perfectly (Kaufman 1979), the impact of this behavior in the present study seemed only slight. Such adjusting occurred after the examinee said he or she was finished, and the timing of the task had ended.

An overall Performance difference between OCD and control subjects on perceptual tasks was not found previously by Flament et al. (1985). This was probably due to the fact that the Object Assembly subtest of the WISC-R was not administered in this earlier study. Although it is one of the least statistically reliable subtests on the WISC-R, the Object Assembly task seems to be a rather consistently difficult subtest for the children with OCD.

Until now, discussion of cognitive test characteristics and test-taking behavior in OCD has highlighted detrimental impact on performance. Kaufman (1979) indicated that there may also be an advantage of compulsivity for test performance. Verbal scores "may be elevated substantially by children who give a string of responses of varying quality . . . who respond to probing with a variety of ideas . . . or with much elaboration" (p. 39). Although these behaviors were observed among the subjects with OCD, no verbal score enhancement was found. It may be that many of the controls (who were drawn primarily from middle-class suburbs of Washington, DC) also have a compulsive style in responding to verbal tasks, perhaps due to educational training.

Suggestions for Cognitive Testing of Obsessive-Compulsive Children

Distractibility, checking behavior, and excessive concern about cleanliness are useful diagnostic observations, but these behaviors can interfere with a valid cognitive assessment. To obtain the most accurate cognitive or academic evaluation possible, a number of aspects of the testing situation should be modified. The testing environment should be as clear as possible, with no clutter. A variety of pencils and pens should be available in case of phobia or superstition about a particular implement. One patient, for example, was highly distracted by the examiner's pen because he was worried that he might get ink on his hands. Extra time should be allowed for the psychological assessment. On the Verbal subtests, many of the obsessive-compulsive subjects' answers may be long-winded. On the Performance subtests, the obsessive-compulsive subjects' distractibility, perfectionistic tendencies, or rumination may lengthen the time needed to complete the various tasks. In addition to obsessive-compulsive behaviors, anxiety and depression may adversely impact on test performance and may be best dealt with by briefing the examinee before the start of testing so that each will know that it is "normal" to miss a number of items.

Despite its low reliability, the Object Assembly subtest should be administered to anyone suspected of having OCD. Aside from the results mentioned above, that obsessive-compulsive subjects do poorly on this test, it also provides a situation for observation of compulsive behavior. Similarly, Coding can also be useful for observing rituals.

Perhaps most important, cognitive scores that indicate mental functioning below previous levels of functioning should be interpreted cautiously because they are likely to be underestimations of actual ability.

Summary

In summary, obsessive-compulsive children and adolescents did not show exceptional intellectual ability, nor did they manifest homogeneously compulsive cognitive style. Subtle cognitive differences between obsessive-compulsive and control subjects—including a slightly decreased performance score, occasional wide verbal-performance differences, and a subgroup with marked impulsivity—suggest a heterogeneous population and do not support preconceptions about continuity between OCD and compulsive cognitive style.

References

Coursey RD: The dynamics of obsessive-compulsive disorder, in Obsessive-Compulsive Disorder. Edited by Insel TR. Washington, DC, American Psychiatric Press, 1984

Dunn LM, Markwardt FC: Peabody Individual Achievement Test Manual. Circle Pines, Minn, American Guidance Service, 1970

Flament MF, Rapoport JL: Childhood obsessive-compulsive disorder, in Obsessive-Compulsive Disorder. Edited by Insel TR. Washington, DC, American Psychiatric Press, 1984

Flament MF, Rapoport JL, Berg CB, et al: Clomipramine treatment of childhood obsessive-compulsive disorder: a double-blind controlled study. Arch Gen Psychiatry 42:977–983, 1985

Flament MF, Rapoport JL, Whitaker A, et al: Childhood obsessive-compulsive disorder and affective disorders: clinical, longitudinal, therapeutical, and biological lines. Paper presented at the International Meeting on Affective Disorders, Jerusalem, April 18–20, 1987

Gittelman R, Klein D: Hillside Behavior Rating Scale. Psychopharmacol Bull 21:898–899, 1985

Hart RP, Kwentus JA, Wade JB, et al: Digit symbol performance in mild dementia and depression. J Consult Clin Psychol 55:236–238, 1987

Johnson MH, Magaro PA: Effects of mood and severity of memory processes in depression and mania. Psychol Bull 101:28–40, 1987

Kaufman AL: Intelligent Testing with the WISC-R. New York, John Wiley & Sons, 1979

Sattler JM: Assessment of Children's Intelligence and Special Abilities (2nd ed). Boston, Allyn and Bacon, 1982

Wechsler D: Manual for the Wechsler Intelligence Scale for Children (rev). New York, The Psychological Corporation, 1974

Chapter 4

Behavioral Assessment Techniques for Childhood Obsessive-Compulsive Disorder

Carol Zaremba Berg, M.A.

Standardized behavioral assessment techniques for childhood obsessive-compulsive disorder (OCD) are limited in comparison to measures
developed for adult patients. However, the recent growth of psychopharmacological and behavioral treatments and the higher-than-ex-
pected prevalence of OCD has spurred the development of reliable
measures in pediatric populations to assess obsessive-compulsive behavior and to document treatment change. Measures discussed here
include self-report inventories, structured clinical interviews, ob-
server rating scales, and direct behavioral observations. The usefulness and pitfalls of the latter methods, developed for or utilized in our
ongoing clinical studies, will be addressed as well as reliability and
validity of scales where available.

Inventories and Rating Scales

Several techniques for measuring childhood OCD have been derived
from instruments designed for adults with OCD (Emmelkamp 1982;
Insel et al. 1983; Stekette and Foa 1985; Yaryura-Tobias and Neziroglu
1983). These adult measures are reviewed briefly to provide perspective on the broader availability of research information. Although all

41

have the goal of symptom identification and quantification, each has its area of incompleteness or being "less than perfect." No one instrument is good enough to use alone, and some combination of clinical evaluation of patient and family together with structural interviews and scales is recommended.

One of the most widely used adult scales has been the Leyton Obsessional Inventory (LOI) (Cooper 1970). The LOI, a card-sort task, consists of 69 obsessive-compulsive symptoms and trait items that a subject rates yes (present) or no, then further rates 65 cards for resistance (severity of symptoms) and interference (disability of symptoms) to daily activities. Advantages found with the LOI are satisfactory test-retest reliability (Cooper 1970), change with drug treatment (Allen and Rach 1975), principal components analysis establishing five factors (Murray et al. 1979), and good correlations with the written form (Snowden 1980). As Cooper initially stated, this instrument was designed for "houseproud housewives" rather than obsessive patients, was never intended to selectively identify a disorder (as opposed to a trait), and does not adequately cover obsessive symptomatology (Yaryura-Tobias and Neizroglu 1983). "False positives" for OCD are thus to be expected.

The 44-item Leyton Obsessional Inventory—Child Version (Berg et al. 1986) was adapted from the LOI for adults. This instrument, therefore, also measures the number of obsessive symptoms with yes/no responses as well as the degree of resistance to symptoms and the interference with daily activities with weighted responses (Appendices 1 and 2). The 44-item Leyton was shortened because time was a factor both with the younger subjects' anticipated inability to attend for longer periods of time and with the known slower response time of obsessive patients. Thirteen symptom items were dropped, four trait items were retained, and seven new items were incorporated. Items were added that were more appropriate to our younger population concerning schoolwork and magic games; wording was simplified for younger subjects. The items are printed on separate cards, which the child places in a yes or no slot of an answer box. Questions address persistent thoughts, checking, fear of dirt and/or dangerous objects, cleanliness, order, repetition, and indecision. The positive responses are then rated for resistance on a 5-point scale from "my thoughts and habits are quite sensible and reasonable" to "what I do bothers me a lot and I try very hard to stop." The responses are rated for interference on a 4-point scale from "my habit does not stop me from doing a lot of things I want to do" to "this stops me from doing a lot of things and wastes a lot of my time."

The 44-item Leyton significantly differentiated obsessive patients from normal controls with yes responses, resistance scores, and interference scores, and patients from psychiatric controls on resistance scores and interference scores. Test-retest reliability was good (Berg et al. 1986). The instrument was sensitive to drug-induced improvement (Flament et al. 1985). The 44-item Leyton yes responses, resistance scores, and interference scores correlated significantly with global clinician ratings (Obsessive Compulsive Rating Scale, Comprehensive Psychopathological Rating Scale—Obsessive Compulsive subscale, NIMH Global and Obsessive Compulsive subscales) only after drug treatment and not at baseline (Berg et al. 1986). Possible explanations were the initial secrecy and denial that is common in patients with OCD and may have increased the discrepancy between patients' self-assessment and clinician observations. A later analysis, based on 38 patients 13 to 19 years of age, demonstrated baseline correlations of .28 to .69 ($p < .08$ to .001) between the Leyton responses and clinician ratings (Obsessive Compulsive Rating Scale, Comprehensive Psychopathological Rating Scale—Obsessive Compulsive subscale), indicating further validity of the 44-item Leyton. Thus it has been shown that adolescents are as capable of reporting their symptomatology with similar accuracy to observations by trained clinicians as are adults.

Advantages of the 44-item Leyton are that it provides a measure of severity and interference as well as a number of different symptoms. To date, this is the only available instrument to measure OCD in children having demonstrated reliability and validity. The card-sort method, in addition, provides an opportunity for rich clinical observations, offsetting this more labor-intensive approach. For instance, a child may spend several minutes arranging the cards or box in an exact position or ponder on the lack of a "sometimes" slot because of indecision. The children are frequently surprised that someone actually knows about symptoms like theirs, which they may have tried so hard to hide, or they follow their own behavioral change from one week to the next during testing sessions. The disadvantages are the specificity of some questions and the lack of ratings of broader obsessive-compulsive patterns, which, of course, must supplement the use of this instrument.

A 20-item Leyton Obsessional Inventory for adolescents was adopted from the 44-item Leyton for use in an epidemiological survey of an entire high school enrollment (5,000 students) of a semirural county (Berg et al., in press) (Appendix 3). Items were selected by examining the scores of 26 obsessive patients and age-matched normal controls (significantly higher mean yes score for the patients and at least 25 percent above the means score of controls, higher interference scores for the patients, and representation of the major categories of obsessive-compulsive symptoms). This version was reformatted as a pencil-and-paper questionnaire since Snowden (1980) found the adult card-sort and written inventory to be comparable. However, due to the limitations, only the interference ratings were used. In the second stage of the study, clinicians interviewed high scorers on the 20-item Leyton and normal controls to determine validity of the instrument and to examine prevalence of OCD in the normal adolescent population (Flament et al., in press).

This version provided age and sex norms for adolescents 13 to 18 years of age and demonstrated good psychometric properties overall. Although it also demonstrated good sensitivity and specificity, its predictive value was only 18 percent due to a large number of false positives. Despite the lower predictiveness, however, the 20-item Leyton was extremely useful in identifying a "high-risk" group within which a 0.4 percent lifetime prevalence of OCD was found in a general adolescent population (Berg et al., in press).

An 8-item teacher Leyton is now being evaluated at the National Institutes of Health with hyperactive children on high doses of stimulant medication who may develop obsessive-compulsive thoughts and behaviors. Items are rated on a 4-point scale (0 = not at all to 3 = very much) (Appendix 4). With hyperactive children, these behaviors are apparent and, at times, distressing to both parents and teachers. They appear to be ego-syntonic to the children, however. For instance, an impulsive child who could not sit still began cleaning his closet every day and writing facts in a progressively structured manner in class but felt nothing was unusual. Younger populations and hyperactive children have more difficulty reading and comprehending the questions than do our younger obsessive population. For these and other reasons, a teacher-screening questionnaire for "true" OCD would be useful to address other behaviors and signs that teachers can notice, such as red and raw hands, frequent requests to go to the bathroom, and repeated erasing on tests and homework.

Another widely used adult inventory is the Maudsley Obsessive Compulsive Inventory (MOCI) (Hodgson and Rachman 1977). The MOCI is a 30-item true/false inventory that was designed specifically to assess obsessive-compulsive complaints. Advantages of the MOCI include the ease of administration (it is a self-report inventory listed on a single sheet) and the principal components analysis that reveals five components (checking, cleaning, slowness, doubting-conscientiousness, total obsessional score). The disadvantages are the lack of a rumination component and the lack of validation of the slowness and doubting scales (Hodgson and Rachman 1977). Difficulties with both inventories include variability with self-ratings (due to secrecy and denial inherent in the disorder) and the possibility of a single incapacitating symptom resulting in a low score. Clark and Bolton (1985) compared 11 obsessive adolescents with 10 nonobsessive, anxious adolescents on the LOI and MOCI and found only the MOCI total score to be a discriminating factor. The lack of differences on the Leyton was attributed to lack of sensitivity of the LOI, the low symptom severity of the patients, and minimizing of their disturbance.

The Yale-Brown Obsessive Compulsive Scale (Y-BOCS) (Goodman et al., submitted for publication) consists of 19 items, with the first 10 items assessing the core symptoms of OCD. Items are rated on a 5-point scale (0 = none to 4 = extreme). Only these 10 items comprise the total score. The other nine items consist of five items explaining associated features of OCD (also using a 5-point rating of 0 = none to 4 = extreme), two items assessing global severity and improvement (rating 0 to 6), and one item each for reliability and for insight. The "obsessions and compulsions" checklist for current and past thoughts and behaviors is the beginning format with inclusion of all possible symptom responses with a target symptoms list. The rating scale was designed to rate the "severity" of symptoms and to assess patient response to treatment (with the intended use as a semistructured interview). This format allows for the maximum exploration of behaviors, including patient reports as well as the clinician's judgment and insight. The Y-BOCS demonstrated good interrater reliability in a study involving four raters and 40 patients with OCD at various stages of treatment (Goodman et al., submitted for publication), as well as good validity and sensitivity to drug change based on 81 patients with OCD (Goodman et al., submitted for publication). Reliability and validity studies are currently being conducted with the Obsessive-Compulsive Disorder Clinic of the Yale University School of Medicine, Department of Psychiatry. The Y-BOCS is likely to receive wide use; it is currently being employed in an ongoing multicenter trial of clomiperamine in OCD.

The comprehensiveness of the probing for symptoms, the exactness of the severity ratings, and the interaction of patient and clinician are the obvious advantages of the Y-BOCS. In addition, it has been designed for documenting the specificity of treatment change. A disadvantage may be the length of time for completion. However, the outcome remains to be seen.

The Children's Yale-Brown Obsessive Compulsive Scale (CY-BOCS) (Goodman et al., unpublished) consists of virtually the same items and format with minor wording modification for younger children (Appendix 5). For instance, obsessions are referred to as "thoughts that keep going over and over in your mind . . . things you're afraid of, things that shouldn't bother you so much." Compulsions are "habits you wish you could stop but can't." Reliability and validity are being established. The usefulness, as with the adult measure, is its comprehensiveness of symptoms and severity rating and the interactive nature with the patient and clinician. As previously mentioned, because patients with OCD are reluctant to report their symptoms, the interviewing clinician should be familiar with obsessive-compulsive behaviors as well as utilize the parent reports. The same clinician and same parent informant should be used over the treatment period, ensuring that reports are consistent over time.

The Obsessive Compulsive Rating Scale (OCR) (Rapoport and Elkins, unpublished), designed as a brief clinician's rating, is a 4-item scale addressing preoccupation with rituals/obsessions, the number of rituals, interference with activities, and resistance time. It is rated on a 5-point scale (none to very severe) (Appendix 6). The OCR is useful due to its brevity, its high correlations with the previously mentioned obsessive scales, and its sensitivity to drug change (Flament et al. 1985). It too, however, must be used in conjunction with other measures.

Structured Clinical Interviews

Structured and semistructured diagnostic clinical interviews are essential research measures for assessing childhood psychopathology. They ensure completeness of information (normal functioning as well as psychopathology) and comparability across studies and centers. None of these interviews was designed specifically with OCD in mind, and each has advantages and disadvantages.

The Diagnostic Interview for Children and Adolescents (DICA) (Herjanic and Campbell 1977; Welner et al. 1987), a structured interview, contains questions about obsessions and compulsions based on DSM-III (American Psychiatric Association 1980) criteria that require a yes/no response. For instance, "Have you ever been troubled by unpleasant or silly thoughts or pictures in your mind which keep coming back to your mind and you can't seem to push them away or forget about them?" or "Do you often find yourself doing things that seem unnecessary like touching things over and over or washing over and over?" Probe questions follow to ascertain age of onset, duration, and degree of distress and senselessness. The DICA establishes a lifetime diagnosis, can be administered by lay interviewers, has standardized scoring criteria, and has established reliability and validity for major diagnoses. A disadvantage is that although the degree and type of probing by interviewers (rather than staying with the yes/no responses) may obtain useful clinical information, it may also skew the response patterns. In addition, the DICA was not constructed to assess symptom severity, making it less sensitive to treatment change and requiring supplemental information before a definite diagnosis can be established.

The Schedule for Affective Disorder and Schizophrenia for School-Age Children—Epidemiologic Version (K-SADS-E) (Orvaschel and Puig-Antich, unpublished), a semistructured interview, records past and current episodes of psychopathology in children and adolescents based on DSM-III-R criteria. The section on OCD presents the DSM-III-R description with a prompt that ratings should reflect the worst episode. The obsessive-compulsive responses are yes/no, with no prompting a skip to the next question and yes leading to probes for symptom suppression, duration, subjective distress, life impairment, and symptom chronology. Questions are phrased only as guides for the rater to obtain information; interviewers must use clinical judgment in asking questions and in rating responses.

The K-SADS-E should be used only by individuals trained in the psychiatric assessment of children and adolescents as well as trained and familiar with the structure of the interview. The authors recommend interviewing first with the parent and then with the child, and finally achieving summary ratings from all sources of available information. Although it provides a lifetime assessment, it is a limited tool for specific areas of psychopathology, is not sensitive to treatment change, and does not include areas such as academic functioning. While this fourth version has recently been documented, early drafts have been used extensively and have established diagnostic reliability (Orvaschel et al. 1982).

The Schedule for Affective Disorder and Schizophrenia for School-Age Children—Present Episode (K-SADS-P) utilizes the same format as the K-SADS-E, but assesses the severity of an ongoing episode of psychiatric disorder and symptoms of the week prior to the interview (Chambers et al. 1985). The K-SADS-P is useful to assess clinical change over time, with the K-SADS-E providing a lifetime assessment. Again, a current version is available with DSM-III-R documentation; earlier versions provided reliability (Chambers et al. 1985).

The Interview Schedule for Children (ISC) (Kovacs 1983, unpublished), a semistructured interview, contains sets of symptom questions for psychopathology and then gives severity ratings. A strong asset of this interview is the manner in which questions are written in "kid" language, with probes for the clinicians' judgment and formatted for parent and child responses. For example, "What do you do when _____ comes to mind? Does it make it hard to _____ (eat out, visit with people, finish things) because you can't be sure that _____."

Severity scores are subjective, again relying on the interviewer's judgment. Obsessional thinking, compulsive behavior, and compulsive personality disorder are considered in an addendum and added to the main interview for further exploration of these areas.

The ISC provides a current diagnosis of psychopathology but provides the interviewer with a more informal style of interviewing. However, it also should be used only by individuals trained in psychiatric assessment of children and adolescents because the probes and severity rating are based on clinical judgment. While the interview could be used to assess global changes before and after treatment, no data are currently available to document this. This is a potentially important instrument, particularly to address the vexed area of compulsive personality disorder in contrast or in addition to OCD.

Behavioral Measures

Other behavioral assessments have great clinical utility. A behavioral diary during a given time period (usually a week) by the patient and the parents should include all obsessive thoughts and compulsive behavior, with notations of frequency and duration of behaviors. Antecedents and consequences of behaviors should be recorded as well as previously unreported behaviors. Rituals—such as the number of hand washings, time spent showering, and amount of time spent checking—can be quantified to establish treatment change.

The "subjective units of discomfort" (SUDS) (Wolpe 1985) are patient ratings of their degree of distress or anxiety from 0 ("no anxiety or distress") to 100 ("the most anxious or distressed you have ever felt"). After rituals are defined, the SUDS can be used to formulate a hierarchy of distressful behaviors to establish behavioral treatment goals. The SUDS was responsive to treatment change in obsessive adults when sampling was done pre- and postintervention (Steketee et al. 1982) and can be used for frequent time sampling within a treatment session to monitor decrease in anxiety with in vivo exposure. While this measure seems subjective and vague, patients frequently are already monitoring their behavior on some internal scale and will frequently describe their distress or avoidance of a situation or a behavior on a "scale of 1 to 10."

General Observations

Our information gathering about a child includes parent and, at times, teacher general observations. Parents can contribute developmental and chronological information such as age at onset, duration of symptoms, and treatment. For many children this disorder has been so painful that they want to forget those behaviors and at times "just can't remember." In contrast, parents who are frustrated and distressed by these repetitive behaviors are usually most anxious to discuss their child. Talking with the parents often provides the best descriptions of behavior that the child may not express or be aware of.

Since many children are secretive about their behaviors, peers and teachers may not be aware of their difficulties. Some children find they do not have to perform rituals at school and are only affected when at home (which involves the family). Although we find our ward teacher and home schoolteachers to be excellent observers of patients' behaviors, we do not typically contact the home schoolteacher in order to discourage the child from "using" his or her disorder for special privileges. If the symptoms are involved with school and support is needed, then cooperation is sought.

Compulsive Personality Disorder

Compulsive personality disorder has been a confounding issue in the diagnosis of OCD (see Chapter 2). Does a compulsive personality contribute to the disorder? Is it a separate entity or secondary complication? The compulsive personality addendum from the ISC, constructed to meet DSM-III criteria, is currently being used with our obsessive-compulsive adolescent patients as part of a study of these phenomena. Leonard (unpublished) has devised a structural interview for children based on DSM-III-R criteria for compulsive personality disorder. Preliminary data suggest excellent reliability. (The interview is available from Dr. Henrietta Leonard on request.)

A promising area for exploration is teacher ratings. Teachers' observations could be clinically useful and have been untapped until now. A teacher, for example, might note the child who repeatedly erases his paper to achieve perfection, places books and papers in a certain order, spends a lot of time in the bathroom, has red hands, or fears touching certain items. Although these may be typical behaviors in a mild form for many, the teacher's input would be of value for the children who suffer in silence. It would be of interest to construct a scale to validate the teacher's observations with the child's self-report.

Conclusion

No one instrument or technique is satisfactory for assessment or to measure treatment change in childhood OCD. An assessment battery containing ratings from the child, family, and clinician give a breadth of responses valuable for differential diagnosis, for more comprehensive treatment, and for better assessment of treatment effects. Despite all of the current technology, however, we have found the most useful question is to ask, "Do you have these thoughts or behaviors?" and to obtain a thorough clinical description. Children, for the most part, are good self-reporters and are honest about their feelings of frustration and the senselessness of their behavior. Their increasing sense of isolation, exhaustion, anger, and pain from their washing, checking, and repetitions of behavior provides, at times, the motivation to "play it straight" to help themselves and renew appropriate interactions with others.

References

Allen JJ, Rach PH: Changes in obsession-compulsive patients as measured by the Leyton inventory before and after treatment with clomipramine. Scot Med J 20:41–45, 1975

American Psychiatric Association: Diagnostic and Statistical Manual of Mental Disorders, 3rd ed (DSM-III). Washington, DC, American Psychiatric Association, 1980

Berg CJ, Rapoport JL, Flament M: The Leyton Obsessional Inventory—Child Version. J Am Acad Child Psychiatry 25:84–91, 1986

Berg C, Whitaker A, Davies M, et al: The survey form of the Leyton Obsessional Inventory—Child Version—norms from an epidemiological study. J Am Acad Child Psychiatry (in press)

Chambers WJ, Puig-Antich J, Hirsch M, et al: The assessment of affective disorders in children and adolescents by semi-structured interview: test-retest reliability of the Schedule for Affective Disorders and Schizophrenia for school-age children, present episode version. Arch Gen Psychiatry 42:696–708, 1985

Clark DA, Bolton D: An investigation of two self-report measures of obsessional phenomenon in obsessive-compulsive adolescents: research note. J Child Psychol Psychiatry 26:429–437, 1985

Cooper J: The Leyton Obsessional Inventory. Psychol Med 1:48–64, 1970

Emmelkamp PMG: Phobia and Obsessive-Compulsive Disorders: Theory Research and Practice. New York, Plenum Press, 1982

Flament MF, Rapoport JL, Berg CJ, et al: Clomipramine treatment of childhood obsessive-compulsive disorder: a double-blind controlled study. Arch Gen Psychiatry 42:977–983, 1985

Flament MF, Whitaker A, Rapoport JL, et al: Obsessive compulsive disorder in adolescence: an epidemiological study. J Am Acad Child Psychiatry (in press)

Herjanic B, Campbell W: Differentiating psychiatrically disturbed children on the basis of a structural psychiatric interview. J Abnorm Child Psychol 5:127–135, 1977

Hodgson R, Rachman S: Obsessive compulsive complaints. Behav Res Ther 15:389–395, 1977

Insel TR, Murphy DL, Cohen RM, et al: Obsessive compulsive disorder. Arch Gen Psychiatry 40:605–612, 1983

Murray RM, Cooper JE, Smith A: The Leyton Obsessional Inventory: an analysis of the responses of 73 obsessional patients. Psychol Med 9:305–331, 1979

Orvaschel H, Puig-Antich J, Chambers WJ, et al: Retrospective assessment of child psychopathology with the K-SADS-E. J Am Acad Child Psychiatry 4:392–397, 1982

Snowden J: A comparison of written and postbox forms of the Leyton Obsessional Inventory. Psychol Med 10:165–170, 1980

Steketee G, Foa EB: Obsessive compulsive disorder, in Clinical Handbook of Psychological Disorders. Edited by Barlow D. New York, Guilford Press, 1985

Steketee G, Foa EB, Grayson JB: Recent advances in the behavioral treatment of obsessive compulsives. Arch Gen Psychiatry 39:1365–1371, 1982

Welner Z, Reich W, Herjanic B, et al: Reliability, validity and parent-child agreement studies of the Diagnostic Interview for Children and Adolescents. J Am Acad Child Psychiatry 26:649–653, 1987

Wolpe J: Psychotherapy by reciprocal inhibition. Stanford, Stanford University Press, 1958

Yaryura-Tobias JA, Neziroglu FA: Psychological Diagnostic Assessments in Obsessive Compulsive Disorders: Pathogenesis-Diagnosis-Treatment. New York, Marcel Dekker, 1983

Appendix 1
Leyton Obsessional Inventory—Child Version

Thoughts
1. Do you often feel like you have to do certain things even though you know you don't really have to?
2. Do thoughts or words ever keep going over and over in your mind?
3. Do you ever have the idea that your parents or brothers or sisters might have an accident or that something might happen to them?
4. Have you had thoughts or ideas of hurting yourself or people in your family—ideas that come and go without any good reason?

Checking
5. Do you have to check things several times?
6. Do you ever have to check water taps, light switches after you have already turned them off?
7. Do you ever have to check doors, cupboards, or windows to make sure that they are really shut?

Dirt and Contamination
8. Do you hate dirt and dirty things?
9. Do you ever feel that if something has been used or touched by someone else, it is spoiled for you?
10. Do you dislike touching someone or being touched in any way?
11. Do you feel that sweat or spit is dangerous and can be bad for you or your clothes?

Dangerous Objects
12. Are you worried that pins, bits of hair, or sharp things might be left lying about?
13. Do you worry that things might get broken and leave harmful pieces?
14. Do knives, hatchets, or other dangerous things in your home make you nervous?

Cleanliness and Tidiness
15. Do you worry a bit about being clean enough?
16. Are you fussy about keeping your hands clean?
17. Do you ever clean your room or your toys when they are not really dirty in order to make them extra clean?
18. Do you take care that your clothes are always neat and clean whatever you are playing at?
19. Do you have special places where you put your things down?

20. When you put things away at night, do they have to be put away just right?
21. Are you very careful that your room is always neat?

School Work

22. Do you get angry if other children mess up your desk?
23. Are you very careful to have neat papers and neat handwriting?
24. Do you ever do papers over just to make sure that they are perfect?
25. Do you spend a lot of extra time checking your homework to make sure that it is just right?

Order and Routine

26. Do you like to do things right on time?
27. Do you have to undress or dress in a certain order?
28. Does it bother you if you cannot do your homework at a certain time or in a certain order?

Repetition

29. Do you ever have to do things over and over a certain number of times before they seem quite right?
30. Do you ever have to count several times or go through numbers in your mind?
31. Do you ever have trouble finishing school work or chores because you have to do something over and over again?
32. Do you have a favorite or special number you like to count up to a lot, or do things just that number of times?

Overconscientious

33. Do you often have a bad conscience because you've done something no one else thinks is bad?
34. Do you worry a lot if you've done something not exactly the way you like?
35. Do you always give a poor report in class even when you planned just what to say before?
36. Do you have trouble making up your mind?
37. Do you go over things a lot that you have done because you aren't sure that they were the right thing to do?

Hoarding

38. Do you keep a lot of things around in your room that you don't really need?
39. Is your room crowded with old toys, string, boxes, games, clothes, just because you think they might be needed some day?

Meanness

40. Do you save up your allowance or money that the family gives you?
41. Do you spend a lot of time counting your allowance and arranging it?

Magic Games

42. Do you have special games you play for "good luck" like not stepping on or near cracks in the street or sidewalk?
43. Do you move or talk in just a special way, to avoid bad luck?
44. Do you have special numbers or words to say, just because it keeps bad luck or bad things away?

Appendix 2
Instructions for Administration of LOI-CV: Card-Sort Format

1. Check that you have:
   a. Complete set of obsessional (1–44) cards
   b. Five "resistance" statement cards marked 1–5 on the back
   c. Four "interference" statement cards marked 1–4 on the back
   d. One "yes-no" postbox
   e. Scoring sheet
2. Cards should be arranged in numerical order with questions facing up.
3. Put the subject's name, age, status, the date and time of starting, and your name on the top of the scoring sheet.
4. Arrange the seats of yourself and the subject so that you are facing each other across a table.
5. Say to the subject "I want to get your replies to a number of questions about your thoughts and habits and how you feel about various things. We find that a good way to do this is to give you the questions on a card, and for you to answer by putting them in the 'Yes' or 'No' box. Read each question carefully, and then make a fairly quick decision about whether to answer 'yes' or 'no.' You may find yourself wanting to answer not exactly 'yes' and not exactly 'no' but in this case put it in the slot which is most nearly correct for you. Try to give your answer without a long debate with yourself. Everybody comes out differently on these questions, and there is no 'right' or 'wrong' number of 'yes' or 'no' answers."

6. Put the cards in front of the subject with the questions up.
7. Ask the subject to start. Answer any questions by repeating the question on the card and by saying "I want to know how you feel about it—what does it mean to you. If you don't know or cannot decide, then guess."
8. When the subject is finished, score the "yes" responses. Remove the box, and set out the "resistance" statement cards. Say to the subject, "Now I would like you to show me how you feel about some things to which you answered yes. You may think that to do these things is quite sensible and reasonable (point to card) or just habit, or you may feel that you do not want to do some of these things and in fact try to stop yourself from doing them. Please look at these questions again, and place each one in front of the card which fits your feeling about it most nearly." Make sure that the subject has read and understood each statement card. Then give the subject the "yes" cards and ask him to place them below each card.
9. When the subject is finished, score the weighted reply next to the number of the questions.
10. Collect the cards again, and set out the "interference" statement cards and say to the subject "Now I would like you to show whether any of these things you do interferes with other things, or wastes your time at all" and explain the card statements as above and score them on the sheet in the same way. When the subject is finished, score the time. Collect the cards and put them back in order.

Appendix 3
The 20-Item Leyton Obsessional Inventory

1. Do you often feel like you have to do certain things even though you know you don't really have to?
2. Do thoughts or words ever keep going over and over in your mind?
3. Do you have to check things several times?
4. Do you hate dirt and dirty things?
5. Do you ever feel that if something has been used or touched by someone else it is spoiled for you?
6. Do you ever worry about being clean enough?
7. Are you fussy about keeping your hands clean?
8. When you put things away at night, do they have to be put away just right?

9. Do you get angry if other students mess up your desk?
10. Do you spend a lot of extra time checking your homework to make sure that it is just right?
11. Do you ever have to do things over and over a certain number of times before they seem quite right?
12. Do you ever have to count several times or go through numbers in your mind?
13. Do you ever have trouble finishing your school work or chores because you have to do something over and over again?
14. Do you have a favorite or special number that you like to count up to a lot or do things just that number of times?
15. Do you often have a bad conscience because you've done something even though no one else thinks it is bad?
16. Do you worry a lot if you've done something not exactly the way you like?
17. Do you have trouble making up your mind?
18. Do you go over things a lot that you have done because you aren't sure that they were the right things to do?
19. Do you move or talk in just a special way to avoid bad luck?
20. Do you have special numbers or words you say, just because it keeps bad luck away or bad things away?

If yes:
　0—This habit does not stop me from doing other things I want to do.
　1—This stops me a little or wastes a little of my time.
　2—This stops me from doing other things or wastes some of my time.
　3—This stops me from doing a lot of things and wastes a lot of my time.

Appendix 4
NIMH Teacher Rating of OCD

STUDENT:

GRADE:

RATING PERIOD:

TEACHER:

TODAY'S DATE:

BEHAVIORAL OBSERVATIONS:	NOT AT ALL	JUST A LITTLE	PRETTY MUCH	VERY MUCH
1. Checks things several times				
2. Spends extra time checking work to make sure it is just right				
3. Does things over and over a certain number of times before they seem quite right				
4. Has trouble finishing school work because he has to do something over and over again				
5. Has trouble making up his mind				
6. Goes over and over letters and numbers with writing instrument				
7. Overly neat and clean				
8. Meticulous: pays close attention to detail				

Appendix 5
Yale-Brown Obsessive Compulsive Scale

GENERAL INSTRUCTIONS FOR ADMINISTRATION INCLUDING
DEFINITIONS OF OBSESSIONS AND COMPULSIONS FOR
CHILDREN ARE AVAILABLE WITH THE TEST PACKET

(published with permission, W.K. Goodman, 1987)

OBSESSIONS AND COMPULSIONS CHECKLIST

PATIENT NAME: _____   DATE: _____

	CURRENT	PAST
AGGRESSIVE OBSESSIONS		
• Fear might harm others		
• Fear might harm self		
• Violent or horrorific images		
• Fear of blurting out obscenities or insults		
• Fear of doing something embarrassing		
• Fear will act on other impulses (e.g., rob bank, shoplift, cheat cashier) . . .		
• Fear will be responsible for things going wrong (e.g., company will go bankrupt because of patient)		
• Fear something terrible might happen (e.g., fire, burglary, death or illness of relative/friend, miscellaneous superstitions)		
• Other		
CONTAMINATION OBSESSIONS		
• Concerns or disgust with bodily waste or secretions (e.g., urine, feces, saliva)		
• Concern with dirt or germs		
• Excessive concern with environmental contaminants (e.g., asbestos, radiation, toxic wastes)		
• Excessive concern with household items (e.g., cleansers, solvents, pets)		

	CURRENT	PAST

- Concerned will get ill . . . . _____   _____
- Concerned will get others ill
  (Aggressive) . . . . _____   _____
- Other . . . . _____   _____

SEXUAL OBSESSIONS
- Forbidden or perverse sexual
  thoughts, images, or impulses . . . . . . _____   _____
- Content involves children . . . . _____   _____
- Content involves animals. . . . . _____   _____
- Content involves incest . . . . _____   _____
- Content involves homosexuality . . . . _____   _____
- Sexual behavior toward others
  (Aggressive). _____   _____
- Other . . . . _____   _____

HOARDING/COLLECTING OBSESSIONS
. . . . _____   _____

RELIGIOUS OBSESSIONS
. . . . _____   _____

OBSESSION WITH NEED FOR SYMMETRY,
EXACTNESS, OR ORDER
. . . . _____   _____

MISCELLANEOUS OBSESSIONS
- Need to know or remember . . . . _____   _____
- Fear of saying certain things. . . . . . . _____   _____
- Fear of not saying things just right. . _____   _____
- Intrusive (neutral) images . . . . _____   _____
- Intrusive nonsense sounds, words, or
  music . . . . _____   _____
- Lucky/Unlucky numbers . . . . _____   _____
- Colors with special significance . . . . . _____   _____
- Other . . . . _____   _____

SOMATIC OBSESSION/COMPULSION
. . . . _____   _____

CURRENT   PAST

CLEANING/WASHING COMPULSION
- Excessive or ritualized hand washing _____ _____
- Excessive or ritualized showering, bathing, toothbrushing, or grooming _____ _____
- Involves cleaning of household items or other inanimate objects . . . . _____ _____
- Other measures to remove contact with contaminants . . . . _____ _____
- Other measures to remove contaminants . . . . _____ _____

COUNTING COMPULSIONS
. . . . _____ _____

CHECKING COMPULSIONS
- Checking doors, locks, stove, appliances, emergency brake on car, etc. . . . . _____ _____
- Checking that did not/will not harm others . . . . _____ _____
- Checking that did not/will not harm self . . . . _____ _____
- Checking that nothing terrible will happen . . . . _____ _____
- Checking for contaminants . . . . _____ _____
- Other . . . . _____ _____

REPEATING RITUALS
- Going in/out door, up/down from chair, etc. . . . . _____ _____
- Other . . . . _____ _____

ORDERING/ARRANGING COMPULSIONS
. . . . _____ _____

HOARDING/COLLECTING COMPULSIONS
. . . . _____ _____

CURRENT   PAST

MISCELLANEOUS COMPULSIONS
- Mental rituals (other than checking/ counting) .... _____   _____
- Need to tell, ask, or confess........ _____   _____
- Need to touch.................. _____   _____
- Measures to prevent:
(not checking)   harm to self....... _____   _____
harm to others..... _____   _____
terrible consequences _____   _____
- Other .... _____   _____

CHILDREN'S YALE-BROWN OBSESSIVE COMPULSIVE SCALE (CY-BOCS)

"I'm now going to ask you several questions about those thoughts that repeatedly enter your mind." [Make specific reference to the patient's target obsessions.]

1. TIME OCCUPIED BY OBSESSIVE THOUGHTS
   Q: How much time do you spend thinking about these things? [When obsessions occur as brief, intermittent intrusions, it may be impossible to assess time occupied by them in terms of total hours. In such cases, estimate time by determining how frequently they occur. Consider both the number of times the intrusions occur and how many hours of the day are affected. Ask: How frequently do these thoughts occur? Be sure to exclude ruminations and preoccupations which, unlike obsessions, are ego-syntonic and rational (but exaggerated).]
      0—None.
      1—Mild (less than 1 hr/day), or occasional intrusion (occurs no more than 8 times a day).
      2—Moderate (1 to 3 hrs/day), or frequent intrusion (occurs no more than 8 times a day, but most hours of the day are free of obsessions).
      3—Severe (greater than 3 and up to 8 hrs/day), or very frequent intrusion (occurs more than 8 times a day and occurs during most hours of the day).
      4—Extreme (greater than 8 hrs/day), or near constant intrusion (too numerous to count and an hour rarely passes without several obsessions occurring).

2. INTERFERENCE DUE TO OBSESSIVE THOUGHTS

Q: How much do these thoughts get in the way of school or doing things with friends? Is there anything that you don't do because of them? [If currently not in school, determine how much performance would be affected if patient were in school.]

    0—None.

    1—Mild, slight interference with social or school activities, but overall performance not impaired.

    2—Moderate, definite interference with social or school performance, but still manageable.

    3—Severe, causes substantial impairment in social or school performance.

    4—Extreme, incapacitating.

3. DISTRESS ASSOCIATED WITH OBSESSIVE THOUGHTS

Q. How much do these thoughts bother or upset you? [Only rate anxiety that seems triggered by obsessions, not generalized anxiety or anxiety associated with other symptoms.]

    0—None.

    1—Mild, infrequent, and not too disturbing.

    2—Moderate, frequent, and disturbing, but still manageable.

    3—Severe, very frequent, and very disturbing.

    4—Extreme, near constant, and disabling distress.

4. RESISTANCE AGAINST OBSESSIONS

Q. How hard do you try to stop the thoughts or ignore them? [Only rate effort made to resist, not success or failure in actually controlling the obsessions. How much the patient resists the obsessions may or may not correlate with his ability to control them. Note that this item does not directly measure the severity of the intrusive thoughts; rather it rates a manifestation of health, i.e., the effort the patient makes to counteract the obsessions. Thus, the more the patient tries to resist, the less impaired is this aspect of his functioning. If the obsessions are minimal, the patient may not feel the need to resist them. In such cases, a rating of "0" should be given.]

    0—Makes an effort to always resist, or symptoms so minimal doesn't need to actively resist.

    1—Tries to resist most of the time.

    2—Makes some effort to resist.

    3—Yields to all obsessions without attempting to control them, but does so with some reluctance.

    4—Completely and willingly yields to all obsessions.

5. DEGREE OF CONTROL OVER OBSESSIVE THOUGHTS
   Q: When you try to fight the thoughts, can you beat them? [For the more advanced child ask]: How much control do you have over the thoughts? [In contrast to the preceding item on resistance, the ability of the patient to control his obsessions is more closely related to the severity of the intrusive thoughts.]
   0—Complete control.
   1—Much control, usually able to stop or divert obsessions with some effort and concentration.
   2—Moderate control, sometimes able to stop or divert obsessions.
   3—Little control, rarely successful in stopping obsessions, can only divert attention with difficulty.
   4—No control, experienced as completely involuntary, rarely able to even momentarily divert thinking.

Questions on Compulsions (Items 6-10) "The next several questions are about the habits you can't stop." [Make specific reference to patient's target compulsions.]

6. TIME SPENT PERFORMING COMPULSIVE BEHAVIORS
   Q. How much time do you spend doing these things? [When rituals involving activities of daily living are chiefly present, ask]: How much longer does it take to complete your usual daily activities because of the habits? [When compulsions occur as brief, intermittent behaviors, it may be impossible to assess time spent performing them in terms of total hours. In such cases, estimate time by determining how frequently they are performed. Consider both the number of times compulsions are performed and how many hours of the day are affected. Count separate occurrences of compulsive behaviors, not number of repetitions; e.g., a patient who goes into the bathroom 20 different times a day to wash his hands 5 times very quickly, performs compulsions 20 times a day, not 5 or $5 \times 20 = 100$. Ask]: How often do you do these habits? [In most cases compulsions are observable behaviors (e.g., hand washing), but there are instances in which compulsions are not observable (e.g., silent checking).]
   0—None.
   1—Mild (spends less than 1 hr/day performing compulsions), or occasional performance of compulsive behaviors (no more than 8 times a day).
   2—Moderate (spends from 1 to 3 hrs/day performing com-

pulsions), or frequent performance of compulsive behaviors (more than 8 times a day, but most hours are free of compulsive behaviors).

3—Severe (spends more than 3 and up to 8 hrs/day performing compulsions), or very frequent performance of compulsive behaviors (more than 8 times a day and compulsions performed during most hours of the day).

4—Extreme (spends more than 8 hrs/day performing compulsions), or near constant performance of compulsive behaviors (too numerous to count and an hour rarely passes without several compulsions being performed).

7. INTERFERENCE DUE TO COMPULSIVE BEHAVIORS

Q: How much do these habits get in the way of school or doing things with friends? Is there anything that you don't do because of them? [If currently not in school, determine how much performance would be affected if patient were in school.]

0—None.

1—Mild, slight interference with social or school activities, but overall performance not impaired.

2—Moderate, definite interference with social or school performance, but still manageable.

3—Severe, causes substantial impairment in social or school performance.

4—Extreme, incapacitating.

8. DISTRESS ASSOCIATED WITH COMPULSIVE BEHAVIOR

Q: How would you feel if prevented from carrying out your habits? [Pause.] How upset would you become? [Rate degree of distress patient would experience if performance of the compulsion were suddenly interrupted without reassurance offered. In most, but not all cases, performing compulsions reduces anxiety. If, in the judgment of the interviewer, anxiety is actually reduced by preventing compulsions in the manner described above, then ask]: How upset do you get while carrying out your habits until you are sure they are done?

0—None.

1—Mild, slightly anxious if compulsions prevented, or only slight anxiety during performance of compulsions.

2—Moderate, reports that anxiety would mount but remain manageable if compulsions prevented, or that anxiety increases but remains manageable during performance of compulsions.

3—Severe, prominent, and very disturbing increase in anxiety if compulsions interrupted, or prominent and very disturbing increase in anxiety during performance of compulsions.

4—Extreme, incapacitating anxiety from any intervention aimed at modifying activity, or incapacitating anxiety develops during performance of compulsions.

9. RESISTANCE AGAINST COMPULSIONS

Q: How much do you try to fight the habits? [Only rate effort made to resist, not success or failure in actually controlling the compulsions. How much the patient resists the compulsions may or may not correlate with his ability to control them. Note that this item does not directly measure the severity of the compulsions; rather it rates a manifestation of health, i.e., the effort the patient makes to counteract the compulsions. Thus, the more the patient tries to resist, the less impaired is this aspect of his functioning. If the compulsions are minimal, the patient may not feel the need to resist them. In such cases, a rating of "0" should be given.]

0—Makes an effort to always resist, or symptoms so minimal doesn't need to actively resist.

1—Tries to resist most of the time.

2—Makes some effort to resist.

3—Yields to almost all compulsions without attempting to control them, but does so with some reluctance.

4—Completely and willingly yields to all compulsions.

10. DEGREE OF CONTROL OVER COMPULSIVE BEHAVIOR

Q: How strong is the feeling that you have to carry out the habits? [Pause.] When you try to fight them what happens? [For the more advanced child ask]: How much control do you have over the habits? [In contrast to the preceding item on resistance, the ability of the patient to control his compulsions is more closely related to the severity of the compulsions.]

0—Complete control.

1—Much control, experiences pressure to perform the behavior, but usually able to exercise voluntary control over it.

2—Moderate control, strong pressure to perform behavior, can control it only with difficulty.

3—Little control, very strong drive to perform behavior, must be carried out to completion, can only delay with difficulty.

4—No control, drive to perform behavior experienced as completely involuntary and overpowering, rarely able to even momentarily delay activity.

"The remaining questions are about both the thoughts and the habits. Some ask about different things."

11. INSIGHT AND OBSESSIONS AND COMPULSIONS
Q. Do you think the ideas or habits really make sense? [Pause.] What do you think would happen if you didn't carry out the habits? Are you afraid something might really happen? [Rate patient's insight into the senselessness or excessiveness of his obsession(s) or compulsion(s) based on beliefs expressed at the time of the interview.]

0—Excellent insight, fully rational.

1—Good insight. Readily acknowledges absurdity or excessiveness of thoughts or behaviors but does not seem completely convinced that there isn't something besides anxiety to be concerned about. Voices lingering doubts.

2—Fair insight. Reluctantly admits thoughts or behavior seems unreasonable or excessive, but wavers. May have some unrealistic fears, but no fixed convictions.

3—Poor insight. Maintains that thoughts or behaviors are not unreasonable or excessive.

4—Lacks insight, delusional. Definitely convinced that concerns and behavior are reasonable, unresponsive to contrary evidence.

12. AVOIDANCE
Q: Have you not been doing things, not going places, or not been with anyone because of your repeated thoughts or out of concern you will carry out such habits? [If yes, then ask]: How much do you avoid? [Rate degree to which patient deliberately tries to avoid things. Sometimes compulsions are designed to "avoid" contact with something that the patient fears. For example, excessive washing of fruits and vegetables to remove "bugs" would be designated as a compulsion, not as an avoidant behavior. If the patient stopped eating fruits and vegetables, then this would constitute avoidance.]

0—No deliberate avoidance.

1—Mild, minimal avoidance.

2—Moderate, some avoidance clearly present.

3—Severe, much avoidance; avoidance prominent.

4—Extreme, very extensive avoidance; patient does almost everything he can to avoid triggering symptoms.

13. DEGREE OF INDECISIVENESS
    Q: Do you have trouble making decisions about little things that others might not think twice about (e.g., which clothes to put on in the morning)? [Exclude difficulty making decisions which reflect ruminative thinking. Ambivalence concerning rationally based difficult choices should also be excluded.]
    0—None.
    1—Mild, some trouble making decisions about minor things.
    2—Moderate, freely reports significant trouble making decisions that others would not think twice about.
    3—Severe, continual weighing of pros and cons about nonessentials.
    4—Extreme, unable to make any decisions. Disabling.

14. OVERVALUED SENSE OF RESPONSIBILITY
    Q: Do you blame yourself for things you can't really change or can't do much about? Do you feel to blame for what happens to others?
    0—None.
    1—Mild, only mentioned on questioning, slight sense of over-responsibility.
    2—Moderate, ideas stated spontaneously, clearly present; patient experiences significant sense of over-responsibility for events outside his reasonable control.
    3—Severe, ideas prominent and pervasive; deeply concerned he is responsible for events clearly outside his control. Self-blaming farfetched and nearly irrational.
    4—Extreme, delusional sense of responsibility (e.g., if an earthquake occurs 3,000 miles away patient blames himself because he didn't perform his compulsions).

15. PERVASIVE SLOWNESS/DISTURBANCE OF INERTIA
    Q: Do you have difficulty starting or finishing things because you have to do things so carefully? Do many routine activities take longer than they should? [Distinguish from psychomotor retardation secondary to depression. Rate increased time spent performing routine activities even when specific obsessions cannot be identified.]
    0—None.
    1—Mild, occasional delay in starting or finishing.

2—Moderate, frequent prolongation of routine activities but tasks usually completed. Frequently late.

3—Severe, pervasive, and marked difficulty initiating and completing routine tasks. Usually late.

4—Extreme, unable to start or complete routine tasks without full assistance.

16. PATHOLOGICAL DOUBTING

Q: Do you find that you're unsure of your memory or that you don't trust your own eyes or ears?

0—None.

1—Mild, only mentioned on questioning, slight sense of self-doubt.

2—Moderate, ideas stated spontaneously, clearly present; patient bothered by significant self-doubt. Some effect on performance but still manageable.

3—Severe, uncertainty about perceptions or memory prominent; self-doubt frequently affects performance.

4—Extreme, uncertainty about perceptions constantly present; self-doubt substantially affects almost all activities. Incapacitating (e.g., patient states "my mind doesn't trust what my eyes see").

[Items 17 and 18 refer to global illness severity. The rate is required to consider global function, not just the severity of obsessive-compulsive symptoms.]

17. GLOBAL SEVERITY: Interviewer's judgment of the overall severity of the patient's illness. Rated from 0 (no illness) to 6 (most severe patient seen). [Consider the degree of distress reported by the patient, the symptoms observed, and the functional impairment reported. Your judgment is required both in averaging the data as well as weighing the reliability of accuracy of the data obtained. This judgment is based on information obtained during the interview.]

0—No illness.

1—Illness slight, doubtful, transient; no functional impairment.

2—Mild symptoms, little functional impairment.

3—Moderate symptoms, functions with effort.

4—Moderate–Severe symptoms, limited functioning.

5—Severe symptoms, functions mainly with assistance.

6—Extremely severe symptoms, completely nonfunctional.

18. GLOBAL IMPROVEMENT: Rate total overall improvement present SINCE THE INITIAL RATING whether or not, in your judgment, it is due to drug treatment.

   0—Very much worse.
   1—Much worse.
   2—Minimally worse.
   3—No change.
   4—Minimally improved.
   5—Much improved.
   6—Very much improved.

19. RELIABILITY: Rate the overall reliability of the rating scores obtained. Factors that may affect reliability include the patient's cooperativeness and his natural ability to communicate. The type and severity of obsessive-compulsive symptoms present may interfere with the patient's concentration, attention, or freedom to speak spontaneously (e.g., the content of some obsessions may cause the patient to choose his words very carefully).

   0—Poor, very low reliability.
   1—Fair, factor(s) present that definitely reduce reliability.
   2—Good, factor(s) present that may adversely affect reliability.
   3—Excellent, no reason to suspect data unreliable.

Items 17 and 18 are adapted from the Clinical Global Impression Scale (Guy W: ECDEU Assessment Manual for Psychopharmacology: Publication 76-338. Washington, D.C., US Department of Health, Education and Welfare 1976).

Appendix 6
NIMH Obsessive Compulsive Scale (ward staff)

Name _____ Date _____ Study Phase ____ Rater _____

OBSESSIVE-COMPULSIVE RATING

	None	Mild	Mod.	Marked	Very Severe
Preoccupations with rituals or obsessions	1	2	3	4	5
Number of different rituals	1	2	3	4	5
Degree of interference with personal (ward) activities	1	2	3	4	5
Amount of time spent resisting compulsive urges & behavior	1	2	3	4	5

Section III

Associated Measures

Chapter 5

Neuropsychological Testing of Obsessive-Compulsive Adolescents

Christiane S. Cox, M.S.
Paul Fedio, Ph.D.
Judith L. Rapoport, M.D.

Because of the increasing evidence for a new biological factor in obsessive-compulsive disorder (OCD), the noninvasive measures of neuropsychology are of great interest. However, the data are meager. Neuropsychological test deficits in obsessive-compulsive patients were first reported by Flor-Henry and his collaborators (1979), who administered the Halstead Reitan battery to a series of 11 obsessive-compulsive adults. A profile analysis suggested bilateral frontal impairment with greater involvement of the left than right hemisphere in 10 of the 11 patients. In addition, 5 of the patients demonstrated evidence of bilateral temporal dysfunction and 2 showed compromised parietal functions bilaterally. Insel et al. (1983) failed to replicate these findings in their sample of 18 obsessive-compulsive patients using the same battery of tests. However, more than half of their patients manifested spatial-perceptual disturbances on all aspects of the Tactual Performance Test and a difference exceeding 15 points between the Verbal IQ and Performance IQ. In contrast, a pilot study of 16 obsessive-compulsive adolescents (Behar et al. 1984) found striking spatial-perceptual abnormalities suggestive of frontal dysfunction.

Since 1976, we have compared the neuropsychological test performance of obsessive-compulsive children and adolescents and matched controls extending the Behar study. We speculated that our group with uniformly early onset OCD would yield a more homogeneous pattern of neuropsychological performance. Tasks were chosen to yield information about frontal, temporal, and parietal functioning. In addition, several experimental tasks were designed to restrict initial stimulus input to one hemisphere, permitting assessment of the relative efficiency of each hemisphere in processing verbal and visuo-spatial material.

At this time, 42 obsessive-compulsive adolescent patients and 35 matched normal controls have been tested. Individuals were excluded if they had Full Scale IQs less than 85, if they would not cooperate with the testing program, or if they had psychotic symptoms, primary depressive illness (patients with secondary depression were included), or definite neurological disease. Controls were matched by age (± 1 year), sex, race, handedness, and IQ (within 15 points). A description of subject characteristics appears in Table 1.

Tests and Procedures

All neuropsychological tests and procedures were administered in a single session of approximately 3 hours. The tests were chosen to

Table 1. Subject characteristics of 42 obsessive-compulsive adolescents and 35 controls.

Measure	Obsessive-compulsive	Controls
Age (yrs)		
Mean ± SD	14 ± 2.7	14 ± 2.6
Range	8 – 18	8 – 18
Sex		
Male	30	26
Female	12	9
Handedness		
Right	34	31
Left	8	4
Intelligence Quotient*		
Verbal		
Mean ± SD	109 ± 12.5	116 ± 10.3
Range	82 – 128	96 – 136
Performance		
Mean ± SD	104 ± 14.0	116 ± 10.5
Range	77 – 136	96 – 135

*Wechsler Adult Intelligence Scale or Wechsler Intelligence Scale for Children.

assess attention; auditory, visual, and haptic perceptual processes; verbal and visuo-spatial learning and memory; spatial orientation and judgment; and the ability to observe test rules. Detailed speech and language testing was not included in this assessment but was obtained independently by another investigator. The following tests were administered:

Stylus Maze Learning. This spatial memory task is thought to be sensitive to frontal and parietal damage. The maze consisted of a 10 × 10 array of metal contacts embedded in a black plastic square matrix (Milner 1965). Using a metal tipped probe, subjects had to learn, by trial and error, an invisible pathway connecting the start and goal buttons. Correct moves were signaled by a low tone (250 Hz), whereas a high tone (1,000 Hz) signaled horizontal directions; diagonal moves were against the rules. Testing was discontinued after 10 trials or two errorless runs. Route-finding and rule-breaking errors were tallied separately for each trial.

Wisconsin Card Sorting Test (Heaton 1981). Four stimulus cards —one red triangle, two green stars, three yellow crosses, and four blue circles—were placed in front of the subject, who was then handed a deck of 64 response cards and instructed to place each one in front of a stimulus card. Subjects were informed only whether each response was right or wrong and had to deduce the correct sorting principle by themselves. The same sorting principle remained in effect for 10 consecutive correct sorts, after which the principle changed without warning. The test was discontinued after all 64 cards had been sorted. The number of correct consecutive sorts was used as a measure of the number of categories achieved. For instance, if a subject completed sorts to color, form, and number, and then gave seven consecutive correct responses according to color before the deck ran out, the subject was given a score of 37. Correct responses, perseverative responses, perseverative errors, nonperseverative errors, and unique errors were scored as outlined by Heaton (1981).

Money's Road Map of Direction Sense (Money et al. 1965). This spatial test reflects an ability to mentally rotate in space. Both frontal and/or caudate lesions may impair performance. Subjects were presented with a simulated street map on which two routes were indicated. The first one had four turns and was used for practice. The second one had 32 choice points and was divided into two sections, each with 16 turns. Subjects were instructed to imagine traversing the route and to indicate a left or right turn at each choice point. In the first part, the direction of travel was congruent with the subject's body orientation; in the second part, the direction was reversed and therefore travel proceeded in a direction rotated 180 degrees from the subject's body orientation. The map remained in a fixed position in front of the subjects, who were not allowed to alter their position in order to facilitate left-right judgments. The sequence of turns along the routes was random, with an equal number of right and left turns. The time taken to complete each section and the number of correct responses in each direction were recorded.

Visual recognition thresholds for words and patterns. This test was included to look for lateralized differences in perceptual sensitivity. The stimuli were presented in a four-field tachistoscope. High-frequency three-letter words were printed vertically, and complex designs were used. A recognition threshold was determined for center and then for left and right visual fields by an ascending method using 3-msec increments. For lateral field testing, the stimuli were delivered in a prearranged, random order to the left or right field. The subject spelled or read the words. A six-choice recognition paradigm was used for the designs (Rosenthal and Fedio 1975).

Rey-Osterrieth Complex Figure (Osterrieth 1944). This test of memory and constructional abilities is sensitive to right parietal damage. Subjects were asked to copy a complex geometric figure. After completion, the drawing was removed. The subjects had to fill out a handedness questionnaire for 3 minutes, at which time they were asked to reproduce the figure from memory. Subjects were not forewarned that reproduction of the figure would be required. Both the time needed to draw the design and accuracy were recorded.

Rey Auditory-Verbal Learning List A (Rey 1941). This test may be sensitive to dominant hemisphere lesions. A list of 15 high-frequency, high-imagery words was presented aurally, in a fixed order, at the rate of one word every 2 seconds. Immediately after presentation, the subjects were required to repeat as many words as possible in any order. Five trials were administered. After a delay of 1 hour, recall was requested. This was followed by a recognition procedure in which subjects had to select among four words the one that came from the list. The distractor words were either semantic, phonemic, or unrelated foils.

Auditory task: monaural condition. Subjects were instructed to repeat six monosyllabic words, delivered in a staggered order to the left and right ear via stereophonic earphones. Six trials were administered, the lead word being delivered to the left or right ear for the same number of times. Words were separated by an interval of 500 msec.

Auditory task dichotic condition. Six monosyllabic words were delivered as pairs to the left and right ear ($\pm$ 20 msec onset time). The words for each pair were matched on the basis of initial phoneme. All stimuli were high frequency words. A free-recall paradigm was used, and the number of words recalled from the left and right ear over six trials constituted the overall score. Both monaural and dichotic conditions were preceded by a practice trial (Kimura 1967).

Dihaptic encoding task. This experimental task was included to look for lateralized dysfunctions. The subjects were required to palpate a pair of three-dimensional, six-pointed forms simultaneously with the index and middle fingers of each hand. At the conclusion of the 10-second exploration time, they had to select from a visually presented array of 10 items the forms they had felt with each hand. Five trials were administered to all subjects; 19 obsessive-compulsive subjects and 15 controls were given 25 trials (Fedio et al. 1979).

Data analysis. Analysis was carried out using the BMDP biomedical statistical program package created by the University of California (1986). Analysis of variance and covariance, with or without repeated measures, was carried out, as applicable.

Results

Although the obsessive-compulsive patients scored well within the average range of intellectual functioning, their Verbal and Performance IQs were significantly lower than that of the controls ($F = 11.23$, 1/75 df, $p < .01$). In general, spatial-perceptual abnormalities were striking, but there were also hints of frontal lobe dysfunction.

Stylus Maze. As shown in Figure 1, obsessive-compulsive subjects committed significantly more route-finding errors than control subjects ($F = 18.39$, 1/75 df, $p < .001$). The group $\times$ trial interaction was not significant, indicating that both groups learned the route at a comparable rate; the obsessive-compulsive patients simply committed more errors to begin with and never reached the low error rate of the controls. As a group, the obsessive-compulsive patients also broke more rules during the 10 trials that were administered ($F = 5.63$, 1/75 df, $p < .05$). Rule-breaking errors represented a significantly larger percentage of total errors for males than for females ($F = 7.36$, 1/73 df, $p < .01$). However, the sex × group interaction was not significant.

Wisconsin Card Sorting Test. The obsessive-compulsive subjects achieved significantly fewer correct consecutive sorts (Table 2) than the controls ($F = 5.03$, 1/72 df, $p < .01$). However, there was no significant difference in the number of perseverative and nonperseverative errors that the two groups committed.

Money's Road Map of Direction Sense. This generated more left-right errors among the obsessive-compulsive patients than controls ($F = 11.02$, 1/75 df, $p < .01$). The largest discrepancy between obsessive-compulsive subjects and controls occurred when the left-right judgments had to be made in an inverted direction. This is seen in Figure 2; subjects had to imagine they were travelling in a direction incongruent with body orientation (group × direction interaction: $F = 8.71$, 1/75 df, $p < .01$).

Rey-Osterrieth Complex Figure. Because the obsessive-compulsive patients took significantly more time than the controls to reproduce the Rey-Osterrieth figure ($t = 2.94$, 76 df, $p < .01$), copy time was used

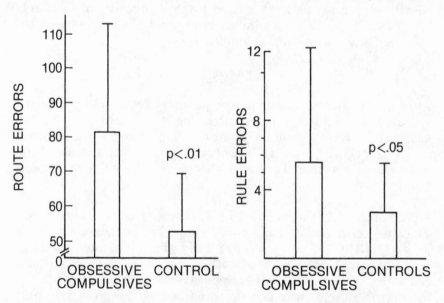

Figure 1. Means and standard deviations for the route-finding and rule-breaking errors committed by 42 obsessive-compulsive and 35 control subjects taking the Stylus Maze test.

Table 2. Neuropsychological test scores for 42 obsessive-compulsive adolescents and 35 controls

| | Mean ± SD | | | | |
	OCD	Controls	*F*	df	*P*
Road map					
Correct moves	25.9 ± 5.8	29.5 ± 3.8	11.02	1/75	.01
Direction by groups			8.71	1/75	.01
Stylus maze					
Route errors	82.0 ± 33.9	53.9 ± 20.8	18.39	1/75	.001
Rule breaking errors	5.6 ± 7.0	2.5 ± 3.0	5.63	1/75	.05
Wisconsin card sort					
Consecutive correct sorts	37.9 ± 12.2	43.9 ± 8.6	5.03	1/72	.05
Rey-Osterrieth figure					
Copy, correct score	26.8 ± 5.2	29.8 ± 3.2	13.88	1/74	.001
Percentage loss	39.5 ± 18.5	29.5 ± 17.4	5.87	1/75	.05
Visual thresholds					
Words (all 3 fields)	33.1 ± 14.9	26.1 ± 12.9	5.02	1/70	.05
Shapes (all 3 fields)	9.5 ± 3.8	8.2 ± 2.8	3.66	1/69	.07
Auditory verbal learning					
Total over 5 trials	51.3 ± 10.7	55.0 ± 7.0	3.16	1/74	.08
Trials by groups			2.37	4/296	.06
Dichotic listening					
Total accuracy	17.2 ± 5.3	16.4 ± 6.2	1.27	1/63	ns
Dihaptic Recognition accuracy	5.1 ± 1.8	5.3 ± 1.4	0.21	1/60	ns

as a covariate in the analysis of copy and memory scores. A significant group effect ($F = 13.88$, 1/74 df, $p < .001$) and task effect ($F = 291.52$, 1/75 df, $p < .001$) were found, but no significant interaction emerged indicating that the obsessive-compulsive patients were less efficient in reproducing the design either from a model or from memory. Because the initial production of the figure was not as accurate for the obsessive-compulsive subjects, memory performance was expressed as a percentage loss score (copy-memory/copy × 100), thus taking into account the quality of the initial production. Again, a significant group difference emerged ($F = 5.87$, 1/75 df, $p < .05$). Whereas control subjects lost an average of 29 percent of the information between copy and 3-minute delayed recall, the obsessive-compulsive patients revealed an average of 39 percent loss.

Tachistoscopic thresholds. The obsessive compulsive subjects required significantly longer exposure duration (in milliseconds) than

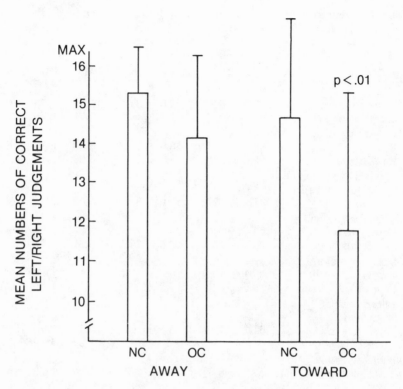

Figure 2. Means and standard deviations of correct left-right judgments made on the Money Road Map of Direction Sense by 42 obsessive-compulsive (OC) and 35 control (NC) subjects in the direction congruent (away) and incongruent (toward) to body orientation.

the controls to identify three-letter words projected to the central (mean: 24.5 and 18.9, respectively), left (38.5 and 31.1), and right (36.4 and 28.2) visual fields ($F = 5.02$, 1/70 df, $p < .05$). The analysis revealed, as expected, a highly significant field effect ($F = 98.26$, 2/140 df, $p < .001$). Thresholds were significantly lower in center field than in either lateral field (Scheffe $p < .01$, for both center vs. left and center vs. right). In addition, subjects in both groups exhibited the usual right visual field advantage for verbal material (Scheffe $p < .05$). There was no significant group × field interaction.

The remaining tasks. Rey verbal learning and delayed recall, monaural and dichotic listening, and dihaptic encoding–visual recognition showed no significant group differences (Table 2).

Relation to clinical impairment. There was no significant correlation between any of several measures of severity of obsessive-compulsive symptomatology and any of the neuropsychological variables for the obsessive-compulsive group. Specifically, we looked at scores in relation to (a) global impairment, measured by the National Institute of Mental Health (NIMH) Global subscale for functional impairment (Murphy et al. 1982); (b) obsessive-compulsive behavior rating carried out by physicians and ward staff using the Obsessive Compulsive Rating Scale (Rapoport et al. 1980), the Comprehensive Psychopathological Rating Scale–Obsessive Compulsive subscale (Thoren et al. 1980), and the NIMH obsessive-compulsive subscale (Rapoport and Elkins, unpublished); and (c) self-rating of obsessive-compulsive behavior using a modified version of the Leyton Obsessional Inventory (Berg et al. 1986; Cooper 1970). Interestingly, normal controls who endorsed a high number of responses on the Leyton Obsessional Inventory obtained low right-hand scores on the dihaptic task (correct score $r = .53, p < .05$; reversals $r = .50, p < .05$). The same was true for a high resistance score (correct score $r = -.66, p < .01$; reversals $r = .45, p < .05$). A high interference score was not only associated with a poor haptic right-hand performance (correct $r = .55, p < .05$; reversals $r = .56, p < .01$), but also with a high error rate on the Road Map in either direction of travel (direction congruent with body orientation $r = .58, p < .001$; rotated orientation $r = .39, p < .05$) and a poor Rey Figure copy score ($r = -.38, p < .05$).

Discussion

Selected neuropsychological tests revealed significant group differences, and these differences were not correlated with measures of severity of obsessive-compulsive symptomatology. This argues against the interpretation that the obsessive-compulsive subjects were so preoccupied by intrusive thought or rituals that they were unable to concentrate on the tasks at hand. These findings replicate and extend the report of Behar et al. (1984).

The tasks that yielded group differences have been shown, in previous research, to be sensitive to frontal and/or caudate lesions. Milner (1965) reported that patients, following frontal lobe resection for treatment of intractable epilepsy, committed significantly more errors, especially rule-breaking errors, on the Stylus Maze than patients who had undergone left or right temporal lobe removals. Fedio et al. (1979) have also shown that Huntington's patients with significant caudate atrophy on computed tomography (CT) scan, as well as subjects at-risk for Huntington's disease but showing no atrophy on CT scan, made significantly more errors on the Stylus Maze than controls.

Milner (1963) also showed that patients with dorsolateral and medial frontal lesions performed more poorly on the Wisconsin Card Sorting Test than patients of similar age and IQ but with lesions in other areas of the cortex.

The differential pattern of impairment displayed by the obsessive-compulsive patients on the Road Map has also been found with Huntington's patients and subjects at-risk for Huntington's disease. The patient groups committed the majority of the errors on that portion of the map where travel proceeded in a direction incongruent with body orientation. This indicates that the patients did not have difficulty with simple left-right orientation because they could make correct discriminations on the part of the route that was congruent with their body orientation. However, when subjects had to imagine themselves in a position shifted 180 degrees, their performance deteriorated. Brouwers et al. (1984) demonstrated that this defect in manipulating egocentric space was not simply a function of progressive cognitive failure in Huntington's patients because Alzheimer's patients, who were also impaired on this task, did not exhibit the same pattern. Other researchers have shown that deficits in egocentric spatial judgment tend to be associated with frontal and/or caudate lesions rather than lesions in other basal ganglia structures (Potegal 1971) or parietal regions (Butters et al. 1972; Semmes et al. 1963).

The tasks chosen to assess possible hemispheric differences in perceptual and cognitive processing yielded few robust differences, with the exception of tachistoscopic recognition thresholds and Rey-Osterrieth Complex Figure copy and percentage loss scores. The fact that obsessive-compulsive patients required longer exposure duration to identify three-letter words in all three fields and showed a trend in the same direction when random shapes were used as stimuli makes it unlikely that obsessive-compulsive patients experienced a specific verbal deficit, especially in the presence of normal verbal learning, verbal memory, and dichotic listening scores. Patients who have undergone right temporal lobe removal for intractable epilepsy also showed overall elevated thresholds (Rosenthal and Fedio 1975), albeit more pronounced for the random shapes. The results of the threshold procedure, taken together with the marginal performance of the obsessive-compulsive patients on the Rey-Osterrieth Complex Figure, suggest a subtle right hemisphere dysfunction.

The present study thus concurs with Flor-Henry et al.'s (1979) earlier work in finding impairment in frontal regulatory function.

However, the bilateral temporal dysfunction that Flor-Henry et al. documented in half of their patients is not found in our sample of obsessive-compulsive children and adolescents who, as a group, tended to exhibit only subtle signs of right hemisphere dysfunction. Independent evidence supporting central nervous system pathology and implicating basal ganglia function has been gathered recently by Baxter et al. (1987), who compared local cerebral glucose metabolic rates with positron emission tomography in adult obsessive-compulsive patients, unipolar depressed patients, and normal controls. Glucose metabolic rates were found to be significantly elevated in the caudate nucleus and orbito-frontal regions. Behavioral improvement during drug treatment correlated significantly with an increase in the ratio of caudate glucose utilization rate/whole hemisphere glucose utilization rate.

To strengthen the position that the impairments in neuropsychological functioning exhibited by the obsessive-compulsive patients are related to the disorder and not to some nonspecific maturational lag factor, it is necessary to demonstrate stability of the findings over time. A 2- to 7-year follow-up study (see Chapter 2) is summarized here briefly and presented in detail elsewhere (Cox et al. in preparation).

At follow-up the Stylus Maze, the Road Map, and a Complex Figure were readministered. Although all subjects performed significantly better at second testing (test-retest: Stylus Maze, $p < .001$; Road Map, $p < .05$; Complex Figure, $p < .001$), the obsessive-compulsive patients were still impaired relative to controls on the Stylus Maze and the Road Map ($p < .01$ and $p < .05$, respectively). Administration of an alternative form of the Complex Figure showed a trend for group differences in the copy score ($p < .06$) but not the percentage loss score. The degree of neuropsychological impairment was, again as at initial exam, unrelated to any measure of severity of obsessive-compulsive symptomatology.

In conclusion, as a group, obsessive-compulsive adolescents are impaired only on a selected subset of neuropsychological tests. On tasks of auditory perception and attention, verbal learning and memory, and dihaptic encoding and recognition, the obsessive-compulsive subject's performance is either very close to or indistinguishable from that of controls. Moreover, tasks demonstrating both group differences and stability of those group differences over time have been shown in other studies to be sensitive to frontal and/or caudate lesions. Since the impaired performance was not correlated significantly with any of the measures of clinical impairment, the differences between the obsessive-compulsive group and the controls do not seem secondary to nonspecific disability, but rather to reflect stable patterns of cerebral dysfunction associated with OCD. These findings support the model of Wise and Rapoport (see Chapter 19) in which frontal lobe–basal ganglia dysfunction is proposed as etiologic in OCD. Brain-imaging techniques such as those employed by Baxter et al. (1987) will be of great interest in addressing these neuropsychological findings.

References

Baxter L, Phelps M, Mazziotta J, et al: Cerebral glucose metabolic rates in obsessive compulsive disorder compared to unipolar depression and normal controls. Arch Gen Psychiatry 44:211–218, 1987

Behar D, Rapoport JL, Berg CJ, et al: Computerized tomography and neuropsychological test measures in adolescents with obsessive compulsive disorder. Am J Psychiatry 141:363–369, 1984

Berg CJ, Rapoport JL, Flament M: The Leyton Obsessional Inventory—Child Version. J Am Acad Child Psychiatry 25:84–91, 1986

BMDP Statistical Software. Los Angeles, University of California Press, 1986

Brouwers P, Cox C, Martin A, et al: Differential perceptual-spatial impairment in Huntington's and Alzheimer's dementia. Arch Neurol 41:1073–1076, 1984

Butters N, Soeldner C, Fedio P: Comparison of parietal and frontal lobe spatial deficits in man: extrapersonal vs personal (egocentric) space. Percept Mot Skills 34:27–34, 1972

Cooper J: The Leyton Obsessional Inventory. Psychol Med 1:48–64, 1970

Fedio P, Cox CS, Neophytides A, et al: Neuropsychological profile of Huntington's disease: patients and those at risk, in Advances in Neurology: Huntington's Chorea. Edited by Chase TN, Barbeau A, Wexler NS. New York, Raven Press, 1979

Flor-Henry P, Yeudall LT, Koles ZJ, et al: Neuropsychological and power spectral EEG investigation of the obsessive compulsive syndrome. Biol Psychiatry 14:119–130, 1979

Heaton RK: Wisconsin Card Sorting Test Manual. Odessa, FL, Psychological Assessment Resources, 1981

Insel TR, Donnelly EF, Lalakea ML, et al: Neurological and neuropsychological studies of patients with obsessive compulsive disorder. Biol Psychiatry 18:741–751, 1983

Kimura D: Functional asymmetry of the brain in dichotic listening. Cortex 3:163–178, 1967

Milner B: Effects of different brain lesions on card sorting. Arch Neurol 9:90–100, 1963

Milner B: Visually-guided maze learning in man: effects of bilateral hippocampal, bilateral frontal and unilateral cerebral lesions. Neuropsychologia 3:317–338, 1965

Money J, Alexander D, Walker HT: A Standardized Road Map Test of Direction Sense. Baltimore, Johns Hopkins University Press, 1965

Murphy DL, Pickard D, Alterman IS: Methods for the quantitative assessment of depressive and manic behavior, in The Behavior of Psychiatric Patients. Edited by Burdock EL, Sudilousky A, Gershon S. New York, Marcel Dekker, 1982, pp 355–392

Osterrieth PL: Le test de copie d'une figure complex. Arch de Psychologie 30:206–356, 1944

Potegal M: A note on spatial-motor deficits in patients with Huntington's disease: a test of a hypothesis. Neuropsychologia 9:233–235, 1971

Rapoport JL, Elkins R: NIMH obsessive compulsive scale (unpublished), p 104

Rapoport JL, Elkins R, Mikkelson E: Clinical controlled trial of chlomipramine in adolescents with obsessive compulsive disorder. Psychopharmacol Bull 16:61–63, 1980

Rey A: Examen clinique en psychologie dans les cas d'encephalopathie traumatique. Arch de Psychologie 28:286–340, 1941

Rosenthal LS, Fedio P: Recognition thresholds in central and lateral visual fields following temporal lobectomy. Cortex 11:217–229, 1975

Semmes, J, Weinstein S, Ghent L, et al: Correlates of impaired orientation in personal and extra-personal space. Brain 86:747–772, 1963

Thoren P, Asberg M, Cronholm B, et al: Clomipramine treatment of obsessive compulsive disorder. Arch Gen Psychiatry 37:1281–1285, 1980

Chapter 6

Psycholinguistic Testing in Obsessive-Compulsive Adolescents

Christy L. Ludlow, Ph. D.
Celia J. Bassaich, M. A.
Nadine P. Connor, M. A.
Judith L. Rapoport, M. D.

Language impairments have been reported in adult patients with obsessive-compulsive disorder (OCD) (Flor-Henry et al. 1979) and interpreted as indicating left hemisphere dysfunction in the temporo-parietal region. However, poor aphasia test performance could be due to other abnormalities.

First, poor performance could result from OCD interfering in some particular fashion with all cognitive functions, including language (Insel et al. 1983; Persons and Foa, in press; Reed 1977; Sher et al. 1983). Lorenz and Cobb (1954) compared the formal language characteristics of adults with OCD with those of normal speakers during restricted discourse. The patients with OCD had reduced percentages of substantive articles (nouns), adjectives, and prepositions, and increased percentages of verbs, adverbs, and pronouns. Since the authors only included patients whose language ability retained normal coherence and grammatical form, they concluded that these results

We thank Carol Berg, Jeanette Herman, and Hope Lake, who assisted with the data compilation and analyses.

reflected patients' preoccupations with actions and relationships and the quality of such relationships rather than a language deficit. Reed (1977) found that these patients were not impaired on memory tasks, although they tended to check frequently on the accuracy of past events. He suggested that OCD interfered with patients' discriminations between real and imagined events, explaining their need to check on previous occurrences. Persons and Foa (in press) explored whether the cognitive mechanisms of indecisiveness, slowness, and fear were found in adults with OCD only on tasks involving their fears or whether they reflected a general deficit in information processing. The results demonstrated that obsessive thinking can be characterized as excessively complex and not limited to thinking about feared topics. More than half of the adults with OCD studied by Insel et al. (1983) were impaired on the Tactual Performance Test from the Halstead-Reitan Battery. Although this deficit was relatively specific, these authors discussed the possibility that this could be reflective of the fear of patients with OCD to touch items particularly when they are blindfolded, rather than a specific perpetual deficit suggestive of right parietal lobe dysfunction. They also noted that this was a time-related task and that several of the Wechsler Adult Intelligence Scale (WAIS) subtests on which the patients were impaired were also timed tasks. Since patients with OCD are known to be slow and indecisive, these results could reflect these patients' cognitive disorder. In contrast, Beech and Liddell (1974) reported that patients with OCD had particular difficulties on decision-making tasks. However, a slowness to respond could not explain these findings because the patients did not differ from normal controls on a simple speed test, the Digit Symbol test of the WAIS. However, Persons and Foa (in press) have suggested that the general reduction in cognitive functioning of patients with OCD may be seen only when tasks require considerable information processing, which would not include the Digit Symbol test.

Deficits seen in patients with OCD could be nonspecific and found in many psychiatric disturbances. In a previous study of 9 obsessive-compulsive adolescents, we employed dichotic listening tasks (Rapoport et al. 1981). The findings suggested a lack of normal laterality for speech perception similar to that seen in several psychiatric conditions, including affective disorders (Wexler and Heninger 1979), and may not reflect a specific difference in cognitive functioning associated with this syndrome. Further, electroencephalogram alterations have been found in the patients with OCD that are similar to those seen in primary depressive disorder (Rapoport et al. 1981).

An alternate interpretation of impaired language test performance in patients with OCD is that some underlying neurological dysfunction is responsible for both the OCD and the language test performance. In this view, deficits in language test performance could provide information relevant to the type and location of brain dysfunction in this syndrome (Behar et al. 1984; Elkins and Rapoport 1980; Flor-Henry et al. 1979). Although patients with OCD do not display consistent deficits on IQ tests (Templar 1972), deficits have been found on certain tests (Insel et al. 1983). Flor-Henry et al. (1979) studied 11 patients with OCD on a battery of neuropsychological tests and found a pattern of performance on cognitive tests suggestive of left frontal lobe dysfunction. The patients' performances were significantly lower than those of normal controls on a variety of tests including: Wepman-Jones Aphasia Screening Test; the Raven's colored progressive matrices; Symbol Gestalt; Halstead category; minute estimation; tactual performance in both hands; the Seashore rhythm test; Purdue pegboard performance with both hands; WAIS Digit Span; and WAIS Digit Symbol.

The differing results of Flor-Henry et al. (1979), Behar et al. (1984), and Insel et al. (1983) may also reflect language processing variation across age groups. Flor-Henry et al. studied older inpatient adults with a chronic history of OCD whereas Behar et al. (1984) studied adolescents and Insel et al. studied mild to moderately impaired adult outpatients with OCD.

Our purpose was to investigate the neurolinguistic functioning of obsessive-compulsive adolescents to determine whether their pattern of performance on psycholinguistic tasks was suggestive of either a specific or nonspecific psychiatric disorder or localized neuropathology. If language-processing deficits in OCD are secondary to disturbed information processing, then these patients should evidence deficits in speed of information processing. Further, their performance deficits should be related to the severity of their OCD. On the other hand, if both OCD and associated language performance deficits are associated with a regional brain dysfunction, then the language deficits of patients with OCD should be similar to aphasia resulting from brain lesions. Finally, if language-processing deficits in OCD are nonspecific and similar to those seen in many psychiatric disorders, then the patterns of deficits may be similar to that previously found in Tourette's syndrome without OCD (Ludlow et al. 1982).

Methods

Subjects

Psychiatric evaluations, family interviews, and extensive medical and neurological histories determined whether patients met the DSM-III (American Psychiatric Association 1980) definition for severe primary OCD (see Chapter 2). Individuals were excluded from the language testing if their Wechsler Intelligence Scale for Children (WISC) Full Scale IQ score was below 85, or if they would not cooperate with the testing program.

Subjects consisted of 24 (17 male) consecutive obsessive-compulsive adolescents with a mean age of 14.4 years (range, 10–18). Patient reports and observations of writing activities confirmed that 18 were right-handed, 5 left-handed, and 1 ambidextrous. The mean (± SD) WISC IQs for the group were 106 ± 13.5 (Full Scale), 106.2 ± 12.4 (Verbal), and 104.4 ± 14.5 (Performance).

In addition, 24 normal controls were selected, each matching a particular obsessive-compulsive patient in age, sex, and handedness, and within the same IQ range. None of the normal controls had a history of a speech or language disorder, learning difficulties in school, or a neurologic or psychiatric illness.

Language Assessment Procedures

Since OCD was expected to produce subtle deficits in language performance, tests were selected and adapted to assess complex aspects of auditory comprehension, speech expression, oral reading and comprehension, and written expression. Three aphasia tests were adapted for this purpose.

1. *The Neurosensory Center Comprehensive Examination for Aphasia* (NCCEA) (Spreen and Benton 1969) is a standardized language assessment battery for measuring language deficits in aphasic adults relative to the normal adult population. Normative data are available for each of the 18 subtests for children and adolescents between the ages of 5 and 13 (Gaddes and Crockett 1975) and for young adults (Spreen and Benton 1969). These normative data provided the mean and standard deviation for normal performance at a subject's particular age level allowing for computation of Z scores relative to normal for each of the patients and controls on each of the NCCEA subtests. Only some NCCEA subtests were selected for this study because many are not sensitive to mild deficits in language function.

2. *The Token Test* (DeRenzi and Vignolo 1962) was developed to detect subtle deficits in language comprehension following brain injury. Ten tokens are presented—five squares and five circles of five different colors: white, yellow, red, blue, and green. Sentences are spoken at a uniform rate and intonation, each requiring the subject to perform a specific action with particular tokens. The sentences are without redundant information, requiring subjects to understand every word to perform the actions correctly (e.g., "Put the green circle

under the blue square"). This test is sensitive to deficits in language comprehension accompanying injury to the left hemisphere (DeRenzi and Vignolo 1962; Swisher and Sarno 1969). The original version contains five parts, the first four parts differing in sentence length and amount of information. Part 5 is the most complex part and contains sentences that vary in their syntactic form and that contain different prepositions, verbs, adverbs, nouns, and adjectives (e.g., "After picking up the red circle, touch the blue square"). For this investigation, four experimental versions of Part 5 of the Token Test with equivalent material were developed to assess four different language functions: auditory language comprehension, language expression, oral reading, and reading comprehension.

3. *The Boston Naming Test* (Borod et al. 1980) includes line drawings of 85 nouns presented in order of decreasing frequency in English. A stimulus tape was developed with click signals for presentations of drawings every 7 seconds. Both the clicks and the subject's responses were tape-recorded. The subject's responses were transcribed, and the time between each presentation click and a subject's response was measured with a stopwatch for correct responses. The nouns contained in the Boston Naming Test were printed on index cards and presented for an Oral Reading Adaptation of the Boston Naming Test, using the same click stimulus tape.

Language Measures

Auditory comprehension was measured from Part 5 of the Token Test, previously described. The percentage of nouns, verbs, prepositions, adjectives, and adverbs correctly recognized in commands was scored.

Three tests were employed to assess *oral expression*. On the Description of Use subtest, subjects explained how an object is used. This measured the retrieval of specific verbs. The NCCEA Sentence Construction Test required the subject to construct a sentence containing specific words in 20 seconds. The faster the construction of a grammatically correct sentence with an acceptable meaning, the greater the number of points earned per item. Another test of oral expression, the Reporter's Test (DeRenzi 1978) assessed the construction of sentences equivalent to those contained in the Token Test. For the Reporter's Test, an adapted version of Part 5 of the Token Test was developed equivalent to the other three forms used in this investigation in syntactic form and content. For this test, the examiner silently produced actions similar to correct responses to Token Test commands. Subjects described what the examiner did following each complete action (e.g., "You put the red circle under the blue square"). The use of complete and grammatically correct sentences was emphasized. Training was provided on at least one item before beginning the test. Three scores were computed from tape-recorded transcriptions: the percentage of nouns, verbs, prepositions, adjectives, and adverbs correctly produced; the percentage of the sentences without grammatical errors; and the percentage of sentences with nouns and verbs produced in the correct sequence.

Two measures of *oral reading* and one measure of *reading comprehension* were obtained. For the Oral Reading Adaptation of the Boston Naming Test, subjects read aloud the names of 85 items written on index cards that were presented at the point of click on the stimulus tape. The percentage correct (based on 85 items) was computed. For the Oral Reading Adaptation of Part 5 of the Token Test, subjects read aloud the Token Test commands printed on an index card. The percentage of words read correctly was computed. Subjects demonstrated reading comprehension by performing the action with the tokens after reading a command aloud. The percentage of nouns, verbs, adjectives, and adverbs for which understanding was correctly demonstrated was scored.

Three *writing* subtests were selected from the NCCEA: Visual-Graphic Naming, Writing Names, and Writing to Dictation. For the first two tasks, eight objects were presented and subjects' written responses were scored for whether the name was recognizable (Visual Graphic Naming) and for spelling accuracy (Writing Names). The Writing to Dictation subtest included two sentences written to dictation. Each word was scored for spelling accuracy.

Four tests of *naming* and word retrieval were included: The NCCEA Tactile Naming Subtest on the Right; the NCCEA Tactile Naming Subtest on the Left; the NCCEA Word Fluency subtest; and the Boston Naming Test. For the Tactile Naming subtests, 16 objects were presented to one hand behind a visual barrier without the subject seeing the object. The Word Fluency subtest from the NCCEA required the subject to produce as many words as possible within 1 minute, beginning with the same letter. The letters F, A, and S were used. This task assesses word retrieval based on knowledge of the written form, and has been found sensitive to brain pathology (Borkowski and Benton 1967). Z scores were computed for each subject on these NCCEA subtests using normative data (Gaddes and Crockett 1975; Spreen and Benton 1969).

Subject response time was measured on four tasks: the NCCEA Tactile Naming Subtest on the Right; the NCCEA Tactile Naming Subtest on the Left; the Boston Naming Test; and the Adapted Oral Reading Version of the Boston Naming Test. For the Tactile Naming subtests, the examiner's cue of when the object was presented and the subject's response were tape-recorded. The mean response time was measured for correct naming responses. Mean response time was also measured for correct responses from tape recordings of the Boston Naming Test and the Adapted Oral Reading Version by measuring the time between the stimulus presentation click and the subject's response.

Short-Term Memory

To assess short-term memory, three NCCEA subtests assessed the speech repetition of orally presented material. The Sentence Repetition subtest contained 22 sentences of increasing length. The number of sentences correctly repeated was scored. The Digit Repetition Forward subtest contained 14 digit strings of increasing length from two to nine digits. Immediate repetition of each string was required. The total number of digits repeated in the correct order was scored. Similarly, the Digit Repetition Backwards subtest required subjects to reverse the order of the digits during repetition of 14 strings increasing in length from two to eight digits. The total number of digits produced in the correct reverse order was scored.

The Memory for Sequence subtest of the Goldman-Fristoe-Woodcock Auditory Skills Battery (Goldman et al. 1974) was selected as an auditory short-term memory task with a motor response. Fourteen strings of between two and eight unrelated single-syllable words were presented on audiotape. Following each string presentation, picture cards of the words presented were provided, and the subject ordered the cards. The percentage of cards correctly arranged was computed. To assess the effects of stimulus and response modality, three experimental versions were developed equivalent to this auditory-motor recall task. The Visual Motor task provided picture cards of the same items used for the Auditory Motor task, ordered in different strings. After viewing a string of pictures, the subject, who was provided with the picture cards, put the cards in the same order as they were presented. The responses were scored according to the number of cards correctly ordered. The Auditory Verbal subtest required the subject to repeat strings of words presented on audiotape. The Visual Verbal subtest required the subject to say the words represented by a string of picture cards, after the pictures were withdrawn. For these latter two tests, both the percentage of words recalled and the percentage of words that were recalled in correct sequence were scored.

Dichotic Listening Speech Perception Test

Dichotic listening is a competitive listening task where equivalent but different speech stimuli are presented simultaneously to both ears.

The subject is asked to report all stimuli. In the majority of normal adults, there is a higher percentage of correct reporting for items presented to the right ear than to the left ear (Kimura 1961). Syllables presented to the ear contralateral to the hemisphere dominant for language are perceived more accurately than those presented to the ear contralateral to the nondominant hemisphere. The left hemisphere is dominant for language in 90 to 96 percent of persons who are right-handed and 70 to 85 percent of those who are left-handed (Branch et al. 1964). To determine whether the patients with OCD would exhibit a normal pattern of right ear advantage, a dichotic listening task for the perception of speech syllables was constructed with the vowel a and varying initial stop consonants—p, t, k, b, d, and g. Tape-recorded syllables whose onsets were perfectly aligned by computer were obtained from Dr. Charles Berlin (Kresge Hearing Research Laboratory, Louisiana State University Medical Center, New Orleans). The difference in recording levels of the two channels were less than 1 dB on half-track low-noise tape. Each of the six consonant-vowel syllables (pa, ta, ka, ba, da, ga) was paired with the other five, yielding 120 pairs presented to each subject. A prerecorded 1,000 Hz calibration tone was set at a 80 $\pm$ 2 dB sound pressure level reading when a sound level meter was fixed by a coupler to each earphone. The stimuli were played on an Ampex A6-350 tape recorder.

The earphones (TDH-49) were mounted in circumaural cushions and were repeatedly reversed following presentation of 30 dichotic pairs. The channel-to-ear orientation for each half of the stimulus tape was counter-balanced across listeners. At the time of testing, all subjects had normal audiometric thresholds (20 dB hearing level, ANSI) in each ear between 500 and 4,000 Hz. The percentage of syllables presented in the right and left ears correctly reported was computed, yielding left and right ear scores.

To measure the degree of right ear advantage independent of performance level, the "e" laterality index developed by Repp (1977) was used. The percentage correct in the left ear was subtracted from the percentage correct in the right; this result was divided by the sum of the percentages correct in the right and left ears. A positive value indicated a right ear advantage; a negative value reflected a left ear advantage.

Measures of Obsessive-Compulsive Disorder

To determine whether psycholinguistic function was related to the severity of patients' OCD, psychiatrists administered a modified version of the Leyton Obsessional Inventory (Berg et al. 1986) on screening for admission to the study, providing scores for number of symptoms, resistance, and interference. Three other ratings of the degree of disability secondary to OCD were National Institute of Mental Health (NIMH) Global and Obsessive Compulsive subscales and a ward rating (see Chapter 4), administered during hospital stay by a psychiatrist, the nursing staff, and another psychiatrist.

Computed Tomography (CT) Scans and Cerebral Ventricular Measurements

CT scans were obtained on a GE 8800 CT scanner. Cerebral ventricular measurements were made according to the procedure developed by Weinberger et al. (1979).

A rater selected and measured the CT slice with the largest lateral ventricular area using a planimeter. Only the posterior and largest portions of the lateral ventricles were measured. The area was divided by the total intracranial space to obtain a ventricular brain ratio (VBR) as a percentage. This measure is reported in detail elsewhere (Behar et al. 1984).

Results

To eliminate any measures that were highly related, Pearson r correlation coefficients were computed between measures of auditory comprehension and expression. R^2 values greater than .50 indicated that more than 50 percent of the variation on one measure could be accounted for by variation on the other measure. Such measures were redundant and both should not be used in group comparisons. Two measures from the Reporter's Test, the percentage correct and the percentage grammatical, had an r^2 of .69. Therefore, the percentage grammatical score was deleted.

Similarly, within the speed of response measures, the mean response times on the Boston Naming Test and the Adapted Boston Oral Reading Test were highly related ($r^2 = .67$). Therefore, the Oral Reading response time measure was deleted.

On the measures of short-term memory, Auditory Verbal Memory Recall was highly related to Auditory Verbal Sequence ($r^2 = .85$) and Auditory Motor Sequence ($r^2 = .50$). Since both of the latter two tests were related to each other ($r^2 = .48$), Auditory Verbal Sequence and Auditory Motor Sequence were deleted. Similarly, Visual Verbal Recall was highly related to Visual Motor Sequence ($r^2 = .67$) and Visual Motor Sequence was also related to Visual Verbal Sequence ($r^2 = .47$). Therefore, the Visual Motor Sequence measure was deleted.

This resulted in 27 independent measures in which the OCD group and controls were compared. Since the standard deviations of the OCD group were frequently greater than in the controls, a nonparametric procedure, the Wilcoxon test for matched pairs, was used.

Language

The mean language scores of the OCD group and the normal controls are presented in Table 1. A criterion probability of .05 was selected for statistical significance. A significant difference ($p < .013$) between the two groups was found on the total number of words correctly recognized on the Auditory Comprehension Adapted Part 5 of the Token Test. Since the two groups did not differ on the oral production version of the same test, the Reporter's Test, this comprehension deficit was not likely due to visual recognition difficulties. The OCD group did not differ significantly from the normal group on any of the oral production tests. In fact, the mean percentage correct production of

Table 1. Comparison of language test scores of patients with obsessive-compulsive disorder (OCD) and normal controls matched on age, sex, handedness, and IQ scores

Function	Test	OCD group Mean ± SD	Control group Mean ± SD	Z^*	p
Auditory comprehension	Adapted Part 5 of Token Test (% correct)	97.6 ± 2.06	99.1 ± 1.19	−2.48	.013
Oral expression	NCCEA Description of Use (Z Score)	−1.38 ± 1.45	−0.81 ± 1.07	−1.69	ns
	NCCEA Sentence Construction (Z Score)	−0.51 ± 2.48	−0.13 ± 2.11	−.94	ns
	Reporter's Test (% correct)	94.18 ± 4.33	96.41 ± 2.65	−1.51	ns
	Reporter's Test (% in sequence)	97.18 ± 5.32	93.50 ± 14.88	−.36	ns

*The Wilcoxon test for matched samples was used to compute a Z score and its probability.

nouns and verbs in sequence tended to be higher in the OCD group than in the controls.

Reading and Writing

The results of the oral reading, reading comprehension, and writing tests are presented in Table 2. No significant differences were found on the oral reading tests. A significant difference was found between the OCD group and the normal controls on the Reading Comprehension Adapted Version of Part 5 of the Token Test ($p < .04$). Since no deficits were found on the oral reading version of the same test, this reduced performance is probably not due to difficulties in recognizing written forms of words. Rather, the poorer performance of the OCD group is most likely due to language comprehension difficulties similar

Table 2. Comparison of patients with obsessive-compulsive disorder (OCD) and controls on reading and writing tasks

Function	Test	OCD group Mean ± SD	Control group Mean ± SD	n	Z*	p
Oral reading	Adapted Boston Naming (% correct)	97.9 ± 2.15	98.6 ± 1.59	22	−1.11	ns
	Adapted Part 5 Token Test (% correct)	99.2 ± 1.10	99.4 ± 1.05	22	−.57	ns
Reading comprehension	Adapted Part 5 Token Test (% correct)	98.0 ± 1.76	99.14 ± 1.70	22	−2.02	.04
Writing	NCCEA Graphic Naming Naming (Z score)	.17 ± .48	.20 ± .34	24	−.21	ns
	Spelling (Z score)	.17 ± 1.18	.54 ± 1.04	24	−1.82	ns
	NCCEA Writing to Dictation (Z score)	.02 ± .51	.18 ± .31	24	−1.24	ns

*The Wilcoxon test for matched samples was used to compute a Z score and its probability.

to those reflected on the Auditory Comprehension Adapted Version of Part 5 of the Token Test. No significant differences were found between the two groups on any of the writing tests.

Naming

The results of the four naming tasks are presented in Table 3. The patients with OCD were impaired on naming objects presented tactually to either hand. Although the mean values of the OCD group tended to be lower than those of the normal controls on the other naming tasks, none of these approached statistical significance. No reduction in performance was found on the Word Fluency Task, indicating that there was no reduction in vocabulary in the OCD group.

Speed of Response

The results of subjects' speed of response during oral naming and reading tasks are presented in Table 3. The OCD group was significantly slower, having longer response latencies than the normal controls on the Boston Naming Test. However, the OCD group was not slower to respond on items named correctly on either of the Tactile Naming tasks.

Short-Term Memory

The results of the tests assessing short-term memory functions are presented in Table 4. No significant differences were found between the two groups on any of the tests, indicating that the perception and recall of language information through speech was unimpaired as was the memory of visual information presented by picture cards. These findings suggest that deficits seen on other tests were not due to difficulties in the perception or short-term memory of test stimuli.

Dichotic Listening

The results of the two groups on the dichotic listening task are presented in Table 5. The OCD group had significantly lower reporting for the right ear in comparison with the controls ($p < .0015$) and a significantly reduced right ear advantage ($p < .027$). The patients with OCD were no more efficient in reporting consonant-vowel syllables from the right ear than from the left during a competitive listening task and did not demonstrate the left hemisphere superiority for speech perception usually seen in the normal population. Since subjects in the two

Table 3. Comparison of patients with obsessive-compulsive disorder (OCD) and controls on tests of naming, vocabulary recall, and speed of response

Function	Test	OCD group Mean ± SD	Control group Mean ± SD	n	Z*	p
Naming	NCCEA Tactile Naming— Right (Z score)	−.83 ± 1.12	−0.71 ± 1.05	20	−2.38	.018
	NCCEA Tactile Naming— Left (Z score)	−.02 ± .82	0.49 ± .32	19	−2.64	.008
	NCCEA Word Fluency (Z score)	.02 ± 1.02	0.61 ± 1.30	24	−1.57	ns
	Adaptation of Boston Naming (% correct)	76.7 ± 9.54	79.5 ± 9.45	23	−.93	ns
Speed of response	Tactile Naming Right— Mean Response Time (sec)	2.64 ± .77	1.79 ± .32	20	−.11	ns
	Tactile Naming Left— Mean Response Time (sec)	3.21 ± 1.20	2.33 ± .70	19	−.56	ns
	Boston Naming Mean Response Time (sec)	2.41 ± .46	2.16 ± .33	23	−2.24	.025

*The Wilcoxon test for matched samples was used to compute a Z score and its probability.

groups had been matched on handedness and since the Wilcoxon test compared matched pairs, this cannot be accounted for by handedness difference between the two groups. Six of the patients with OCD had reversed laterality scores, indicating that their rate of accurate report-

Table 4. Comparison of patients with obsessive-compulsive disorder (OCD) and controls on tests of short-term memory

Function	Test	OCD group Mean ± SD	Control group Mean ± SD	n	Z*	p
Short-term memory	NCCEA Sentence Repetition (Z score)	−.94 ± 1.37	−.93 ± 1.37	24	−.52	ns
	NCCEA Digits Repetition Forward (Z score)	.75 ± 1.12	.83 ± 1.01	24	−.47	ns
	NCCEA Digits Repetition Reverse (Z score)	.49 ± .85	.67 ± .98	24	−.08	ns
	GFW Auditory Verbal Recall (% correct)	84.09 ± 8.0	85.6 ± 7.4	22	−.52	ns
	GFW Visual Verbal Recall (% correct)	86.55 ± 6.72	88.77 ± 5.66	22	−.84	ns
	GFW Visual Verbal Sequence (% correct)	73.82 ± 13.25	79.18 ± 10.42	22	−1.29	ns

*The Wilcoxon test for matched samples was used to compute a Z score and its probability.

ing was higher in response to stimuli presented to the left ear. Of these 6, 3 were right-handed and 3 were left-handed. Three of the normal controls, all right-handed, also had slight left ear advantages.

Relationships with Severity of OCD and Ventricular Brain Ratio

The 27 measures of language processing, naming, short-term memory naming, and dichotic listening, were correlated with three measures of severity and impairment from OCD and with the VBR. There were, therefore, more than 100 computed correlations. Only five correlations were significant, and two of these were in the opposite direction

Table 5. Comparison of patients with obsessive-compulsive disorder
(OCD) and controls on dichotic listening tests

Function	Test	OCD group Mean ± SD	Control group Mean ± SD	df	Z*	p
Dichotic listening	% correct right ear	58.29 ± 14.54	72.43 ± 10.95	1,40	−3.18	.0015
consonant-vowel syllables	% correct left ear	51.62 ± 13.72	48.14 ± 18.65	1,40	−.49	ns
	Right Ear Advan-tage**	0.06 ± 0.18	0.23 ± 0.24	1,40	−2.21	.027

*The Wilcoxon test for matched samples was used to compute a Z score and its
probability.
**Repp (1977)

from that predicted. Therefore, no significant relationship between
clinical ratings of impairment and language performance was obtained.

Discussion

Since the OCD group was not impaired on any of the tests of short-term
memory when words were presented visually or auditorily, no perceptual processing difficulties were found in OCD when stimuli were
spoken or presented visually. Further, on the language testing, the
OCD group had no difficulty (a) repeating sentences or digits presented auditorily, (b) writing the names of objects presented, or (c)
writing to dictation. Their normal performance on these tasks suggests
that they had a normal vocabulary and spelling skills and that their
disorder did not interfere with the perception and recognition of
words or objects.

The patients with OCD were not impaired on the two timed language tests—the Word Fluency test and the Sentence Construction
test—which depend on a normal speed of response for a good score. On
the Word Fluency task, the subjects with OCD could recall as many
words within 1 minute beginning with a particular sound as the normal controls. In sentence construction, subjects produced a sentence
quickly using the words spoken by the examiner. Further, the speed of
recognition of objects presented tactually and named correctly was not
slower than normal. Thus the OCD group did not exhibit an overall
slowing in their speed of response. Their response latency was impaired only on the Boston Naming Test. The OCD group was impaired
in two other naming tests: tactile naming when objects were presented

to the right and to the left hands. Behar et al. (1984) demonstrated that several of the same obsessive-compulsive adolescents had no difficulties with dihaptic perception. However, two studies of adults with OCD (Flor-Henry et al. 1979; Insel et al. 1983) found impaired performance by obsessive-compulsive patients on the Halstead-Reitan Tactual Performance Test, a measure of nonvisual spatial organization. Insel et al. (1983) suggested that deficits on the tactual tasks could reflect the concern of many of their patients with touching objects that have been handled by others. If this were the case, such a disturbance should have interfered with performance on the dihaptic perception test by Behar et al. (1984). Further, when subjects were able to name objects actually presented, their response time was not slower than normal. The poor response on the Tactile Naming tests by the OCD group in this study may reflect difficulty with the naming response required rather than the tactual perception.

Our adolescent obsessive-compulsive patients had impaired performance on two language comprehension tasks: the Token Test of auditory language comprehension and the Reading Comprehension Token Test. Since these patients had no difficulties with the perception of speech or pictures or immediate information retrieval, short-term memory deficits could not account for the patients' impairments on language tasks. The patients' performance on these language tasks, however, were not like patterns seen with language disorder. None of the speech expression tasks incorporating the same material evidenced differences between the OCD group and the controls. None had symptoms of aphasia in their everyday conversation. Even the scores of those patients scoring below the range of the normal controls were well above the scores of brain-damaged aphasic adults on the same tasks (Gaddes and Crockett 1975; Spreen and Benton 1969). Further, there was no reduction in the stored vocabulary of the OCD group as evidenced by normal performance on the Word Fluency task.

Each of the tasks on which the OCD group had a lower performance than normal required mental manipulation or processing of linguistic information. For example, on the Auditory and Reading Comprehension versions of the Token Test, subjects were expected to decode the sentences and then encode a motor response representing the linguistic content of the sentence. The reduced speed of response on the Boston Naming Test, requiring lexical retrieval, demonstrated less efficient information processing in obsessive-compulsive patients even when their response was correct. Thus their processing of information was affected although their linguistic knowledge was not.

These results are consistent with previous studies. Beech and Liddell (1974) reported impaired performance in obsessive-compulsive adults on decision-making tasks, also requiring a manipulation of knowledge. Behar et al. (1984) reported patients were impaired on a maze crossover task requiring subjects to remember a maze configuration and to reverse it mentally. Further, two studies (Beech et al. 1983; Ciesielski et al. 1981) have demonstrated reduced evoked potential amplitudes and increased latencies in obsessive-compulsive patients in comparison with normal controls during decision-making tasks requiring shape discrimination. In both studies, the differences between the OCD group and the controls became more marked as task complexity increased. The results on the dichotic listening task may further reflect a difficulty of obsessive-compulsive patients in adopting an efficient information-processing strategy. Morais (1978) and Morais and Bertelson (1973) demonstrated that ear advantage on dichotic listening tasks can be affected by spatial attentional factors, bringing into question the degree to which right ear advantage depends on brain lateralization for language (Warrington and Pratt 1981). Kinsbourne (1973, 1975) demonstrated how attention to verbal material can shift attentional biases to the left hemisphere (the right side), whereas biases to the left side can shift attention to the right hemisphere. Thus, in interpreting these data, attentional effects must be considered as well as the physiological effects of the more rapidly conducting contralateral pathways to the dominant hemisphere from the right ear. The lack of a significant right ear advantage in the OCD group may indicate that these patients did not adopt an efficient attentional bias of attending to the right ear to perform the task. Since they had the same level of reporting in the left ear as the controls, they did not have an overall reduction in performance on this task.

Our results differ from those of Flor-Henry et al. (1979). We did not find reductions on digit span or language tasks such as naming and word fluency, which are most sensitive to left hemisphere involvement. This may be due, in part, to our rigorous subject selection criteria, eliminating any subject with signs of neurological impairment. Subjects similar to those excluded by us may have been included for study by Flor-Henry et al. (1979) accounting for the larger number of neuropsychological test deficits found by those investigators. Only two relationships in the expected direction were found between performance on the linguistic tasks and clinical severity. The obsessive-compulsive patients showed a wide range disorder, ranging from those who were entirely able to mask their difficulties socially to those who could not function outside a hospital. Surprisingly, no significant relationship was seen between impairment and linguistic testing. Thus speculations that the test deficits were due to the psychiatric disorder remain a reasonable, but unproven, interpretation of the data.

Finally, it should be mentioned that the pattern of language tasks on which the patients with OCD were impaired was quite different from those found in a group of patients with Tourette's syndrome (Ludlow et al. 1982). In that study, patients between 12 and 18 years of age with Tourette's syndrome were administered the same language tests as used in this study and had significant impairments on all subtests requiring speech and language formulation or a written response (i.e., word fluency, sentence construction, reading and writing names, and writing to dictation). Thus the pattern of impaired language performance found in the patients with OCD was dissimilar from at least this group with Tourette's syndrome. This is of particular interest in light of the association between OCD and Tourette's syndrome (Pauls et al. 1986). The difference in linguistic patterns suggests either that Tourette's syndrome may represent a more severe disorder or is a qualitatively different condition.

In summary, our results demonstrated a specific performance deficit of patients with OCD on tasks requiring the manipulation of knowledge presented in one form for expression in another. These information-processing deficits could not be accounted for by perceptual or short-term memory deficits or by the patients' speed of response. Thus one needs to postulate reduced efficiency of cognitive manipulations of information in obsessive-compulsive patients. The language deficits, however, did not resemble any known pattern associated with particular brain pathology. Although the data suggest performance deficits of these patients with OCD are due to the disorder's interfering with complex language processing, what mediates this interference remains unclear.

References

American Psychiatric Association: Diagnostic and Statistical Manual of Mental Disorders, 3rd ed (DSM-III). Washington, DC, American Psychiatric Association, 1980

Beech HR, Liddell A: Decision-making, mood states, and ritualistic behavior among obsessional patients, in Obsessional States. Edited by Beech HR. London, Methuen, 1974

Beech HR, Ciesielski KT, Gordon PK: Further observations of evoked potentials in obsessional patients. Br J Psychiatry 142:605–609, 1983

Behar D, Rapoport JL, Berg CJ, et al: Computerized tomography and neuropsychological test measures in adolescents with obsessive-compulsive disorder. Am J Psychiatry 141:363–369, 1984

Berg CJ, Rapoport JL, Flament MF: The Leyton Obsessional Inventory—Child Version. J Am Acad Child Psychiatry 25:84–91, 1986

Borkowski JC, Benton AL: Word fluency and brain damage. Neuropsychologia 5:145–140, 1967

Borod JC, Goodglass H, Kaplan E: Normative data on the Boston Diagnostic Aphasia Examination, Parietal Lobe Battery, and the Boston Naming Test. J Clin Neuropsychol 2:209–216, 1980

Branch CB, Milner B, Rasmussen T: Intracarotid amytal for the lateralization of cerebral speech dominance. J Neurosurg 21:399–405, 1964

Ciesielski KT, Beech HR, Gordon PK: Some electrophysiological observations in obsessional states. Br J Psychiatry 138:479–484, 1981

DeRenzi E: The Reporter's Test: a sensitive test to detect expressive disturbances in aphasics. Cortex 14:279–293, 1978

DeRenzi E, Vignolo L: The token test: a sensitive test to detect receptive disturbances in aphasics. Brain 85:665–678, 1962

Elkins R, Rapoport JL: Obsessive-compulsive disorder of childhood and adolescence. J Am Acad Child Psychiatry 19:511–524, 1980

Flor-Henry P, Yendall LT, Koles ZJ: Neuropsychological and power spectral EEG investigations of the obsessive-compulsive syndrome. Biol Psychiatry 14:119–130, 1979

Gaddes WH, Crockett DJ: Spreen-Benton aphasia tests, normative data as a measure of normal language development. Brain Lang 2:257–280, 1975

Goldman R, Firstoe M, Woodcock RW: Auditory Skills Battery. Circle Pines, MN, American Guidance Service, 1974

Insel TR, Donnelly DF, Lalakea ML, et al: Neurological and neuropsychological studies of patients with obsessive-compulsive disorder. Biol Psychiatry 18:741–751, 1983

Kimura D: Cerebral dominance and the perception of verbal stimuli. Can J Psychol 15:166–171, 1961

Kinsbourne M: The control of attention by interaction between the cerebral hemispheres, in Attention and Performance, Vol. 4. Edited by Kornblum S. New York, Academic Press, 1973

Kinsbourne M: The mechanism of hemispheric control in the lateral gradient of attention, in Attention and Performance, Vol. 5. Edited by Rabbit PMA, Doric S. New York, Academic Press, 1975

Lorenz M, Cobb S: Language patterns in psychotic and psychoneurotic subjects. AMA Archives of Neurological Psychiatry 72:665–673, 1954

Ludlow CL, Polinsky RJ, Caine ED, et al: Language and speech abnormalities in Tourette syndrome, in Advances in Neurology, Vol. 35. Edited by Friedhoff AJ, Chase TN. New York, Raven Press, 1982

Morais J: Spatial constraints on attention to speech, in Attention and Performance, Vol. 7. Edited by Requin J. Hillsdale, NJ, Lawrence Erlbaum Associates, 1978

Morais J, Bertelson P: Laterality effects in dichotic listening. Perception 2:107–111, 1973

Pauls D, Towbin K, Leckman J, et al: Gilles de la Tourette syndrome and obsessive compulsive disorder: evidence supporting a genetic relationship. Arch Gen Psychiatry 43:80–111, 1986

Persons JB, Foa EB: Thinking processes in obsessive-compulsive disorder. Behav Res Ther (in press)

Rapoport JL, Elkins R, Langer DH, et al: Childhood obsessive-compulsive disorder. Am J Psychiatry 138:1545–1554, 1981

Reed GF: Obsessional personality disorder and remembering. Br J Psychiatry 130:177–183, 1977

Repp BH: Measuring laterality effects in dichotic listening. J Acoust Soc Am 62:720–737, 1977

Sher KJ, Forst RO, Otto R: Cognitive deficits in compulsive checkers: an exploratory study. Behav Res Ther 21:357–363, 1983

Spreen O, Benton AL: Neurosensory Center Comprehensive Examination for Aphasia (rev ed). Victoria, British Columbia, University of Victoria, 1969

Swisher LP, Sarno MT: Token test scores of three matched patient groups: left-brain damaged with aphasia; right-brain damaged without aphasia; non-brain damaged. Cortex 5:264–273, 1969

Templar DT: The obsessive-compulsive neurosis: review of research findings. Compr Psychiatry 13:375–383, 1972

Warrington EK, Pratt RTC: The significance of laterality effects. J Neurol Neurosurg Psychiatry 44:193–196, 1981

Weinberger DR, Torrey RF, Neophytides AN: Lateral cerebral ventricular enlargement in chronic schizophrenia. Arch Gen Psychiatry 36:735–739, 1979

Wexler B, Heninger G: Alterations in cerebral laterality during acute psychotic illness. Arch Gen Psychiatry 36:278–284, 1979

Chapter 7

Neurological Examination

Martha B. Denckla, M.D.

When the decision was made in 1982 to examine neurologically and with PANESS (Denckla 1985) each patient entering the obsessive-compulsive disorder (OCD) research protocol, there were two rather broad rationales. One was related to the psychopharmacological research trial aspect of the OCD protocol. A baseline neurological status was to be established for each patient so that iatrogenic pharmacologically induced neurological effects (such as dyskinesia or akathesia) might be clearly differentiated from pretreatment neurological signs. The other rationale stemmed from a general interest in neurological "at risk" correlates of psychiatric morbidity—that is, the neurodevelopmental motor correlates of attention deficit disorder with hyperactivity (Denckla and Rudel 1978) and the child psychiatry literature over the past decade reinforcing the concept of neurodevelopmental deficits associated with psychopathology (Mikkelsen et al. 1982; Shaffer et al. 1985; Szatmari and Taylor 1984). Furthermore, OCD has been associated with reported abnormalities in computed tomography (CT), electroencephalogram (EEG), evoked potentials, and positron emission tomography (PET) scans. Altered neurological function following head trauma, encephalitis, and suspect perinatal events have been linked to OCD (Capstick and Seldrup 1977; Hillbom 1960; McKeon et al. 1984; Schilder 1938).

At the outset, over 5 years ago, there was no expectation that a particular subset of neurological findings would stand out and become the focus of theoretical interest. Over the 5-year period of OCD protocol intake, however, the large proportion (eventually 18/44 or 41 percent of those with neurological findings) who had specifically the choreiform syndrome converged on the growing literature in behavioral genetics and clinical epidemiology linking OCD with Tourette's syndrome. The triad of OCD, tics, and choreiform involuntary movements suggested a common basal ganglia localization. Somewhat surprisingly to us, no clear-cut case of Tourette's syndrome emerged among the patients with OCD or their first-degree relatives seen at the National Institute of Mental Health (NIMH) over the past 24 months despite the detailed questioning with respect to personal and/or familial occurrence of tics that was added in systematic fashion to the OCD protocol data collection.

Between 1982 and 1987, 54 patients with OCD, ranging in age from 6 to 20 years, were examined by one neurologist, using, in addition to the conventional standard neurological examination (i.e., strength, tone, reflexes, sensation, cranial nerves), the revised PANESS (Denckla 1985). The PANESS allows neurodevelopmental status referenced to age-expected performance to be determined. Balance, steadiness of posture (including absence of lapses or tremors), gaits, and timed repetitive and alternating movements are recorded in a quantitative format.

Each neurological form was recorded at the time of the examination and later stored, so that each patient was assigned to a category: 0 = normal; 1 = left hemisyndrome; 2 = choreiform syndrome; 3 = neurodevelopmental deficit; and 4 = right hemisyndrome or some set of miscellaneous assorted signs, a "syndrome characterized by the absence of a syndrome" (Touwen and Prechtl 1970). To be in category 3, at least four items had to be scored as "not up to age-expected level of performance" or "failed for age." If neurodevelopmental signs coexisted with criterial signs for categories 1, 2, or 4, placement in one of these other categories took precedence over the simply neurodevelopmental category 3, and the patient was assigned to category 1, 2, or 4.

Of the 54 patients examined neurologically, 10 were normal (i.e., had no positive lateralized developmental "failures-for-age"). Their mean age was 14.4 years (range, 6–18), but only 2 were less than 14 years old. There were 13 patients (mean age, 13.6 years; range, 9–19 with neurodevelopmental signs only. Of the 54, 18 (mean age, 13.4 years; range, 8–17) had choreiform syndrome; 8 of the 54 had left hemisyndrome (mean age, 13.6; range, 9–19). Five had either right-sided or miscellaneous neurological signs other than neurodevelopmental and were identical in mean age and range to the left hemisyndrome group.

The relationship of neurological group to subgroup of OCD symptoms was analyzed by contingency table, using a 2 × 5 format. Due, most probably, to the very small number of purely "obsessive" ($n = 4$) and purely "compulsive" ($n = 8$) patients, all the remainder being considered obsessive-compulsive, no significant neuropsychiatric correlation emerged from the data.

The relationship between neurological group and personal or family history of tics was examined for the 32 for whom this information had been systematically collected. Of 14 patients with choreiform syndrome, 7 had either personal or family history of tics; 2 patients had both. Five of 18 other (nonchoreiform) patients with OCD had personal or family tics; 1 had both. A chi-square test of the relationship between tics and choreiform syndrome was nonsignificant.

The relationship between neurological group and neuropsychological test performance on tests regarded as revealing (a) spatial and (b) planning ability (see Chapter 5) revealed some complex relationships. First, neither age nor sex significantly accounted for differences on tests called "road map" (Money et al. 1965) or "mazes" (Milner 1965). Thus analysis of variance for each test, using neurological status alone, was performed. Choreiform syndrome–OCD patients were more accurate than left hemisyndrome patients, but still worse than controls, on road maps. Left hemisyndrome–OCD patients were impaired relative to controls and all other neurological patients on both maps and mazes.

Of the 54 patients with OCD for whom complete data are available, 45 had some positive neurological findings. The 10 patients free of neurological signs clustered toward the top of the adolescent age range. (Although the mean age of 14.4 and the range of 6–18 appear only slightly different from that of the other groups, the distribution was skewed so that only 2 of these neurological "normals" were under 14 years old and 8 were 16, 17, or 18.) Distributions were more "normal" in the neurologically "positive" groups.

The major result—that 44 of 54 were stigmatized by some set or combination of neurological signs—is in accord with the findings of Hollander et al. (1987), who reported that of 19 adult patients with OCD, 13 had four or more "neurological soft signs." Compared with a control group of 10 adults, the OCD adult group had significantly more total soft signs (mean = 6.2) than did normals (mean = 1.5). Fine motor coordination impairment accounted for most of the difference in total soft signs. Although not only fine motor coordination but also involuntary movements and sensory function were included on Hollander's 20-item examination, the results were not analyzed more finely in terms of categorizing each patient's profile of neurological dysfunction. Furthermore, Hollander et al. did not perform the traditional neurological examination, including cranial nerve functions, strength, tone, and reflexes; hence no "hemisyndrome" designation was possible from their procedure. Their findings do lend support to a neurological risk factor or diathesis underlying OCD, although neurological specificity is not addressed by Hollander et al.

Within our own group of 44 neurologically stigmatized children and adolescents with OCD, three major subgroups emerged for theoretical speculation. To be discussed in reverse order from their frequency are the implications of (a) 8 cases of left hemisyndrome, (b) 13 cases of neurodevelopmental "immaturity," and (c) 18 cases of choreiform syndrome.

Left Hemisyndrome: Theoretical Implications

If left hemisyndrome is a marker for right hemisphere dysfunction of a cognitive nature, then we might expect with a left hemisyndrome a person who has grown up with imbalance between, on the one hand, normal verbal ability and, on the other hand, impaired nonverbal orientation to and perception of the environment to be vulnerable to obsessions or obsessions leading to compulsive actions. Indeed our 8 left hemisyndrome patients with OCD were significantly impaired relative to controls on maps and mazes, both nonverbal/spatial orientation tasks. We might theorize, then, that indeed left hemisyndrome marks the presence of right brain dysfunction; that such unchecked verbal thoughts, running like an audiotape in the brain, might prevail in dominating mental life due to deficient environment processing, orienting the person to nonverbal reality factors. Had we sufficient numbers with "pure obsessional thought" vs. "pure compulsive act" pathology, it would be tempting to speculate that left hemisyndrome cases would be associated with the former far more than with the latter. Since most cases are mixed, however, we are left with only a few intriguing clinical anecdotes of champion ruminators among our 8 left hemisyndrome cases, and the hypothesis that future series may, with larger numbers, show a relationship between "right-impaired-relative-to-left" hemisphere imbalance and an "obsessional thinking" diathesis.

But there is another theoretical possibility confounding and overlapping with this information-processing theorizing about risks in left hemisyndromes/right brain dysfunctions. That is, the right hemisphere has been shown to play a preeminent role not only in extrapersonal spatial orientation narrowly defined but in the more general sense of "orientation" that means fully alert attentiveness (the opposite of which state is "disorientation"). So there is a more general mental alertness-attentiveness dimension in the right hemisphere repertoire that brings to mind the attention deficit disorder. In that sense, left hemisyndrome may simply mark a more extensively involved neurological case essentially similar to the neurodevelopmentally "immature."

Neurodevelopmental Findings: Theoretical Implications

This set of findings—aptly described years ago by Marcel Kinsbourne with the statement, "had the child been younger, the findings would have been normal"—has repeatedly been found to be associated with hyperactivity, inattentiveness (even outside the confines of syndrome diagnosis, as in a normal school sample), and impulsivity/disinhibition. Timed-task slowness and "immature" extraneous overflow movements constitute the reliable bases for calling someone "not up to age-expectations." A ceiling at age 13 or 14 exists, so, as in Hollander et al.'s (1987) report, the persistence of "immature" signs into the late teens and adult life makes the OCD group look much like a group of patients with attention deficit disorder. Motor immaturity correlates with the inattentiveness already mentioned above in the context of discussing left hemisyndrome and suggests impulsive disinhibited patterns of mental activity in this OCD subgroup as well.

Again, on a clinical-anecdotal level, many of the patients with OCD with neurological findings had earlier childhood histories suggestive of attention deficit disorder. Perhaps "disinhibition" is the common denominator linking prepubertal attention deficit disorder with postpubertal OCD, but with different targets for inhibition peculiar to each developmental stage. The neuroanatomic deficit causing disinhibition may be frontal, more specifically right frontal (in some cases extensive enough to give left-sided classic neuromotor signs) or (as in the final section) in the basal ganglia.

To recapitulate: anterior brain regions, particularly on the right side and in close proximity to motor areas, both cortical and subcortical, may be in some way defective in patients with OCD. The contribution to mental life of these anterior areas—generally characterized as attentiveness, reflectivity, and self-control—may be insufficient in OCD and constitute "at risk" status.

Choreiform Syndrome: Theoretical Implications

Turning now to the largest group of neurologically stigmatized patients, the 18 with choreiform syndrome, again the aforementioned concept of disinhibition (and/or diminished self-control mechanisms) applies. A substantial subset of prepubertal patients with attention deficit disorder present with the choreiform syndrome as their neurological associated "marker" (Denckla 1978). Choreiform syndrome may be the "basal ganglia" subtype of attention deficit disorder. It has long been thought that attention deficit disorder may have a variety of neurological localizations along a pathway including frontal, limbic, basal ganglia, and brain-stem areas. Basal ganglia, a system that is characterized as an afferent sensory gating station, is suggested by involuntary movements. Impairment of basal ganglia may lead to inappropriate perseverative behaviors secondary to unmodulated sensory input. Either frontal or caudate (basal ganglia) impairment may diminish modulation of patterned motor responses appropriate to a given environmental context. Basal ganglia are so connected as to derive a role in integrating cognitive, emotional, and motor behavioral "sets." Possible compartmentalization or dissociation of cognitive, emotional, and motor components may allow unstable and/or perseverative motor states to alternate or even coexist. Choreiform instability of posture may be viewed as the outward observable sign of mental instability (as is suggested by the more blatant and progressive chorea and dementia of Huntington's disease). Why "instability" should switch, generally at puberty, to the perseveration of obsessive-compulsive behaviors is an intriguing puzzle.

It is a similar paradox for choreiform and neurodevelopmental cases, prepubertally attention deficit disorder, later OCD. If left hemisyndrome (to recapitulate) is also viewed as simply a more extensive, perceptuo-motorically involved lesion encompassing a frontal "mental" component, then virtually all of youthful OCD can be conceptualized as a switch from lack of fixation to overfixation, from an underfocused to an overfocused mental state. This represents a major challenge for developmentalists to explain.

Without *explaining* the mechanism whereby attentional instability relates to OCD, the literature suggests that damage to the frontal/limbic/basal ganglia circuitry is associated with the symptoms (see Chapter 19).

Last but not least, the past 5 years have seen a burgeoning literature connecting OCD with Tourette's syndrome. If we add choreiform movements and simple tics to the borders of a circle encompassing OCD and complete Tourette's syndrome, we have an interesting pathophysiological complex (Cummings and Frankel 1985; Devinsky 1983). In relatives of patients with Tourette's syndrome, OCD occurs at a constant rate, whether or not the probands themselves have obsessive-compulsive symptoms. The same is true of chronic simple tics or frank Tourette's syndrome (Pauls et al. 1986). Children with Tourette's syndrome report significantly more obsessive symptomatology than do a comparison group; their parents and teachers concur in reporting more obsessive-compulsive symptoms in these Tourette's syndrome children (Grad et al. 1987).

Tourette's syndrome is linked to the basal ganglia because of the association, common to both, of the dopaminergic system. Therapeutic suppression of tics by haloperidol implicates dopaminergic dysfunction in Tourette's syndrome (Caine et al. 1979; Flament et al. 1987). Dopaminergic pathway convergence on the basal ganglia is well-known; hence, it is suggested that Tourette's syndrome has its neuroanatomic basis in some anomaly of the basal ganglia. The involuntary movements of Tourette's syndrome are not preceded by cortical electrical activity, suggesting a subcortical origin of the tics. PET scans have pointed to elevated metabolic rates in the basal ganglia in Tourette's syndrome (Chase et al. 1984). Another recent PET study (Baxter et al. 1987) showed similar basal ganglia hypermetabolism in OCD, although, in addition, left orbital cortex metabolism was elevated. Baseline caudate-to-hemisphere ratio was not elevated in the morbid OCD state, but the drug treatment that ameliorated OCD led to an increase in the caudate/hemisphere metabolic ratio. This suggests that successful treatment restores the caudate portion of basal ganglia to its gating function (behavior appropriately responsive to emotive and environmental inputs). Again, as with choreiform correlates of OCD, the tics of Tourette's syndrome coexisting with OCD suggest some abnormal dissociation such that "upstream" mentation is perseverative and "downstream" motor outflow is unstable. Perhaps PET and other in vivo studies of patients with Tourette's syndrome and OCD will provide the clues critical to the solution of this neuropsychiatric mystery.

References

Baxter LR, Phelps ME, Mazziotta JC, et al: Local cerebral glucose metabolic rates in obsessive compulsive disorder. Arch Gen Psychiatry 44:211–218, 1987

Caine ED, Polinsky RJ, Ebert MH, et al: Trial of clomipramine and desipramine for Gilles de la Tourette Syndrome. Ann Neurol 5:305–306, 1979

Capstick N, Seldrup U: Obsessional states: a study in the relationship between abnormalities occurring at birth and subsequent development of obsessional symptoms. Acta Psychiatr Scand 56:427–439, 1977

Chase TN, Foster NL, Fedio P, et al: Gilles de la Tourette Syndrome: studies with fluorine-18-labelled fluorodeoxyglucose positron emission tomographic method. Ann Neurol (Suppl 1) 15:5175, 1984

Cummings JL, Frankel M: Gilles de la Tourette syndrome and the neurological basis of obsessions and compulsions. Biol Psychiatry 20:1117–1126, 1985

Denckla MB: Minimal brain dysfunction, in Education and the Brain. Edited by Chall JS, Mirsky AF, Relage KJ. Chicago, University of Chicago Press, 1978

Denckla MB: Revised PANESS. Psychopharmacol Bull 21:773–800, 1985

Denckla MB, Rudel RG: Anomalies of motor development in hyperactive boys. Ann Neurol 3:231–233, 1978

Devinsky O: Neuroanatomy of Gilles de la Tourette's Syndrome. Arch Neurol 40:508–514, 1983

Flament MF, Rapoport JL, Murphy DL, et al: Biochemical changes during clomipramine treatment of childhood obsessive compulsive disorder. Arch Gen Psychiatry 44:219–225, 1987

Grad LR, Pelcovitz D, Olson M, et al: Obsessive compulsive symptomatology in children with Tourette's syndrome. J Am Acad Child Psychiatry 26:69–73, 1987

Hillbom E: After-effects of brain injuries. Acta Psychiatrica et Neurologica Scandinavica 35:82–106, 1960

Hollander E, Shiffman E, Liebowitz M: Neurological soft signs in obsessive compulsive disorder (poster presentation). Presented at 140th Annual Meeting of the American Psychiatric Association, Chicago, May 1987

McKeon J, McGuffin P, Robinson P: Obsessive compulsive neurosis following head injury: a report of four cases. Br J Psychiatry 144:190–192, 1984

Mikkelsen EJ, Brown GL, Minichiello MD, et al: Neurologic status in hyperactive, enuretic, encopretic and normal boys. J Am Acad Child Psychiatry 21:75–81, 1982

Milner B: Visually-guided maze learning in man: effects of bilateral hippocampal, bilateral frontal and unilateral cerebral lesions. Neuropsychologia 3:317–338, 1965

Money J, Alexander D, Walker HT: Road Map Test of Directional Sense. Baltimore, Johns Hopkins University Press, 1965

Pauls DL, Towbin KE, Leckman JF, et al: Gilles de la Tourette's syndrome and obsessive compulsive disorder. Arch Gen Psychiatry 43:1180–1182, 1986

Schilder P: The organic background of obsessions and compulsions. Am J Psychiatry 94:1397, 1938

Shaffer D, Schonfeld IS, O'Connor PA, et al: Neurological soft signs and their relationship to psychiatric disorder and intelligence in childhood and adolescence. Arch Gen Psychiatry 42:342–351, 1985

Szatmari P, Taylor DC: Overflow movements and behavior problems: scoring and using a modification of Fog's test. Dev Med Child Neurol 26:297–310, 1984

Touwen BCL, Prechtl HFT: The neurological examination of the child with minor nervous dysfunction. Clinics in Developmental Medicine No. 38. London: S.I.M.P. with William Heinemann and Philadelphia, Lippincott, 1970

Section IV

The Patients Speak

Editor's Note. Because of the paucity of writing by patients with obsessive-compulsive disorder (OCD), I have included in this section the writing of two families and of several teenage patients.

In Chapter 8, a husband tells of his checking compulsions and of his discovery and attempts to get help for his son, who had, at least in part, a similar problem.

Chapter 9 consists of separate essays written by a family in which both the father and the son have the disorder.

Chapter 10 consists of the stories of several individual teenagers and young adults who had obsessive-compulsive problems since childhood, and are now looking back on their earlier years.

The essays speak eloquently to the pain and suffering that OCD brings. They also demonstrate the insight and clarity with which the symptoms are seen, yet without any force of this insight to control the symptoms.

Judith L. Rapoport, M.D.

Chapter 8

Like Father, Like Son

Stephen S.

Living an Obsessive-Compulsive Attack: "Checking"

I'm driving down the highway doing 55. I'm on my way to take a final exam. My seat belt is buckled and I'm vigilantly following all the rules of the road. No one is on the highway—not a living soul.

Out of nowhere an obsessive-compulsive attack strikes. It's almost magical the way it distorts my perception of reality. While in reality no one is on the road, I'm intruded with the heinous thought that I *might* have hit someone . . . a human being! God knows where such a fantasy comes from.

I think about this for a second and then say to myself, "That's ridiculous. I didn't hit anybody." Nonetheless, a gnawing anxiety is born. An anxiety I will ultimately not be able to put away until an enormous price has been paid.

I try to reality-test away this fantasy. I reason, "Well, if I hit someone while driving, I would have *felt* it." This brief trip into reality helps the pain dissipate . . . but only for a second. Why? Because the gnawing anxiety that I really did commit the illusionary accident is growing larger—so is the pain.

The pain is a terrible guilt that I have committed an unthinkable, negligent act. At one level, I know this is ridiculous, but there's a terrible pain in my stomach telling me something quite different.

Again, I try putting to rest the insane thought and that ugly feeling of guilt. "C'mon," I think to myself, "this is really insane!"

But the awful feeling persists. The anxious pain says to me, "You really did hit someone." The attack is now in full control. Reality no longer has meaning. My sensory system is distorted. I have to get rid of the pain. Checking out this fantasy is the only way I know how.

I start ruminating, "Maybe I did hit someone and didn't realize it. . . . Oh my God! I might have killed somebody! I have to go back and check." Checking is the only way to bind the anxiety. I can't live with the thought that I actually may have killed someone—I have to check it out.

Now I'm sweating . . . literally. I pray this outrageous act of negligence never happened. My fantasies run wild. I desperately hope the jury will be merciful. I'm particularly concerned about whether my parents will be understanding. After all, I'm now a criminal. I must bind the anxiety by checking it out. Did it really happen? There's always an infinitesimally small kernel of truth (or potential truth) in all my obsessive-compulsive fantasies.

I think to myself, "Got to check it out. Rush to check it out. Get rid of the hurt by checking it out. Hurry back to check it out. God, I'll be late for my final exam if I check it out. But I have no choice. Someone could be lying on the road, bloody, close to death. I have to check it out." Fantasy is now my only reality. So is my pain.

I've driven 5 miles farther down the road since the attack's onset. I turn the car around and head back to the scene of the mythical mishap. I return to the spot on the road where I "think" it "might" have occurred. Naturally, nothing is there. No police car and no bloodied body. Relieved, I turn around again to get to my exam on time.

Feeling better, I drive for about 20 seconds and then the lingering thoughts and pain start gnawing away again. Only this time they're even more intense. I think, "Maybe I should have pulled *off* the road and checked the side brush where the injured body was thrown and now lies? Maybe I didn't go far enough back down the road and the accident occurred a mile farther back."

The pain of hurting someone else is now so intense that I have no choice—I really see it this way.

I turn the car around a second time and head an extra mile farther down the road to find the dead corpse. I drive quickly. Assured that this time I've gone far enough, I head back to school to take my exam. But I'm not through yet.

"My God," my attack relentlessly continues, "I didn't get *out* of the car to actually look on the side of the road!"

So I turn back a third time. I drive to the part of the highway where I think the accident happened. I park the car on the highway's shoulder. I get out and begin rummaging around in the brush. A police car comes up. I feel like I'm going out of my mind.

The policeman, seeing me thrash through the brush, asks, "What are you doing? Maybe I can help you?"

Well, I'm in a dilemma. I *can't* say, "Officer, please don't worry. You see, I've got obsessive-compulsive disorder (OCD), along with 2.5 million other Americans. I'm simply acting out a compulsion with obsessive qualities." I can't even say, "I'm really sick. Please help me." The disease is so insidious and embarrassing that it cannot be admitted to *anyone*. Anyway, so few really understand it, including myself.

So I tell the officer I was nervous about my exam and pulled off the roadside to throw up. The policeman give me a sincere and knowing smile and wishes me well.

But I start thinking again. "Maybe an accident did happen and the body has been cleared off the road. The policeman's here to see if I came back to the scene of the crime. God, maybe I really did hit someone. . . . why would a police car be in the area?" Then I realize he would have asked me about it. But would he, if he was trying to catch me?

I'm so caught up in the anxiety and these awful thoughts that I momentarily forget why I was standing on the side of the road.

I'm back on the road again. The anxiety is peaking. "Maybe the policeman didn't know about the accident? I should go back and more thoroughly conduct my search."

I want to go back and check more . . . but I can't. You see, the police car is tailing me on the highway. I'm now close to hysteria because I honestly believe someone is lying in the brush bleeding to death. Yes . . . the pain makes me believe this. "After all," I reason, "Why would the pain be there in the first place?"

I arrive at school late for the exam. I have trouble taking the exam because I can't stop obsessing on the fantasy. The thoughts of the mystical accident keep intruding. Somehow I get through it all. The moment I get out of the exam I'm back on the road—*checking* again. But now I'm checking two things. First that I didn't kill or maim anyone and second, that the policeman doesn't catch me checking. After all, if I should be spotted on the roadside rummaging around the brush a second time, how in the world can I possibly explain such an incriminating and aimless action. I'm totally exhausted, but that awful anxiety keeps me checking. A part of my psyche keeps telling me that this checking behavior is ridiculous—it serves absolutely no purpose. But with OCD there is no other way.

Finally, after repeated checks, I'm able to break the ritual. I head home, dead tired. I know that if I can sleep it off, I'll feel better. Sometimes the pain dissipates through an escape into sleep.

I manage to lie down on my bed—welcoming sleep. But the incident has not totally left me—nor has the anxiety. I think, "If I really did hit someone, there would be a dent in the car's fender."

What I now do is no mystery to anyone. I haul myself up from bed and run out to the garage to check the fenders on the car. First I check the front two fenders, see no damage and head back to bed. But . . . did I check it *well enough*?

I get up from bed again and now find myself checking the *whole* body of the car. I know this is absurd, but I can't help myself. Finally . . . finally, I disengage and head off to my room to sleep. Before I nod off, my last thought is, "I wonder what the next set of checking behaviors will be."

My Story

I'm 36 years old and have had OCD since I was 6 years old. My son, age 5, has had the illness since birth. My two brothers most probably have the disease, though less severely. There is a good chance my nephew, age 8, has OCD, as well as my father and my paternal grandmother.

I cannot really describe the torturous pain of the anxiety brought on by an obsessive-compulsive attack. The checking incident I just relayed to you used to happen to me often. Between the ages of 23 and 33 (save one or two brief remissions), this kind of surreal event, an attack, occurred every day. Many times it stayed with me all day long. If it disappeared, a new attack, spawned from the old one, would quickly replace it.

I do not intend to sound dramatic, nor am I soliciting your sympathy or pity. It's simply a fact of life that it's the pain—the deep, searing, neverending pain—that makes this illness so unbearable. I know the pain. So do all the other people with OCD out there who share this illness with me and my family members.

As a parent you must first understand this insidious disease not in terms of its origins or the bizarre behaviors it creates. Instead you begin to understand OCD in terms of the pain it causes its victims. If you can accept your child's pain, the whole illness becomes easier to live with.

Looking back, it seems that the hurt of an obsessive-compulsive attack was more psychologically painful than the death of my father whom I loved. This may be hard for a normal, mentally healthy parent such as yourself to comprehend. Nonetheless, it's sadly true. My sense of loss and grief was trivial compared to any of the hundreds of obsessive-compulsive attacks I have had in my life.

While there were indications from early childhood that I had the disease, it didn't clearly manifest itself until I was 22 years old. My symptoms were typical. I would check the gas oven and door locks, sometimes 20 times, before I could go to bed at night. I would worry about poisoning myself and others with insecticides or cleaning fluids I may have touched. I would drive home from work, thinking that I had left the light on in my office and drive all the way back to see if it was off because "it could start a fire." Sometimes I did this more than once in a given day.

Many of my obsessions and compulsions were based on an extraordinary fear that my aggressive impulses—my anger—would, without my knowing it, surface, or leak out. I always thought I would start a fire by being negligent with cigarettes or kill someone by being a reckless driver. My vigilance was ongoing . . . and exhausting.

Each obsessive-compulsive incident was accompanied by the fantasy that if I didn't act on it, something terrible would happen to me or someone else. Losing my job, being sent to prison, or hurting someone else were average catastrophic fantasies. Making *sure* these outcomes would not occur drove my obsessive-compulsive behaviors.

The energy and time I would exert toward a hundred aimless acts has me shaking my head in disgust right now. I look back and wonder how I lived this way for over 10 years. It was unbearable.

I hid my OCD. I was like an alcoholic hiding his drink. My greatest fear was to be discovered. At times my wife hated me for the illness. I hated myself. But I couldn't help it. The disease controls you, not the reverse.

A parent of a child with OCD must understand the pain of the anxiety and also its controls over one's behavior. Your child has absolutely *no control* over what he or she is doing . . . NONE. Your child's rituals may be totally aimless. They will make no sense to you. You cannot intellectually understand why your child does what he or she does. Don't try to understand in this way because all it will do is frustrate you . . . normal human reasoning and logic does not exist with this disease. The only logic there is, is your child's relentless pain, and his enormous need to bind this pain and his involuntary behavior geared to this end.

In 1973, one year after the first onset, I went into therapy. The psychiatrist was good . . . very good. Over the next 3 years I made some excellent progress with the illness. I learned ways to cope and adapt. If there was an emotional source to the illness, the psychiatrist did as much as could be done to eliminate it.

Shortly thereafter, I went into remission and was fine for about a year or so. Not perfect, but substantially improved. After 5 years in therapy, it became clear that normal life stress events seemed to trigger obsessive-compulsive episodes. After the birth of our first child, the disease struck again. This time it was worse than ever before.

I was able to work and actually performed quite well. But I had to exert so much energy managing the disease day to day that I spent much of the time emotionally and physically exhausted. Everything took me twice or three times as long to do. I'd be doing computer programming for my research and spend hours checking, rechecking, re-rechecking, and re-re-rechecking my programs for accuracy. I would consider the task done but sure enough I was up at 2 a.m. with an OCD attack thinking the program had one or two more errors. I would check another time . . . each check took hours because I'd check what I had just checked and then doubt that I'd adequately checked it. So I had to go back and recheck again . . . and again, and again. It was ludicrous and purposeless. I knew what I was doing made no sense at all. Yet I had no choice but to keep checking things. These aimless acts controlled my life.

I went back and forth in therapy.

My wife couldn't stand my illness. She found it repugnant. I'm not sure I blame her, because in its severe forms it is disgusting. I hated myself for being sick, and hated my wife for her intolerance. Yet inside both hates . . . I knew I couldn't help myself and she couldn't help her reaction. We coped with it in a few ways. First, she would leave me alone while I had an attack. This minimized her exposure to the illness, and my exposure to the family. Second, my therapist served a crucial function. Instead of talking about the disease with my wife, I could relate to the psychiatrist about it. This took much of the pressure off my wife. Third, I hid it from my wife so as not to embarass myself and upset her. I learned to be a great actor. I'd be dying on the inside with rapid-fire obsessional thoughts, and all smiles and congeniality on the outside. This was no solution for me, but I think it helped her some.

The first approach was best—being left alone during an episode. You see, a person with OCD cannot willfully turn off an attack. If I was with someone, even my wife, I was there in physical presence only. My mind was so consumed by the pain and all the obsessional thoughts that I couldn't interact. The consequences were all disastrous, not the least of which was terrible communication. It was best to be left alone.

One of the amazing things about the illness was that it could go on "hold" if I *had to* do something professionally or socially important. For example, if I had to teach a class, I would forget about the current obsession during the class. The second it ended though, I was back into obsessive-compulsive thoughts and behaviors. This was fortunate because it allowed me to function at work and with friends . . . but only barely.

In 1983 after 9 years in therapy, I was on average better, but I was still plagued by the illness. I felt that if there was an emotional etiology to OCD, we had done our best to rid myself of it. My psychiatrist and I discussed various forms of drug therapy. Valium had been used for years to blunt the pain, but it was only marginally helpful. The drug made me feel tired and gave me headaches. I begged him—literally—to consider other forms of medication. It hurt so badly, and the disease disrupted my life so thoroughly that I was reaching for any possible solution—I was desperate and exhausted.

He prescribed imipramine. I started on very low doses, 25 mg, because I had a history of heart disease. Over a 4-month period of time I moved up to 200 mg.

The only way to describe what happened then is through the phrase, "all of a sudden." All of a sudden, in the fifth month on medication, the OCD stopped. I still had obsessive-compulsive thoughts, but I forgot them almost instantaneously. This horrendous illness fled to the recesses of my mind.

At first I didn't trust it. I thought it might be a placebo effect or that I had gone into remission again (still a possibility). But the effect kept lasting and got even stronger.

The drug "leveled" me. Before starting the drug, I had a manic quality to my behavior—extreme highs and pretty low lows (mostly when I had an OCD attack). When I was on a high, I was most vulnerable to an attack. The drug seemed to minimize the variance in these mood states. With the highs gone, so was much of the vulnerability.

Imipramine seemed to stop all the catastrophobic thinking. Problems became manageable, not insurmountable. It seemed to put my perceptions back in order. For the first time in over a decade, the world—its risks and its potential hurts—were put back into perspective.

Attacks went from every hour of every day to once a week. I stayed this way for about 4 months. Then they became even less frequent, once a month. Now they occur once every 2 or 3 months. I will still get obsessional thoughts, but the pain is no longer attached to them.

How do I feel? Great! I don't mean to sound maudlin, but I have been given a new life. The most important thing was that the pain, that relentless and driving hurt, is gone.

Today I'm on a maintenance dose of imipramine, 100 mg. I never thought it would come to an end. For the last 2 years it has. I still pray that the pain will never come back to hurt me.

The problem, unfortunately, is that as I began to improve, my 4-year-old son got sick.

My Son's Story

I went to Father's Night at my son's preschool. He was playing with a Fisher-Price toy, a schoolhouse. But his play was strange. He stood before the toy, jumped up and down, and flapped his arms as if excited with the toy (we later labeled this behavior, "flapping"). His muscles from head to toe contracted and relaxed over and over again. He would grunt and contort his face as if he was exerting great effort. When the jumping stopped, he would put his arms together and wiggle his fingers just above eye level (we later labeled this behavior "wormies"). Somehow the finger movement was a form of self-stimulation. The grunting and muscle contraction, relaxation sequence would continue during "wormies" as well. He did this nonstop for 35 minutes. I could not disengage him. No matter what I tried, he simply wouldn't stop.

Occasionally he would bring a toy, person, chair, or desk into the play . . . but these self-stimulating behaviors and the self-induced muscle contractions continued. When I tried to disengage him, I was met with repeated and rigid resistance. He *had to* do this bizarre behavior. He also had to play with the toy "his" way . . . any change I introduced was vehemently rejected.

That night I spoke with my wife. We had a hunch that something wasn't right.

We reviewed his behavior over the past year. We noted his excitability and extremely low attention span. He could not sit still, nor could he focus on a given task. It would literally take him 15 minutes to put his socks on since he got so distracted by other things. We discussed how he would wiggle his fingers or dangle strings in front of his eyes for long periods of time (labeled "stringing"), while doing muscle contractions and grunting. Resistance to change and new experiences were all too easy to identify. If we told him he was going to McDonald's for lunch and the plans changed, he would throw a short but intense tantrum. We remembered instances of him at age 2 flapping with his arms and jumping up and down in front of fans and spinning record players. His obsessions with counting, serializing, and the repetition of questions he already had heard the answers to 100 times before were also easily recalled. He would throw a fit at age 2 if an object was not in its "proper" location on his night table. Loud noises seemed to bother him more than they would a normal child his age, and in general things in his environment scared him. He had a sleep disorder. He would be put to bed at 8 p.m. and lie there for 3 or 4 hours before nodding off. What was he thinking about?

And then we realized what was *not* there!

Except for rare instances he never played with toys. He showed no interest in his peers. At times he was unable to calm himself. When he would get upset he would cry, "Mommy, calm me down!" We couldn't engage him in any age-appropriate activity. When we got him involved in some normal play—say block building—he would bring stringing, wormies, and flapping, along with the muscle contractions, into the play.

Frame of reference—context—can do funny things to one's perception. As we began to identify all the puzzle's pieces, we knew we could no longer chalk all this up to developmental lag or immaturity. We desperately wanted to, but we couldn't. Something was fundamentally wrong. And he was getting worse . . . steadily. Often, we look back and ask ourselves, "How could we have waited so long to get help?" The question is really a statement of "How could we have been so negligent." The reasons lie in a few places.

Denial is one. What parent wants to face the fact that their child is handicapped? At the same time, he was so young—just 4 years old— that it was easy to rationalize away much of his aberrant behavior: "He'll grow out of it." "It's only temporary." "He's a boy and boys mature slower than girls."

In addition, he had so many positive attributes. His intelligence was clearly apparent. His language skills were consistently improving. His attitude was generally good. He expressed a wide range of affect— sadness, smiles, silliness, boredom, and much laughter. A strong need to please his parents, especially Mommy, was developing. He manifested an insatiable level of curiosity about spatial location—"Krogers is next to Wendy's? Right Mommy?" He was gentle and kind . . . perhaps to a fault. He would hug and kiss. Expressions of anger were rare. When I told him, "Jeffrey, you make Daddy smile," he responded, "Daddy, you make me smile too." While he didn't play at all with peers, he readily engaged adults.

Yet, when a child dangles strings in front of his eyes 4 hours a day and tells you he can't help himself, or asks, "Mommy, why do I play with strings?" the rationalizations soon wear painfully thin. Our child was sick.

Off to the Doctors

Many times in my life I have said to myself, "If I only knew then what I know now!" How true this is when I look back at our experience with Jeffrey and my personal ordeal.

Our first contact was a bright and empathic psychologist. His orientation was highly cognitive and developmental. All that means is that he was less likely to attribute childhood psychological maladies to poor parenting and more likely to attribute them to a lack of organic or biochemical maturity in the brain, informational-processing errors of the mind (due to slow growth and development), and so forth.

He was wonderful—caring and sensitive. He felt that Jeffrey was very bright, his language adequate though not great, perhaps hyperactive and/or prone to attention deficit, though he didn't fit this diagnostic category exactly. He suggested we take Jeffrey to a speech therapist to work on his low attention span and general distractibility. We did this immediately. But the focus of his prescription was to wait . . . "Let's keep on evaluating him and give him time to grow. Wait it out a while so we can get a clearer picture."

The string play and repeated questions continued to grow in complexity and intensity. The string play was now coupled with more grunting and muscle contraction . . . as much as 5 hours a day. We told Jeffrey that the string play was undesirable, and that we would like to do other things with him. So what did Jeffrey do? He started to go up to his room. He would slam shut the door and "string" for hours on end. My son needed string play like a drug addict needs a heroin fix. He couldn't stop it . . . and I think he really wished he could because he knew it made Mommy and Daddy unhappy.

Endless streams of repetitious questioning marked the day. He learned how to count and that became a new obsessional activity— "Mommy, when I'm 5 years old, Joanne [his older sister] will be 8. Mommy, when I'm 6 years old, Joanne will be 9." This went on and on with everyone he knew. The psychologist was kept updated but told us to be patient. What the hell was our son doing?

The problem was that Jeffrey, and for that matter any 4-year-old, does not possess the intellectual sophistication to accurately self-report what he's feeling and thinking. The guessing game as to what was wrong with our child went on. I began to wonder if Jeffrey would be able to go to school, learn to read, or hold a job when he grew up.

We made videotapes of Jeffrey's stereotypic behaviors (stringing, flapping, wormies, etc.). This turned out to be a diagnostic savior. Why? Because none of the health professionals we consulted seemed to honestly believe he played with strings all day long. Yes, they intellectually believed us, yet they didn't seem to experience the same sense of urgency about the problem. When Jeffrey was put before any health professional he was so interested in what was going on (the surroundings, equipment, offices, etc.), that whatever drove him to "string" and "flap" seemed to wane at these times. So he looked relatively normal during his countless evaluations.

Consistent with this, the child psychiatrist who saw Jeffrey next didn't seem too concerned. After all, here was a bright and inquisitive kid. Yet when he saw the videotape, he knew something was very wrong. . . . His interest was piqued, so to speak. And the same reaction occurred with Jeffrey's pediatrician. His kind patience and sincere sympathy was quickly turned into fast action after viewing the videotape. And act he did. With the psychologist's and psychiatrist's concurrence, the pediatrician felt a neurological workup was needed. An appointment was made on almost an emergency basis. This meant that the soonest we could get in to see the pediatric neurologist was in 4 weeks.

With a child you love, *waiting* is an impossible state of affairs. Time takes on a totally different dimension with a sick child growing sicker. You want answers not tomorrow or the next day, but *immediately*! Uncertainty with a sick child breeds a level of fear second to none. To be told that your next appointment is in 3 weeks, that the speech evaluation is in a month, and "We're sorry, the child psychiatrist can't see any new patients until after the first of the year," adds unbearably to a parent's sense of helplessness.

To a lost and frightened parent, each doctor's appointment represented another chance to find "the answer." While we were not so naive as to think there was only one answer, we nonetheless felt, hoped, dreamed, whatever, that the *next* doctor would make *the* key diagnostic breakthrough. The bigger the doctor's name and reputation, the higher the anticipatory high. The more equivocal, uncertain, and confused the health professional was after the assessment, the lower the lows.

A well-known pediatric neurologist said that my son might well be hallucinating during his string play. When I told him that Jeffrey relayed no fantasies during the string play, he discarded my comment.

I went further and said that during the string play Jeffrey didn't seem to lose touch with his environment. For example, I told the neurologist that Jeffrey would stop the string play momentarily to inquire about a salient remark someone else made—"Jeffrey, time to get your coat on to go to the doctors for your booster shot." That information was dismissed.

When I told him Jeffrey had a wide range of mood and affect (schizophrenics often have blunted or dulled affect), he nodded and plowed ahead with his diagnosis.

When I told him I had OCD, he smiled and moved on. When I asked him how many 4-year-old schizophrenic children he had seen, he responded that he had seen only one in the last 6 years of medical practice.

When I told him that I read that it was hard to diagnose schizophrenia at such a young age, he agreed and went on to tell me that my son, nevertheless, was schizophrenic. We later learned that OCD and schizophrenia are often confused.

When I asked him why he ruled out hyperactivity/attention deficit disorder, he said that Jeffrey didn't fit the pattern, and in particular he couldn't "string" for hours on end if he had this disorder.

This just wasn't adding up. Nonetheless, we had to find out for ourselves if Jeffrey really was schizophrenic. So we went to the medical library and checked out every book on childhood schizophrenia and psychosis. We called the psychologist and psychiatrist and other medical professional friends who were familiar with the case and asked them for their assessment.

Jeffrey didn't seem to fit any of the descriptions given in the literature . . . but the literature is less than definitive. All the medical people we spoke to seemed to disagree with the pediatric neurologist's assessment. The disagreement ranged from mild to definitive. Although there was some consensus that schizophrenia was absent, the thought of having a potentially psychotic child never left us.

The Ups and Downs With Drugs

Jeffrey was first put on Dexedrine, a stimulant that has been used to treat attention deficit disorder and hyperactivity since the 1930s. This was given because of Jeffrey's hyperactivity, not for OCD.

Jeffrey had a terrific first hour response to this drug. He stopped flapping and stringing for the first time in 1½ years. Then, 2 hours later, the roof fell in.

Within a few hours, his behavior reverted back. But it was now profoundly exacerbated. Five hours of string play became all-day string play. The grunting and deep muscle relaxations were equally intensified. It seemed like he was doing this to relieve himself of enormous energy and/or anxiety.

My wife, her resolve to help this child strengthening proportionally with each increase in the severity of his illness, would interrupt his behavior for hours at a time—a physically and emotionally draining activity. She thought of every possible alternative that could catch the child's interest beyond strings. She explored every medical alternative. She worked 24 hours a day on this problem. She also shut out the rest of her life.

She couldn't help it, but there was nothing else left for the rest of us. The only topic she would converse on was Jeffrey. The standing joke was that my wife was studying for her Medical Boards in Child Psychiatry. But, like so many jokes, it was based on hurt and suffering.

Naturally, the other children suffered. Our 7-year-old daughter didn't like the differential standards of behavior that emerged in our home. Different demands and expectations were made of her that couldn't be made of Jeffrey. "That's not fair," she would complain. She, too, felt alone. "Daddy, why do you always play with Jeffrey and not with me?" She was right.

We told her he was ill. She understood, but nevertheless felt abandoned. She wanted a brother to play with . . . yet Jeffrey couldn't really play. One day she came into our bedroom crying, "I feel *so bad* for Jeffrey."

Perhaps compared to all of us, she learned to cope best with his behavior. She learned to accept and work around his limitations. She never stopped trying to engage him in any way possible. She developed patience for his rigidity and even lovingly cajoled him to try age-appropriate activities. She never stopped trying to solve her own ambivalence.

For me, the most amazing thing was that I never hated Jeffrey for doing this to our family. Not once did I get angry at him. Frustrated by the situation? Yes. Feelings of impotence and loss of control? Yes. But never rage toward my child. Never wishful fantasies of him being dead. None of this. Why? Because as an obsessive-compulsive myself, I know all too well what it's like not being able to control your own behavior. It's almost as devastating as the pain itself. And I knew Jeffrey had absolutely no control over what he was doing. Parents of children with OCD must never forget this.

My illness also helped me to tolerate my momentarily departed wife. She too had no control over her rescue mission.

Jeffrey continued to deteriorate. My wife began getting conflicting directions from the pediatrician and the psychiatrist on how to medicate Jeffrey. No one was at fault per se. We had brought several consultants into the picture. In effect we had hired a team of professionals without a manager/coach. The medical professionals, in deference to each other's turf, were reluctant to take on a coordinating role. The result was poor case management.

A new specialist from our local university hospital and his associates brought us crucial organization and new planning. The family history that the specialist took was incredibly detailed. There was an informal multispecialty team in addition to a variety of other professional resources available. This created a truly comprehensive care modality. All available hypotheses, reasonable and not so reasonable, were considered. They spent a great deal of time with Jeffrey. And, a child psychiatry resident was available to meet with my wife and me on a weekly basis to monitor what was going on.

Equally critical was the shift of responsibility for case management from my wife as the quarterback/patient advocate to the psychiatry resident. Quality medical care demands thoughtful planning and a balance between objectivity and emotion. My wife and I were too close, too involved, and too frantic to add much thoughtfulness and objectivity at this stage. The responsibility the medical resident took on was both appropriate and badly needed for everyone concerned.

The medical resident's role deserves more attention because it serves as a role model for physicians trying to work with parents of handicapped children. His patience and caring for my wife and me was incredible. Sometimes my wife would call him with a different question 5 days in a row and he was there to answer patiently each one, no matter how ridiculous it was. He would go to the library and find articles for us to read. He *always* had Jeffrey's best interests at heart even when it meant he had to firmly disagree with things we wanted to do. His ability to use resources was amazing. He'd call anyone if they possessed information we needed. His medical expertise and guidance was invaluable as we got deeper into psychopharmaceutical medications. He and his supervising physicians worked with us every step of the way. He always treated us with dignity and respect even when his crowded schedule and academic demands made us a drain on his time and energy. In essence, his behavior defines how cases like this should be medically and interpersonally managed.

The specialist and the resident felt that attention deficit/hyperactivity disorder was still the primary diagnosis. But they felt that a secondary diagnosis of OCD might be in order. Most important, they came to this conclusion after seeing Jeffrey and prior to taking my OCD history—they didn't know I was one. They were interested in the obsessive patterns to Jeffrey's questioning. They were also willing to say, "I'm not confident of any of this yet." Honesty, even if it didn't give us the "answer," was better than the neurologist's dogma.

They became especially interested in my OCD history and in particular my recovery and maintenance on imipramine. However, they decided to exhaust the most researched and safest medication first.

The university hospital team decided to try another central nervous system stimulant—Cylert. Jeffrey's behavioral and attitudinal problems worsened. Of note was that the amount of anxiety he was experiencing became frighteningly clear for the first time. A nuclear magnetic resonance brain scan (like a computed tomography scan) showed no pathology. Biochemical tests came back normal. Hearing and vision tests told us these were *not* problem areas.

Still, Jeffrey wouldn't stop stringing. He couldn't. How badly he must have been hurting inside. His question, "Mommy why do I play with strings," was again posed. He asked me and his mother, "Did you play with strings when you were little?" He asked his baby-sitter the same question.

Two things happened simultaneously. The psychiatry resident by now concluded that the stimulants were a complete disaster. He decided to move to the next class of drug intervention, tricyclics. The medical resident prescribed imipramine for Jeffrey, a drug I had been successfully treated with for 3 years.

On a Friday night exactly 6 months into the odyssey, we gave Jeffrey his first 10-mg pill of imipramine. He became quite tired and went to sleep.

The next morning he woke up and came downstairs for breakfast. *There was no string play!* For the first time in 1½ years (save the 1 hour respite from the first Dexedrine pill), Jeffrey was not stringing, doing wormies, or flapping.

The drug didn't work just once, but every 2 or 3 hours we administered it. More amazing was that his symptoms returned, though much less intensely, about 20 minutes before the drug had fully worn off. And, 20 minutes into the next administration of imipramine, the weakened rituals stopped. Jeffrey would occasionally try to conduct his stereotypic behaviors, but he seemed less interested in them. His hyperactivity and poor attention span improved—he actually sat still for periods of time. To us this was a miracle in our lives.

We and the psychiatric resident began to wonder if Jeffrey had had OCD from birth (in addition to some degree of hyperactivity and attention deficit disorder).

Adults with OCD carry out their ritualized and aimless behaviors to bind their piercing anxiety. While there may be a "kernel of truth" in each obsession, those with OCD in their more rational moments know that what they're doing is totally senseless. What drives us to do this is the pain—the ceaseless anxiety that if we don't do it some unimaginably horrible event will occur.

Now why can't ritualized play with a string be a 4-year-old's version of checking compulsion, hand washing, or whatever obsessive-compulsive symptoms we typically attribute to adult victims? Why can't ongoing muscle contraction be identical to the anxiety *reduction* benefits of deep muscle relaxation techniques? Couldn't serialized thinking and obsessions with number sequences and relationships be identical to an obsessive-compulsive adult trying to create an orderly and predictable environment? Isn't my son's rigidity to change and fear of the novel and unknown identical to an obsessive-compulsive adult's attempting to order the environment? If a child is feeling extreme anxiety, wouldn't loud noises and changes in his environment cause him even greater discomfort?

Some Additional Thoughts for Parents

Reading

Reading is one of the great ways to cope with the devastation of this illness. Anyone who is the parent of an obsessive-compulsive child will have most of their questions answered through what is available in the literature. Although there isn't a lot, there is some.

Reading buys you even more. You learn that you're not alone. You learn a vocabulary that assists you in putting this disease into a meaningful conceptual framework—it helps you understand. You realize that medical researchers know about this nightmare and are trying to do something about it. The availability of medications, prescription drugs, that have been researched and can help some victims are vividly described. And so is the bad news.

Not everyone is helped by the drugs. The disease is as awful as I described it earlier—in fact it can be so debilitating that it requires hospitalization.

One great piece of news is already in the literature. It *may not* be your fault that you or your child has OCD. Early toilet training, a disciplined home environment, an unresolved Oedipal complex, and endless demands that your child clean up her "disgusting" room may not be and is probably not the cause of OCD.

OCD, like diabetes, may be physiological; it may even be inherited from one generation to another as suggested in my family's case. However, OCD manifests itself as a psychological disorder. For my wife and me this was a great relief. The problem now was getting Jeffrey's teacher and others to understand this.

Telling Others

So how do you tell people that your family is struck with a serious illness? How do you explain to people that the cause of this psychological malady may well be physical?

We began with Jeffrey's preschool teacher. She is an exceptional individual, but like so many people has her particular way of viewing the world. She has been trained to explain the vast majority of developmental problems in children in emotional terms—poor nurturing, sibling rivalry, and an emotionally impoverished home environment. In many instances this is totally valid. Yet it made her reluctant to accept that this child may have a physiological deficit. She also had difficulty accepting that a 4-year-old child was being medicated. In fact, she didn't accept any of this and viewed the problem as "emotional."

She is correct in that serious emotional problems will result from OCD. But just as important is where they begin and what helps. By holding on to her emotional hypothesis, she made my wife feel awful and the sole cause of Jeffrey's maladies. Having a handicapped child is difficult enough. Having someone sit in judgment of your parenting practices—when you know in your heart you have loved your child as much as is humanly possible—is unbearable.

It wasn't until the preschool teacher learned that I have the disease that she began to back off. And what the preschool teacher believed was not unique. The same pattern of events occurred with many members of our families.

We learned that the best way to tell others was to present *all* the facts. It's not entirely their fault that they don't understand the illness. It is poorly publicized and like many emotional illnesses denied, ignored, or hidden in a closet. One way around this is for parents of children with OCD to share the facts with others. At times this is very difficult. It means we have to admit a handicap; that we and the emotional extension of ourselves, our child, are handicapped. It means we have to admit to a disease that is like a psychological form of leprosy. It means we have to reveal very personal things about ourselves that normally we wouldn't. All of this is very difficult . . . but we have no real choice if we love our children enough to help them manage their OCD.

Today, Jeffrey is being maintained on imipramine. A similar and perhaps more helpful drug, clomipramine, is being held as a back-up medication. L-Tryptophan, an amino acid that is presumed to increase brain serotonin, seems to help him also.

Since he was put on these two drugs, most of Jeffrey's symptoms have disappeared. His language development has blossomed. He is playing with his sister and little brother. Peer play is still absent, as well as playing with toys. He is calmer and shows better coordination and attention span. He goes places with me, although with difficulty. He even took a 2-day trip with me and his uncle, and did beautifully. He is showing letter recognition, skills with numbers, and excellent intellectual development. He watches TV, sometimes for 30 minutes at a time. His anxiety has waned dramatically. But he still has a long way to go.

Panic thoughts over Mommy's whereabouts still seem to intrude into his psyche. He cannot draw or manage scissors. His resistance to trying new things remains, although this is somewhat improved. He sleeps beautifully at night . . . really for the first time in his life. But the real magic is that he doesn't have to play with the strings anymore.

We have learned to better manage Jeffrey over the past year. We now go to great lengths to prepare Jeffrey for any change in the status quo. This makes him less rigid and resistant to the new and different. We never surprise him with anything because his first response is fear and anxiety. We have also learned to give in to him on small issues, especially when his disease seems to be forcing him to behave in a troubled fashion. On the big issues we can't let him get his way—disease or no disease. He too has to learn to accommodate himself to us.

We work as much as possible with his strengths. Since his intelligence is a trump suit, we do whatever we can to facilitate its development. He likes this, and gains pleasure from it. Currently, maps are of great interest to him, so we have put maps all over his room. We make a conscious effort to reinforce his interpersonal strengths. He shares beautifully, for example, and we let him know how proud we are of this.

But a lingering uncertainty remains. Jeffrey has good days and bad days. I wish I could for the moment turn the clock ahead 15 years and see how this will end.

My wife has come to accept his handicap. Her roller-coaster ride is coming to an end. We're all the better for this. She has come to realize that unless she has herself emotionally intact, there is no way she can help Jeffrey or the rest of the family. When Jeffrey's having a bad day, she has learned to disengage herself from him. I take over primary child-care responsibility until her patience is recharged. It's easier for me to tolerate his OCD symptoms because I share his illness. She'll never understand fully because she has never had the pain.

Postscript

As I mentioned earlier, other members of my family seem to be OCD victims as well. My brother has had a remarkable response to imipramine. He said, "I never thought I would live my life without the pain and anxiety of all my 'dread' thoughts." [*Editor's note:* In general, imipramine is not helpful for OCD. This family is a dramatic exception. See Chapter 13 on drug treatment.]

Chapter 9

Zach and His Family

Zach's Mother

When we saw Zach trying to pick things up without using his hands, we both felt a growing fear, almost a panicked feeling. This feeling was quickly accompanied by anger. He was only 6 years old.

Our new baby was 1 month old and so I was seeing our pediatrician regularly. He encouraged me not to assume the worst. It might be a reaction to the baby. As the rituals increased, like ripples from a stone dropped into a pool of water, we all agreed Zach needed help. We consulted a child psychiatrist. Zach was dealing with his obsessions and compulsions with total denial. He seemed to believe that no one saw anything. He, at times, couldn't use his hands, might touch the ground after so many steps, or would take a little back-kick after so many steps. At one time, he lay down on the floor of a shopping mall and drew a line around his body with his finger. He seemed to be defining his territory, protecting himself from some unseen danger or evil. Zach washed his hands. He washed and washed and washed. He wouldn't touch his shoes or his glasses. His sleeves always hung down over his hands. He used the sleeve as a protective shield when he had to touch something. And then he washed some more.

The washing of his hands began to take longer. Sometimes it was 1 minute, sometimes 2 or 3 minutes. He developed a routine that involved sticking his thumbs up in to the faucet and then swinging his hands back and forth under the water until his whole body was moving with an uncontrolled force. Then he couldn't dry his hands. They would be raw and chapped, but he wouldn't dry them. Often he would finish washing his hands, then turn around and start all over again.

Sometimes this behavior would cause Zach to miss the school bus or an activity or even a party.

Zach began to exhibit many of the characteristics of his father, Sam. He was angry, tense, and often depressed. They are both perfectionists and show anger if they do anything wrong or imperfectly. All of these symptoms saddened me. I felt at a loss to help Zach. The psychiatrists said that Zach was continuing to totally deny the OCD. I believed I was doing everything I could to help him, but I still felt frustrated and saddened by his inability to control his own mind and his own body. And really I could do nothing to help at all. I knew what not to do to make him feel worse. I didn't question his behavior, demand that it cease, tease him, badger him, or otherwise shame him. But that provided little satisfaction as I watched him suffer. Sometimes I would feel very down as I watched two people I love so out of control and so unhappy.

I worried about Zach's sister and brother. I especially worried about his sister who was old enough to sense that something was not right. She watched all the strangeness around her without understanding it, without understanding how pervasive it really was. She asked why Zach washed his hands so much. I tried to explain that it was something he *had* to do, that he had a special feeling he couldn't make go away any other way. She accepted it. But I could see that Zach's strange behavior made her uncomfortable. In moments of great anger she would tease him about it. A terrible gap existed between Zach and his siblings. He was a loner even at home. He developed a loathing for his sister because she didn't share his problems. As his brother grew older, he resented him as well. He blamed everything on them and always wished his sister ill.

Zach was afraid of everything. He stayed close to home. He chose to be alone a lot. He became very dependent on me. I felt I had to protect his secrets. But I yearned for a normal, carefree childhood for him. I also yearned for a normal family with typical relationships.

We were fortunate to hook-up with the OCD clomipramine study at the National Institutes of Health. We had reached an impasse. Although the psychiatrists might help Sam and Zach to deal with their lives, they were unable to "heal" them of their OCD.

Before Zach left for Washington, DC, to be hospitalized for evaluation for that program, 2½ years after we had noticed his first symptoms, Sam shared his own story with Zach. Zach was, I believe, elated at having a comrade. I think it took away much of his shame and maybe even some of his fear. In looking back over the last 15 years, I am amazed at how living with rituals has become a natural part of . . . life. I try not to get angry, frustrated, or impatient. I am glad to have an understanding of what is happening. I hope . . . believe . . . that major progress in helping those who suffer with OCD is close. Zach has had a good response to the clomipramine. His rituals are still there, but they have been greatly reduced. Zach is not nearly as depressed as he used to be. He has begun to play with his friends and to accept imperfections with himself. This, of course, has made me very happy.

Sam's response to the drug has not been as clear-cut. But we patiently await changes. We now talk about his response to the clomipramine, about side effects, and about rituals and OCD. Lifting the veil off his "deep dark secret" has given us a new relationship. It has made us much stronger. It has given us much greater strength, too, to deal with Zach's problems and to propose solutions to new problems as they come up.

Zach

I am now 9 years old. When I was 6, I started picking up things with my elbows because I thought I would get my hands dirty if I picked things up with my hands. By the time I was 7 I was washing my hands 35 times a day. For the next 2 years my fear of getting my hands dirty grew worse. Until I started on medicine, my life was wrecked, unpleasant, and crippled by my compulsion.

When I was 6, I started doing all these strange things when I swallowed saliva. When I swallowed saliva I had to crouch down and touch the ground. I didn't want to lose any saliva . . . I had to sweep the ground . . . and later I had to blink my eyes if I swallowed. I was just frustrated because I couldn't stop the compulsions. Each time I swallowed I had to do something . . . for a while I had to touch my shoulders to my chin. I don't know why. I had no reason. I was afraid. It was just so unpleasant if I didn't. If I tried not to, all I got was failure.

I tried to tell my Mom. I told her I had to do it. She said, "You're doing some strange things, why do you do it?" I said, "'cause I don't want to lose any saliva," and she said, "Maybe you'll want to talk about it later." I don't want to lose any saliva and there's no good reason.

I just don't want to. I was afraid to tell anybody. People would think I was crazy or something. I didn't want to tell Dr. Kaufman. I was nervous when I first came to him and then I just didn't want to talk about it. It just bothered me to talk about it. I felt ashamed. I didn't want anyone to know. I wanted it to be just for me to know, no one else.

It wrecked my life. It took away all my time. I couldn't do anything . . . if you put it all together maybe an hour and a half or sometimes three hours a day.

I had bathroom problems too. I had to take some toilet paper and rip them up a lot of times into little pieces . . . teeny pieces that had to be just the right size . . . about a millimeter. They had to be torn perfect and then I'd flush them away.

I had to do all kinds of things with my fingers and my mouth. I had to touch all my fingers to my lips a few times if I swallowed saliva. Swallowing was one of the first things too. There were the elbows first. I was afraid of getting my hands dirty. My mind said they were dirty. My mind said I had to wash them. My mind said "wash them, they're dirty." They felt dirty, and after I went to the bathroom everyone has to wash their hands, only mine always felt dirty.

I would forget one thing after another . . . after I changed one pattern, I would completely forget it. I remember one part of one pattern. I had to touch the ends of my thumbs to where the water came out of the faucet.

And some other things I don't remember. I couldn't turn the water off with my hands. I was late for school a lot. The medicine worked. I didn't have to do all these things. Gradually one went away and then the next and then the next. My mom says I seem happier. I have a lot more time to do things. I'm always going to hate my sister but not as much. I don't hate her as much now. Maybe that's from the medicine.

I knew something was very wrong. I kind of thought it's going to go away tomorrow. It's going to go away the next day or the next day or sometime and it never went away and I kind of gave up hope and kept on doing them. I didn't really have an explanation. I imagined that God picked me because He gave me some other gifts so he had to give me some problems too, so he just gave me that. I'm in gifted classes and I'm a good athlete and I'm fast and strong and I'm perfect.

Well, almost perfect, as close as you can get. And I have a bowel movement problem and a nevus trunk and seven operations and my beauty marks.* (Everyone has a few of them but I just have more than most people.) I know a kid who had 20 operations. My mom says he's perfect. Everyone has some problem whether it's a stammer or they can't walk. I have a lot of things that are very good. I've had a more exciting 9 years than most people. I wouldn't mind not having the nevus trunk and all the beauty marks and the bowel movement problem but I like myself the way I am. I wouldn't want to be anybody else.

*[Editor's note: Zack has had a number of premalignant pigmented nevi removed surgically from his trunk and around the anal area. He also has unrelated intestinal problems.]

Zach's Mother/Sam's Wife

From our first meeting, Sam seemed very intense, terribly afraid to "let go" and strangely secretive. I often thought, however, that I was imagining peculiarities that weren't really there, that I was trying to put together pieces of a puzzle when, in fact, there was really no picture to assemble. But, there was an indefinable "something," and, as time passed I knew it was true, illusive but truly there. It *was* like a puzzle.

It was usually easy to find reasons, or at least excuses, for Sam's behavior. I believed he was very nervous. Twitches would come and go. But there's nothing criminal about a twitch. Sam never acknowledged their existence, but I assumed he was embarrassed and chose not to say anything. But there were other eccentricities. Sam would page through a book or magazine as if looking for a certain word. He would look with an obsessive intensity. If I asked him what he was doing, or even spoke, my inquiry would be met with silence. But I also detected a controlled rage. Why?

I often noticed Sam write something down on a piece of paper and then throw the paper away. I always thought that he believed I didn't see him doing it. This was always a very determined act. If I pointedly asked, he would ignore me or try to make a joke of it.

My curiosity became overwhelming. I thought the words he had written held the answer to his strange behavior. Twice I went into the garbage and collected all the paper scraps. I put them together like a jigsaw puzzle. What I found only mystified me more. The first phrase was "past, past, past." The second said, "Zeus is worthless." I never told Sam what I had done. Nor did I ask what it might mean. I was sure he would respond with anger.

The strange behaviors would come and go. But if one disappeared it seemed to be replaced with another. I kept hoping it would all just go away. Sam was often depressed. Sometimes he would go into an intense deep depression. Those seemed to come at times when we had no serious problems. When, in fact, we did have a serious problem to deal with, Sam always pulled himself together and coped. This made me wonder if he really could control all of this if he wanted to.

I always believed that Sam and I had a solid, happy marriage. I always believed that we communicated well and that we shared our feelings and problems together. But there was always this dark secret, this vague unapproachable subject hanging over us. It was there in happy times and sad times, on vacations, anywhere, everywhere, always.

To me, it constituted a kind of selfishness. I was expected to live with it and never question it, never acknowledge it, never understand it. But I knew it was there and often it took over. There was always the fear that it would raise its head and I never knew what precipitated it. It also represented to me an involvement with oneself that was self-centered, egocentric, and selfish. Sam was so introspective, so involved with his own "craziness," that I often felt neglected, left out, forgotten. I am a patient person. I waited. I sensed that this was all beyond Sam's control. I just hoped for some confession, some explanation of what was going on.

We had been married 10 years. I had become pregnant with our third child. I had watched Sam ride his roller coaster and I had learned to adjust to his needs, his moods, his peculiarities, his secretiveness, to his anger and his self-loathing. I had at times entertained the thought that he was having an affair and couldn't deal with the guilt, or that he hated me but couldn't deal with a broken family situation. But I knew that really it was "something" coming from inside. He had reached a new low. He was terribly depressed and angry. He was totally involved with himself and seemed to withdraw deeper into a shell each day. He was almost totally noncommunicative.

I was frightened both for myself and for our children. I was angry that "we" were expecting another child, but Sam's spirit was not a part of our family. It was somehow totally involved with himself. He was possessed.

I thought of people to go to for help: his parents, our rabbi, our family doctor. I dismissed each and every thought, knowing Sam would be furious with me if I spoke to anyone about him. I finally decided to write down all my thoughts, all my feelings, and give them to Sam. I also demanded that he go for professional help. I threatened to leave him if he didn't cooperate. I had hit a brick wall. I could no longer ignore it, excuse it, try to understand it, or believe it would just go away. I could no longer stand the secrecy, the exclusion, the self-involvement, the peculiar behavior, or the depression and anger. I was angry and I was frightened. I felt helpless and I felt I was watching Sam drown without trying to reach for any lifeline. I was truly afraid he might commit suicide.

Sam consulted with a psychiatrist and entered psychoanalysis. His illness was given a name. Doors began to open and little by little some light shone through. Slowly, Sam opened up. I began to learn the history of his behavior and how it controlled him. At times, knowing made it no easier to deal with. He still would get depressed and angry. He still seemed self-centered and I still felt excluded. But now I had some hope as well as an explanation and believed that the psychiatrist would help him to learn to live with his affliction. I hoped that the psychoanalysis would help Sam to understand and deal with his anger. The depression no longer reaches the depths it used to. The rituals have become as familiar and natural to me as my husband's face.

Zach's Father

Try not to think about pink elephants for a while. Try to think about something else, anything else, something that will assuage the uneasiness, perhaps block out completely all thoughts.

Segregate your thoughts of pink elephants in a tiny corner of your mind. Surround them with other thoughts. Concentrate—hard.

Now, at the same time, do something else. Read a book. Drive a car. Ride a bicycle. Concentrate on both things at the same time. Oh, and if a random, uneasy thought of a pink elephant—or of death, perhaps, though one never knows for certain what the thought will be—should happen to escape the prison you have set up, should come barreling into your consciousness, ward it off, blot it out, hold up a cross to the Dracula. Ritualize.

Quick, think of something pleasant. Think of good times. Repeat in your mind those mantras you say to yourself over and over. Life. Life is good. Concentrate. Wait! Don't stop pedaling your bike. You'll fall. Life. Life is good. Say it, over and over. Say it in your mind until you get it absolutely right. Life. Life is good. Look where you're going. You're coming to an intersection. Life. Life is good. I am alive. Faster. The light is red and you haven't got it quite right yet. Life. Life is good. Life, life is good. The intersection. Red light, almost. Life, life is good. Life is good! Life is good! Life is good!! Twitch. Got it! Stop! Made it. I'm okay, for now, for a few seconds, until it starts again.

Have you ever seen the juggler who gets a dozen or so plates spinning on the end of narrow sticks? He starts with one and then he adds more and more, always being careful that none of the plates stop spinning and falls, racing from one to the other to re-spin them, all the time trying to start more and more plates spinning. He must get tired doing that.

Be careful as you read that book or newspaper or magazine. One never knows what terrible things lie on the next page or the next paragraph or the next sentence. Be careful. Read slowly. Concentrate on the mantra.

Damn! "Death." Alright, start to offset it. Be careful. Better to go backward over what you've already read. Try to remember where the words are. You can't go forward anyways, because forward is the future and you don't want to contaminate the future with eyes that have just beheld a world of such terrible consequence. Go back over what you've read. Go to the past. You can't really harm the past . . . you don't really believe that . . . only use it to your advantage.

Now what was it you saw, the word *death*? Yes. Alright, careful. *Life* must be here somewhere. Go back more pages. Where did I see it? *Life*, where are you? There's *living*. No, that won't do. It would work for *dying*, but not *death*. *Death* is the most terrible word. It can only be appeased with *life*. And if *death* was capitalized, try to find *life* capitalized also, or find two or three *life*s to even things out. Careful.

No-ooo. Damn! *Died*. Now you've got to find *living* or *alive or lives* or some such word to offset *died* before you can go back to the first problem. What about *lived*? It's not much better than *died*. Implicit in *lived* is that what was alive is now dead. No, it must be one of the others.

Shit! *Deceased*. Now you've got to offset that before you can offset *died* and then offset *died* before you can offset *death*.

You want to scream out in anger and frustration. This is silly. This is stupid. Why am I doing this? Stay calm. Work through it. Carefully. Slowly. There, *alive*. And there, *lives*. Alright, one left to go.

Shit. *Corpse*. I can't go on like this. Why am I doing this? Wait. *Life*. Okay. I'll use that for *corpse*. Now, just one more *life*. Just to be sure.

No!! I can't believe he asked me for a sheet of paper, interrupted me just when I was coming to the end of the search, only had one to go. Now I've got to start over. Be calm. He doesn't know what you're doing. Hide it. Don't let on. Why can't I be normal? All these other people don't have to do these things. I'm tired. I can't keep this up. What was the order in which I saw the words? Maybe I just won't do it. But I have to do it. Try not to look up with your contaminated eyes until you've finished with the good words. What time is it?

Ach! Now I've looked at the clock, time, the future—contaminated it. Now I've got to offset that against something else. But what? The past. That's it. Find a calendar or a book. Here, this old textbook. At the front, there should be a copyright date. Yes, a year long before I was born, so I can use it to free myself of the contamination I effected by looking at the clock without affecting myself. Stare at the year with your eyes. Get ready to zap it with your eyes. Wait. What do the numbers in the year add up? Nineteen. No, I can't believe it. Nineteen was the age of my ex-secretary's son when he was killed in the automobile accident that night she called at 2 a.m., hysterically crying. Block it out. Think mantras. No, find another year, one that adds up to 18, to *chai* to *life* in Hebrew. Yes, here's another book, another year: 18. Relief. Now, don't look at the clock. Don't look at . . . "Just stop," my mother would say, in a cajoling fashion. "People are looking at you. They're wondering why you're doing those things." What things? I'm not doing anything. Just leave me alone. But you know they're watching you, talking about you, belittling you. And you feel like a jerk. You know you look strange. You're weak and it sickens your stomach. You can't stop. There's a feeling, a constant uneasiness.

I get no comfort from religion. My God is stern and demanding, as unforgiving of me as I am of myself. My gods are hard, insisting on perfect penance constantly. Shape up, boy!

I have no tolerance of religion. I have my own magic. It's strong. It's demanding. It's up to me to do what must be done, to faithfully ritualize. I must protect those I care about. I must ward off the incessant evil contamination that is everywhere.

It's so primitive—religion, so childish. It's what I do on a mass scale. Offer sacrifices. Zap people and then write them off. That girl in graduate school never did understand why I never asked her out. I had even asked my friend to test the waters, to see if she was interested, and she had been. He told her I wanted to ask her out, to expect it, and I had wanted to, had looked forward to it. Ah . . . the anticipation of something pleasant. It's dangerous. Don't you remember all of the rituals, the weight of your past machinations? You're walking on eggs. You barely got by with the other rituals. Don't tempt fate. She is pleasure.

Are there demons? Do you hear commands? Don't be silly. It would be a lot easier if I could blame it on devils whispering in my mind, just be a contented schizophrenic. No, that's ridiculous. The rituals are ridiculous. But can't you feel the weight of the sadness, of the impending doom, impelling action?

Ritualize. The feeling. The torment. Never any relief. And disaster waiting all around me, like a vulture on a dead branch, watching me, smiling smugly, waiting for me to indulge a warm feeling.

Okay, I won't listen to the radio today. Not quite right. Okay, I won't listen to the radio today or tomorrow. Still not enough. Increase the power. I won't listen through a week from today. Not enough. Okay, for a month from today. How am I going to remember that? I'll forget. I'll absent-mindedly turn it on before the month is up. Then I'll really have problems. I will undoubtedly go somewhere where a radio is on. Won't that blow the ritual? No, it must be an affirmative action on my part. There must be intent. If I just walked into a store where a radio was playing, that would be passive, not active. Still, a month to remember the ritual. Okay, got to find something else. I won't use a tape recorder today. I won't use a tape recorder through tomorrow. Do I have a tape recorder? Yes, of course, the hand-held one. It won't do to deny myself something I have no access to. There must be a realistic potential to deny myself. I can't deny myself an airplane ride if I'm unlikely to take an airplane today. Ah, but wait. I've already denied myself the use of a tape recorder for 3 more days. Or was it 4? It's so hard to keep track of what I have denied myself and for how long.

Is anyone looking at me? Can anyone guess what I'm doing? No, I don't think so. No one knows what I'm going through. No one can know. The rest of them are normal. I'm probably the only one cursed like this. But I can do something. I have the power to ritualize, to make a difference, if I just appease the feelings.

I'm running out of things to deny myself. Maybe I'll use elevator denial after all. No, too late. Once you take a pass on a denial, it's not available again until the next ritual. Panic. I'm running out of things. Easy. Concentrate. There must be something else. Board games, maybe. Hold that one. Music boxes. Close to phonographs and tape recorders but different enough to work. Hold that, too.

How did I get started on this in the first place? I didn't see a trigger word like *death* or hear such a word, for that matter—which, of course, would have required that I see someone, preferably the person who uttered the first word, to cleanse the act by saying the word *life*. All I did was have that feeling, that uneasiness, that almost physical need to assuage, to keep things under control.

The rituals are so unforgiving. You've got to work so hard and they won't give you a break. If there is more than one way to view something, the rituals insist that you take the hardest. The gods—the rituals—demand strict obedience. If you don't quite get it, do it over.

Neutral. Unfeeling. Calloused. Cold. Hard. Impervious. It's the only way to maintain my equilibrium. Feel nothing. Not too good. Not too bad. Control. If I have control, I won't have to ritualize as much. Strive for numbness.

I suffer from obsessive-compulsive syndrome. I cannot remember ever not being obsessive compulsive. I cannot imagine life free of obsessive-compulsive behavior. It is as much a part of me as my blue eyes. It is as if I had been born with a birth defect, like the baby that cannot hear that knows no life of sound.

It is with me every waking and every sleeping moment. I ritualize in my dreams. It is my master. There is no escape. I am the legislative, judicial, and executive branches. I "make" the rules, interpret them and enforce them—strictly, brutally, incessantly, without remorse.

My first memories of obsessive-compulsive behavior center about the age of 7. I was playing with a group of children in front of my house. We were playing a variation of a game of "it." We called it "cooties." One person "had the cooties" and all of the others tried to avoid being tagged, of "getting the cooties," of being contaminated. I remember the feeling. It was more than just a game. It was a matter of desperation for me. I just could now allow myself to be tagged, to have all of the contamination flow into me. I ran very fast to escape.

My family called them "superstitions." I don't know if I coined the word or if my mother did. "Just stop," she would say. And I would want to stop. And I would hear the wistfulness in her voice as she ordered/begged me to stop. "Just stop."

Drug abuse starts out as a choice. It may be no easier to stop than obsessive-compulsive behavior but at least the drug abuser has exercised free will. I did not. I just did things because I "had to." I did not understand. I still don't. And this is 31 years later.

I remember thinking, at the age of 7, that by the time I became 15 years old, an incredibly long time in the future, I would stop these things. I would have outgrown them.

I remember my mother telling me about her oldest brother who did similar things, who just finally "outgrew them." I don't know how she knew he outgrew them. She probably thinks I outgrew them, too. I thought about her brother from time to time. I thought more about it when, to my dismay, my son began exhibiting obsessive-compulsive behaviors. I recognized it. I understood it. And I, of all people, was as frustrated and angered by his behavior as my father probably had been over mine. I just wanted him to stop.

There has always been a compelling logic to the rituals. I was always trying to assure or avoid some outcome by my ritualizing. The professed focus would change. But the behavior persisted. Protect myself from contamination. Protect my grades, my sports prowess, my masculinity, my life, my success, people I cared about.

With a change in my focal point would come changes in the stimuli of the rituals. There was a point, for example, when my need was to protect myself from stupid people, that I could not even look at certain people—those who had already failed a grade or were doing poorly. I would prop a book up on my desk at school and put my head down on my arm behind the book so I did not even accidentally catch a glimpse of an untouchable. For every glimpse was a new stimulus, a new invitation for a command performance of rituals. If I finished one ritual and saw an untouchable, I would be required to start again. Over and over and over. It was so tiring.

An 8-year-old cousin of mine died when I was 7 years old. It was sudden. It was frightening. The details were always shrouded in mystery. To this day, I don't know. I never really wanted to know too much. It was traumatic.

It was also, as I think about it, concurrent with my first memories of ritualizing. I don't know whether there was a sort of symbiosis between the rituals and my cousin's death, but it would not surprise me. I dreaded going to my cousin's house—the empty bedroom, the sadness, the pallor, the unspoken. The house seemed antique, shrouded. I did not want to touch anything there. I just wanted to get away. Being there upset me. Thinking about it upset me. Cooties. Pink elephants.

My cousin's very name became an anathema. A classmate of mine with the same name became per se odious. I could not look at her, touch her, think about her without associating it with my cousin. Pink elephants. Twitching.

As a young graduate student, an older, married woman, the wife of the head of a small company where I worked part-time, made a pass at me. I was on the rebound at the time, vulnerable. I probably would not have done anything even if her name had been different from my cousin's. That her name was the same sealed the decision. Better to avoid a moment's pleasure for the terror I would have felt thereafter. Ritualistically, it would have been the union of sex and death. Forever. Avoid it. Better to deny oneself than to suffer such egregious consequences.

I was never exactly sure what the consequences would be—death, eternal damnation, stupidity, failure, errors, contamination. I was not about to tempt the fates to find out.

One distressing aspect of my situation was my certainty that I was the only person on earth who suffered, had ever suffered, would ever suffer as I did—the great ritualist. I could not talk to anyone about my rituals or my fears. I was scared and mortified. That I could not stop ritualizing only served to make me feel more helpless, more ridiculous, more detestable.

I remember once seeing a very good friend of mine doing some things that to my ritually attuned mind seemed oddly akin to my rituals. Could it be? A comrade in arms? I could not ask him. I would have died before I would divulge my secret. To this day, I still wonder.

I do not think it would have made much difference to me anyhow, though I will admit that my recently acquired knowledge that perhaps 2 percent of the population suffers from obsessive-compulsive syndrome had a liberating effect on me. Suddenly I was not the only crazy person around. On the other hand, that knowledge struck me rather like the news that my ex-fiancée and my best old ex-friend had called off their engagement. There was vindication but no joy.

What are they, these rituals? Sometimes I fantasize that they're like a virus, a foreign invader that simply needs to be expunged. Occasionally, more bemusedly than sadly, I would imagine myself being the controlled pawn of observers from outer space. How else could one explain the inability to fight the compulsions that I knew were so senseless?

What are these rituals? My chemistry, I think. Why such chemistry? Genetics, I think. Did the ritualizing cause the self-hate? Or did the self-hate cause the rituals? Why do I do so much cognitive ritualization while others wash their hands? What can washing one's hands do? If I see the word *death* it makes eminent sense to me to negate it by countering it with a glance at the word *life*. Do others try to wash away self-hate?

I have a theory, in the embryonic stage. My theory makes serious presumptions, based on the earliest of memories. I cannot remember very many events, only shards here and there, impressions that make a bell in my mind ring occasionally.

My theory is that, as a child, I could find little solace or comfort for my fears. I strongly resist foisting blame on my parents. My first years are but a black box. It violates my sense of justice and responsibility to lay my troubles on others' doorsteps, like an abandoned child. That is a cop-out. I will take responsibility.

Perhaps there was a sternness. Perhaps there was a sense that others had such pervasive fears of their own that they were incapable of and disinterested in dealing with the fears of a little boy. Maybe the little boy was met with stern looks, or with blame for the world's ills. Maybe the little boy had a sense he was being manipulated, whitewashed. Maybe the little boy decided he could find no comfort from others. Maybe he was chemically incapable of being comforted. Maybe the little boy became very afraid. Perhaps he came to the conclusion that he would need to deal with his fears on his own.

But how can a little boy cope with a little boy's fears by himself? How indeed? Maybe he tries to impose an order on things. Maybe he convinces himself, in desperation, that there is an order of things, because the little boy is his own last resort. But that's ridiculous. There is no order of things. Ah, but there must be an order. It makes sense. It is logical. It is beautiful in its logic. It's simply a matter of uncovering the order, working it out. One must simply learn the rules. It's a great leap of faith, but he's a very scared little boy.

The rules. What are they? Simple. Counter bad with good. Offset. No one will help you. You must do it yourself. Others may not even be aware that the danger exists. Do good.

What's this? Abuse. Why are they giving me such strange looks? Why do I feel like I've done something wrong? What do they mean, stop it? Don't they realize that I must do these things? If I stop doing these things, evil and terrible things will occur, will result. Weak. Why do I feel weak? Why do I feel shame? Why are people looking at me like that? Anxiety. Weakness. Weakness undermines my effectiveness. Twitch. Offset the doubts they are creating. Ritualize. Ritualize. Ritualize your brains out!!!

I am a very successful professional, in a very large city, involved with matters of substantial importance and substantial sums of money, working in a very competitive market. I have a beautiful, loving, understanding wife and three terrific, bright children. Times are good. I am a survivor.

I am 38 years old. I take 300 mg of clomipramine a day. It helps. It takes the edge of terror off the impulses. It helps me fight. So does my anger. I suffer. Sometimes my anger at my rituals is intense. Then I remember that some people are blind, some are deaf, some are paralyzed. I resist feeling sorry for myself. I fight. And I try to understand. I am a survivor. If you don't believe so, count the references to death in here. Despite my fears and anxiety, I wrote this. I will not let them control. I will fight. I am a survivor and proud of it.

Chapter 10

The Children Speak

Richard

All of a sudden, one day in sixth grade, placing my shoes down on the floor perfectly was a necessity. Perfectly is the key word for the beginning of my illness. I had to put my shoes down perfectly. I had to write using extraordinary penmanship, and talk without any slips of the tongue, variations in speech rate, or deviations in tone of speech. My steps had to fall in perfect cadence, with arms moving machine-like alongside my body.

Tests on computer-scored paper were a menace—the circle had to be filled in so perfectly that the tests were never finished.

In sixth grade I had no idea that something was wrong. I thought the slowness was just a part of me, how my personality was. In junior high school I started delivering papers, and then I could see how different I was. I had to look back constantly to see if any papers had dropped off my cart (they never had); I had to go back to each house to see if I had missed a delivery (I never missed). It took me 2 hours to deliver 40 papers; it took other kids 1 hour. Something coerced me to check, to ensure.

These obsessions were like "mosquitoes of the mind." I couldn't make them go away. It wouldn't stop, always there, insistent, itching, a force.

Cleanliness thinking was part of it too. If something was near me or touched me that I thought was "impure" (don't ask me why or how something got to be impure; I don't know why—it just *felt that way*), I was uncomfortable. For instance, in social studies eighth-grade class, there was an "unclean" air conditioner next to my seat. I didn't hear the teacher call on me; he yelled at me; I was sent out. Actually I had to sit in the corner.

High school was counting numbers. I would begin what I thought might be an ordinary day, and then the only thing that would enter my mind would be "6,6,6,6," or "8,8,8,8"; I had no control over these numbers. They had a mind of their own—my mind!

Our marching band had a competition during my numbers time, and I got confused by the numbers, didn't keep up with the steps. We lost the competition and I always felt it was my fault and maybe it was. I was also in the symphonic band. During one competition I could not play my clarinet because I had so many numbers in my mind that I couldn't concentrate on or "hear" the music. I only pretended to play. Maybe no one knew about that time. I often wondered.

Obsessions ruined golf for me too. I tried out for the school golf team. I had been pretty good at golf, but the cleanliness obsession made me uncomfortable with hitting the clubs in the dirt—it would spread the dirt, and make things, including me, "unclean." I knew that to get a clean stroke of the ball you had to hit the ground and create a divot. But I couldn't make myself dig into the earth. I missed the ball a few times and didn't even get on the golf team.

Later in high school, the sexual thoughts were part of it too. I felt guilty that I masturbated. But that wasn't so bad. It was the obsessive thought that perhaps the neighbors had looked into my window and seen me, an end-of-the-world feeling. The neighbors, I was sure, had seen me. I said they couldn't see me because of how my bedroom window was placed. But this disease gets ridiculous at times. *I felt sure* that they had climbed the roof in order to look into my window. My mind almost had to figure out how it could be real because the idea was there all the time.

I thought about dying and what a relief it would be. I could never be *sure* that the neighbors *didn't* see me masturbate. Everything had to be clear-cut, but it never was. Life never is. Now that I am in college, I know that.

My obsessing has evolved and keeps changing. After the perfection, the numbers, and the sex, there has been a more general feeling of depression. My obsessions extended themselves, I think about them as independent agents, into other areas of my life. I worried about what I said to people; the way I was holding different features of my face, like my lips and tongue; and about how I appeared to people.

But the worst part, the part that is now hurting my college life, is the way the obsessions take up so much time and mind space that I have less time to think of friends, of girls. I don't initiate any kind of relationships. The secret for me now, it seems, would be to force myself to start to talk to people. I can't stand feeling so passive and I know it will pay off.

Since I have had times when I was perfectly OK, I do have perspective on how much I am missing when I am sick. I go on and learn, try to learn, how to live with the pain. The pain is one that only those with obsessive-compulsive disorder (OCD) know. Others can't really understand how awful it is. I don't think anyone who doesn't have OCD can ever understand but this may help some.

Arnie

I cannot remember exactly when I first began having problems with obsessive-compulsive behavior. I once had a vague idea that it started around the time of my father's death when I was 6. But I also do seem to remember one night coming down my stairs, even before my father died, and saying to my parents that I was being bothered by the way I had put on my pajamas. My parents told me not to worry about it. So I might have had rituals (like putting on pajamas a certain amount of times) when my father was still alive, if my memory serves me right. But, I still think my father's death had a tremendous impact on my life, and this may have caused my rituals to worsen later in the fifth grade.

I can remember having trouble walking out of my yard when I was between the ages of 6 and 8. I had to walk out of my yard between two marks on the sidewalk, and I avoided certain cracks. If I didn't walk through it right, I would have to do it all over again. Between the ages of 7 and 11 I don't recall too many specific incidents. I'm not saying I wasn't bothered with any rituals, just that they weren't bad enough to be recognized too well. When I was in grade school I would try to avoid thinking certain bad thoughts. In order to do this I would think or say the words of Jesus Christ to stop the bad thoughts. This happened when my rituals were just developing.

Another thing is that during the third and fourth grades I came home sometimes worried sick about a person wanting to "beat me up" after school. He never did hit me but it still increased my anxiety about school in general. This was enough to start my rituals off a little bit more.

It wasn't until the second time I was in the fifth grade that I remember having more rituals than before. I was 12 that year and I remember being teased about doing my rituals in class. For example, I would have to spin around in circles a certain number of times in the coatroom before it "felt right" to come out into the classroom due to a good thought. The people in class who saw me would tease me about my rituals, but I couldn't help it. This was the first time that it started to interfere with me at school, and the first time it was noticeable to other people.

Originally, I tried to cope with my problem on my own. At first I even thought doing my rituals was a normal thing to do. But then I noticed that other people did not do rituals, and then I started to feel that I was different from them because I was the only person with obsessive-compulsive behavior. (At least I didn't know anyone else with the same type of problem.) Because of this feeling, I sometimes thought other people were part robot and part human. I thought I was the only real human alive and that some people were against me or were more powerful than I. But these ideas went away as I got older.

Later on, I knew the rituals weren't the normal thing to do and I looked silly doing them in front of other people. So I did try several times to stop them, but I couldn't. Although I do remember that I was able to stop my rituals for several days when I was about 10 or 11. I also tried to hide my symptoms from other people, but sometimes I couldn't help doing rituals in front of them. The main thing is that I first tried to deal with my problem with obsessive-compulsive behavior on my own, and for a long time, before my mother found a psychologist to help me.

When I was in the fifth grade for the second time, my obsessive-compulsive behavior became a bit more difficult to handle. I might have started doing a little bit more in the fourth or fifth grades. I didn't notice them to be pretty bad until the second time I was in the fifth grade. I was 12 years old and some of the friends I used to hang out with started to turn against me and tease me a lot. I only had a couple of friends to hang around with. I would skip school also and I started to do so in the fourth grade. The reason I did not go to school was because I did not like people teasing me about my rituals.

When I entered the sixth grade things were worse. I gradually started getting worse with my rituals and I skipped school more often. I was withdrawn from most everybody except for a few friends. I didn't talk much either.

All through the sixth grade I had become more and more wrapped up in my rituals. My mom could not get me to see my doctor.

By then, *I was extremely controlled* by my rituals to the point where I was almost completely immobile. I could not move around the house without having to do things over and over.

I especially had trouble going into my yard when I got out of school. It would take me hours to get into my house from outside my yard. I had to go through my gate a certain way and a certain amount of times. I would have to go through my gate almost perfectly in order to make it inside my house. For example, I could only look at certain spots when walking through my gate, and I was not supposed to step on *any* cracks in the sidewalk either. As I was doing this ritual I would be trying to think good thoughts so I would not have to do my rituals over too many times. Sometimes when I got out of school at 3 o'clock I would not get into my house until 4 or 5 o'clock because I would be real anxious and my rituals would be real bad. I would also have more bad thoughts to try to get rid of by doing my rituals over and over.

I had trouble with getting dressed over and over, taking a shower, getting to certain places in my house without thinking bad thoughts, avoiding cracks outside, etc., and all this was very frustrating.

Later on I stopped going to school and my rituals were at the worst they have ever been. It took me from 5 to 30 minutes to get where I wanted to in my house. I would make certain movements with my arms and/or make noises with my mouth to get my bad thoughts out of my mind. Since I was so anxious at this time, my rituals had taken complete control. I stayed in my pajamas all day because I didn't feel like even trying to put on my regular clothes; it took me so long to get dressed (since I did it over and over). This was one reason I stopped going to school; I could not get dressed in time for it.

My rituals were so much a part of my life during this time and they interfered so much that I only had time to do a couple of things during the day. I felt like giving up because I was immobile all day long. It did not seem worth it to go through all my rituals all day long, so I avoided situations that would occupy me for a long time. For example, I would avoid getting dressed in the morning so I would not have to go through my dressing rituals.

I had stopped going to school for weeks, and that's how I ended up in the hospital. When my mom told me about the hospital, I didn't want to go. But, though my family had a tough time getting me into the hospital, I now feel it was a smart move.

People in my family did not understand my problem with rituals at all. They didn't tease me or anything, but they weren't that supportive either. My sisters would yell at me for getting in their way when they watched TV, when I was only trying to get by as fast as I could, with as few rituals as possible.

My sister helped me by getting me inside the house. This was when I could not get through my front gate without my rituals. She would encourage me to get inside and sometimes it helped.

But after a while at the hospital, it got a little better. My family got more supportive and they accepted me easier. After I got out, I did not have hardly any rituals. But when they got worse again, my brothers and sisters did not ignore me, and tried to help out. My mother would yell at me to get in the house when I was having trouble getting inside and that also helped. If anyone told me to stop doing a ritual, it would help a little.

My obsessive-compulsive behavior has changed a lot over the years. From when I was in the hospital in 1979 until now I have learned, accepted, and grown up so much that my rituals are only a small thing in my life. I probably will never get rid of my rituals but they have gotten better.

Working at Montgomery Wards' became a deciding factor in cutting the rituals down. When I work I am so busy that even though I am not finished with a ritual, I have to stop in the middle because I have so much to do. I worried at first that I didn't finish my ritual, but later on I realized it wasn't real necessary and I stopped worrying. Now there aren't any special numbers to count. I used to have to get dressed in the morning a certain number of times; now I hardly have this problem at all.

Some of the Symptoms I Still Have

I try to walk through only one side of doorways and will try not to look at certain spots or think bad thoughts when I walk through it; if I do think bad thoughts or look at certain spots, I will have to back up and do it again only if I am anxious, otherwise I go through the door only once.

I have trouble walking through my kitchen because when I see knives or other sharp objects I get bad thoughts of the knives cutting me. I try to walk through my kitchen again without looking at the knives.

I read things over in a book I have to read for school. I will read sentences or paragraphs over until I think of a good thought.

Instead of trying to stop my rituals (which is virtually impossible), I've tried just to control them. This has worked for me because when I talk about my problems, my rituals aren't too bad and they are then under control. Unfortunately, the medicine didn't help me and neither did group therapy.

I don't think just self-control could have helped my problem because I needed the discipline and support of the staff members I've had and the therapy to get over my problem with rituals.

I have been seeing a psychiatrist since August 1983 who has been pretty helpful in the past 2 years with me in areas such as going to school, having more confidence, and taking more responsibility for myself. I don't talk about my rituals that often with him because basically they are not a problem with me anymore. Also, I feel good to know that when something is bothering me, I have somebody to talk to about it.

I have had problems with depression at certain points in my life that were very serious at some times while less severe at others. When it was very severe I had thoughts of suicide, but this was long ago when I had a low self-esteem and no confidence in myself.

Most of the time, I am pretty happy even though I don't look like it. The reason I don't always look happy is because I constantly worry about everything and even though I am sometimes preoccupied I am still pretty happy. But when I talk about what I worry about or write it down, it usually helps.

I get along with other people pretty well. I am a little shy when meeting people at first, but after I get to know them I become much more relaxed and can talk openly to them. When I was younger I had a hard time telling people when I was angry at them because I thought they would dislike me for it. But now I will usually tell people if I am angry at them and I don't worry about it too much.

I am also pretty friendly to people and I enjoy their company most of the time. I also consider myself a caring, understanding, and sensitive person who is very likable and a person that others enjoy being around.

I'm doing pretty good in my life now. I would say that there has been a big decline in the number of rituals I do and the number of times I do them over the past years. I'm not saying that I don't have any rituals left, just that they don't occur as much as they used to. I used to be controlled by my obsessive-compulsive behavior long ago, but I would say that I am in control now.

Morris

I began having problems with obsessive-compulsive behavior when I was 13. My family had just moved from a rather large city to a small town just 2 years before. Being a shy person, I had a hard time making new friends and going to a different school. I had started on a paper route with more than 100 deliveries to make, and I remember missing a few people on particular night. Some called and complained, and I felt as if I had let a lot of people down. This led to doubts about my way of living . . . of whether or not I was doing things right, or whether I had done them at all. I remember standing in my room at night, mentally reviewing the events of the day, making sure I had done everything I was supposed to do that day. Eventually I became obsessed with thinking over every event of the day that occurred, including whether or not I read the paper or watched TV. Then the compulsive thinking spread to compulsive actions, and it took me much longer to do routine things such as brushing my teeth or taking a shower. This caused me to get to bed later at night, and I was consistently late for school. Doing and thinking about things over and over and being obsessed with cleanliness was very characteristic of my life at that time.

As my problem increased in severity when I was 13, I gradually began to feel more helpless and could not cope. My parents were concerned enough, fortunately, that they got help for me from a psychologist. I would try to hide my symptoms of checking at school, but they were eventually noticed.

After a couple of months, I was no longer just being late for school—I was missing school altogether. I was out of school for more than a month; part of the time was spent in a regular hospital, recommended by the psychologist, but this did no good. I convinced my psychologist that I was well enough to leave the hospital, but once I got home, the problem was at its worst; it has never been that bad since. A shower that once took 10 minutes now took 45 to 60 minutes. It was taking me over 20 minutes just to brush my teeth. Dressing took more than an hour. I couldn't even put my socks on in the morning without checking the bottoms of my feet (for dirt) many, many times. Eventually I dreaded getting up in the morning and facing all the compulsive actions associated with showering and dressing. At one time I got up about 10 or 11 a.m. and was not showered and dressed until 8 p.m. My parents did everything they could, from setting time limits and cutting the water off to having one parent give me a shower—I couldn't do it on my own. It would also take me an incredibly long time to get to bed, both with the compulsive actions associated with washing and brushing my teeth and the compulsive thoughts and worries about the day. Finally, I went to a psychiatric hospital.

As an only child, I had a greater impact on my parents when I developed obsessive-compulsive behavior. They became very concerned over what was happening to me and I sensed their feelings of anger, frustration, sadness, pity, and love. They became angry and frustrated at me because they felt I was not making enough of an effort to change, but felt very sad and had pity for me when they realized I could no longer help myself.

After being hospitalized more than a year, I got better enough to return home and to school. I was taking less time to do things (such as taking a shower), and the compulsive actions and obsessive thoughts had diminished greatly, although I still reread textbooks and rechecked math problems. I spent late nights with homework that should only have taken 2 or 3 hours. Toward the end of high school, I completely recovered, and went on to become increasingly involved in extracurricular activities and graduated in the top 5 percent of my class. This remission lasted until my third year of college, when I wanted to transfer to another school; my grades suddenly dropped. The anxiety over whether I would be accepted at the other school and follow through with my career plans was, I think, why I got sick. The repetitive thoughts now consisted of going over in my mind any important responsibilities I had during the day. My only compulsive action was in reading each sentence in my textbook assignment several times, which prevented me from having enough time to read all of the assignment. The compulsive reading, coupled with procrastination, caused my grades to drop and locked me in a habit of compulsive thinking for the second time in my life. When I got home from college, the thinking spread to compulsive actions (such as putting something away in a drawer). I still had not resumed compulsive washing and haven't since. I hope that my problems will never be as bad as they were when I was 13.

I think that good physical exercise, increased involvement with school extracurricular activities, and interaction with more people, as well as improved grades and improved self-confidence, helped to contribute to my complete recovery the first time around.

The new crisis of poor grades and the anxiety over my future caused the return of the problem, but I'm not really sure what caused it to get worse.

When the problem was at its worst, my parents would set time limits for me to do things and encourage me to prevent myself from getting locked into a repetitive pattern of thinking and checking. Self-control only worked part of the time. Eventually only strict behavior modification at the psychiatric hospital helped lessen the problem. This involved enforcing time limits and not allowing me to spend time alone thinking. Gradually I felt less of a need to engage in certain obsessions and compulsions, and they gradually disappeared after a positive experience in high school.

I have not been able to follow any of the suggestions given by the psychotherapists for the problem. The only thing that helped me was a strict behavior modification program. I needed time limits for showering and toothbrushing! I was not allowed to go in my room by myself and think or to spend too much time studying; I was forced to go out and interact with the other patients.

At one time the thought of killing my parents and/or my dog crossed my mind. Another time the thought of gouging out my eyes with needles crossed my mind more than once. These thoughts troubled me because I had no explanation for them and would in no way *ever* want to even attempt to harm anyone else or myself or any animal. After convincing myself that they were irrational, the thoughts of harm eventually went away. I feel guilty when I have them, and recently, without any explanation, a curse against God has gone through my mind. This usually involves a swear word being associated with God, Jesus Christ, the Lord, etc. This thought has always made me very guilty and angry with myself for I have always considered myself a strong Christian. Yet the more I try to repress it, the more the thought keeps coming back. I have no explanation for these irrational thoughts that come and go, but I detest them all and hope I never have them again.

Most of the time I feel content and cheerful; sometimes when I'm not making progress with this problem, I'm blue, but I was very depressed on only one occasion. I had just gotten a test back with a very low grade, and it looked like I was going to fail a course and that my plans for my future were in jeopardy. (This was during my third year of college.) I felt worthless, and the thought of committing suicide crossed my mind, but I never would actually do it. I haven't had any suicidal thoughts since.

Although I'm a rather shy person and have trouble introducing myself to strangers, I get along very well with other people and enjoy being with others.

I am now out of college for the summer and working at a part-time job, stocking shoes for a department store in town. I still have problems with compulsive thoughts (thinking over responsibilities of the day and the future as well, as to whether or not I've done certain tasks of personal hygiene). In addition, I have a great number of compulsive actions (checking clothes as I put them in a drawer or checking a surface before I set anything on top of it, for example). I get to bed 60 to 90 minutes later than I should and arrive 2 to 7 minutes late for work each morning. About the only way I can cope is forcing myself not to give in to the temptation to recheck or rethink about something, but that is very hard.

Sorting shoes by their stock number and size brings out rechecking, and this slows me up. I don't have any hobbies or social life of any kind. When I'm not at work, I'm at home with my parents. Besides going to an occasional movie, my only leisure activities are reading, watching TV, or listening to music.

A new problem is my superstition with certain numbers that I avoid because I think they bring me bad luck. For example, in the course of my checking something or thinking about something several times, I will make sure I do not repeat something 6 or 13 times, or 60, 66, or 130 for that matter. Even numbers that add up to 6 or 13 or can be multiplied to get them are avoided, such as 32, 76, or 85. Other numbers such as 7 and 33 are also avoided.

Although I can hardly write from a standpoint of a cured obsessive-compulsive person at this time, I believe my ideas for recovery may be at least of some help to some people.

My advice to others with obsessive-compulsive behavior would be to not get discouraged with your problem or accept it as your way of living for the rest of your life. Ask yourself when in the midst of a checking ritual or a string of compulsive thoughts, "Is it really necessary for me to be doing this?" Realize that you're only human, and things are never going to be 100 percent perfect, straight, neat, or clean, so why bother? It will be hard at first, but after a while you will find that you will no longer need these obsessive-compulsive behaviors.

My advice to doctors treating patients with this problem would be to provide encouragement and to remind the patient that no one is perfect and the patient should not try to be.

Francie

I was about 14. I came home from track practice and walked into the house. My mother said, "Guess what's happened now?" She told me that my older brother had been infested with fleas from our cat. This, in turn, reminded me of the time when I was in fifth grade, when my brother had caught lice from a boy he sat next to in school. All of us kids got lice too. I was the one who found them first. My parents thought that I was making it up. I had to keep on showing them and finally they believed me. We had a school check and I was found to have them, of course. I had to be called out of class and sent home. All the other kids knew and they teased me about it. Well, we got the shampoo and it finally blew over. But the day that my mother told me about the fleas it brought it all back. After she told me, I started to think that if my brother had it they were probably everywhere all over the house and in our clothes and things. I was taking science in school and I knew all about germs and how dirty bugs were. I figured that anything I touched would be dirty or something. . . . I figured I'd better go wash my hands, and I did. Then I would touch something and I thought that probably had germs on it too. So I washed my hands again. The first night it wasn't that bad. But in about 2 weeks, it became noticeable. Thanks to the science course, I knew the purifying value of alcohol, rubbing alcohol, and I started using it. I started to shake out my clothes for fear that fleas or their eggs might be in them. Eventually my fears and obsessions grew stronger; I felt that if I ever neglected to do any of my rituals something terrible would happen to me, my family, or even strangers.

At first I tried to hide my habits. But as they grew stronger and more frequent, I couldn't hide them. I didn't care though, because if anyone tried to stop me I'd find a way—even if it meant staying up all night to complete them. My parents sent me to a psychiatrist, which I didn't mind. I didn't understand my problem and I certainly welcomed help to overcome it. But because a lot of people didn't know what exactly was wrong with me, I more or less had to deal with it myself. I just went from day to day living with this obsession, which slowly but surely demanded more and more of my time. So it finally got to the point where I didn't do anything but deal with my problem. I just had to live with it myself.

At the worst, my obsession completely controlled my life. I probably couldn't spend 10 minutes a day not performing some sort of ritual. I didn't do anything like watch TV or go out. I even had let these problems interfere with my body function. I lost weight because I wouldn't let myself eat more than three things a day (like some ice cream would be one, an orange two, and eggs three). I had to hold my bladder in the morning, and for the rest of the day, for about 30 to 45 minutes because this was how long it took me to clean the toilet seat before I would use it. I remember thinking, "I'd rather be dead than live through something like this," but as for seriously thinking about suicide, I'd say no. I don't think that I am or ever was someone who could do something like that.

Now I don't have any "real" problems with it at all. I do a few little things that I consider my quirks, but everybody has some. They're like safety valves to me, but if I can't do them, I don't get all rattled or anything. And they aren't time consuming and they don't lead to more quirks.

Doctors have to coax the patient into letting the doctors help them to let themselves change their "plans," as I did with my psychiatrist. That was the biggest step in my recovery.

Taffy

When I was at my worst my whole day was taken up with rituals. (The number of times I would do a ritual would switch back and forth between an odd number of times and an even number of times.) From the time I got up in the morning until I went to bed it was continuous rituals. I would go back and forth around my bed a certain number of times when I was making it up. I would count a certain number of sheets of toilet paper to use when I was using the bathroom. I would wash my hands several times. I would get a certain number of paper towels to dry my hands with if the bathroom had paper towels. Getting dressed was a major battle—for a few days I almost couldn't come to a stopping place in the number of times I put on my pants and shirt and especially socks and shoes (tying my shoelaces was the worst part of the shoes bit). After getting dressed I would go to breakfast. Walking to breakfast was another chore—go so many steps and come back to the starting point several times, then move ahead so many steps and back several times and on and on till I would finally reach the cafeteria. Then on to school—with the same pattern of pacing back and forth in a certain range and then on ahead and pacing back and forth till I finally would reach the school building.

Classroom rituals consisted of sharpening my pencil several times, getting so many sheets of paper, writing only a certain number of words across the paper. After awhile it got to where I would write only so many letters across the page and I would put a dash after the letter and finish the word on the next line. I would also write a word and erase it a certain number of times until I would wear the eraser down to nothing. At lunch I would pick my fork up and put it back down a certain amount of times. I would pick up my glass and set it back down several times. I would spit out the last bit of food and I would also leave a little bit of each thing I had on my plate. I would push my chair in a certain number of times too. When we all went back down to the cottage, I would pace the floor back and forth. When we had group meeting (where we all talked about how we'd done that day—"group therapy" I guess you could say), I would go through verbal rituals. I would start saying something and repeat it several times, but I wouldn't say a whole sentence, only several words at a time. That was, I guess, the most frustrating ritual I did because I was trapped within the ritual and couldn't express myself freely. I also would make a ritual out of asking people questions a certain number of times—if they didn't answer me it added to my frustration.

I had another ritual that was almost as frustrating as verbal rituals and that was touching people a certain number of times also whenever they touched me or happened to brush up against me. I would sometimes be open about it (touching them back) and then other times I would try to be subtle in my approach to touch them back—depending on if they were hostile or irritated or tried to get away from my touching them. Several people would make a game of it with me to see if I could get them back and of course this infuriated me. There were a couple of people who I ended up getting into a slapping match with over this ritual after they got fed up with me touching them. This list could continue, but I know I've already said plenty so I will stop here.

I was put in a psychiatric hospital at the time that my rituals were at their worst. I did feel like giving up several times and I just became deeper involved in rituals when I felt this way.

How did this affect my family? My brother—it affected him the least, I'd say, because he was in high school at the time and was active in football and church and all the activities involved with these things. He stayed so busy that he didn't have to see much of my rituals. But when he did see them he got mad. He called me a mental case, and that really hurt my feelings. He really didn't know what to think so he just would get mad. Several times when I involved my mother in a verbal ritual (and we both were yelling at each other and I was fighting with her physically to get her to answer me), my brother acted like he was my dad and smacked me and picked me up and dragged me to my room and put me down. I, then screaming at him and telling him to leave me alone and to get out of my room, would slam the door and cry for a good while.

Dad reacted pretty much the same: hostile and irritated. He had a little more patience though. He would intervene sometimes when I would be asking my mother to answer me like I said my brother did, but he would give me a spanking and then send me to my room. This, of course, was when I was getting out of hand and, like I said earlier, when I was fighting my mother physically to get her to answer me. Dad didn't answer me hardly when I would try to involve him in a verbal ritual.

My mother, on the other hand, was affected the most; I've always been closest to her. She was caught in a bind because of our closeness. She would go along with my verbal rituals for awhile to try to help, but I never could stop so she eventually had to pull out. She sometimes even then would give in to my demands. It was the toughest for her because she suffered with me knowing more what I was going through. She tried to help me more than my dad and brother too. She's told me herself that she wished that she could have taken my place and suffered for me because "No one knows except a mother what it feels like to see your child suffering and not be able to do anything about it."

She prayed for me all the time. She said depending on God for support was what kept her going through the whole ordeal.

What helped? Talking and trying to sort out my feelings helped the most in the long run. Verbal rituals made it hard to express my feelings but eventually I would accomplish something. When I would be getting stuck on saying something it made me even worse for whomever (counselor) I was talking to to put a limit on how long they would give me to get out what I was saying. I would end up repeating what I was saying even more. But then on the same token putting a time limit on my physical rituals gave me the boundary I needed, like a counselor saying "By the time I count to 3 I want you to tie your shoes." Also, "If you don't tie your shoes and leave them tied when I count to 3 you won't be able to wear your shoes for the rest of the day."

Self-control couldn't help me—that was the problem; I didn't have enough self-control to stop or I would never have done rituals to start with!

I saw a movie when I was in the hospital one night when we went on an outing. The movie was called *Ragtime*. The main theme of the movie was not so significant as was its effect on me. It was, instead, one particular scene that had its greatest effect. That particular scene was where this black man prayed to God about what he should do (either to blow the building up that he and his hostages were in or surrender to the police, which were the ones that caused the problem in the beginning), and this made me think more about God. I started realizing that I need to lean on God and that's exactly what I did. I started reminding myself that God was helping me and I *believed* that I was in the process of eliminating all of my rituals and I *really was* in the process.

Section V

Treatment

Chapter 11

Behavioral Treatment for Obsessive-Compulsive Disorder in Childhood

Carol Zaremba Berg, M.A.
Judith L. Rapoport, M.D.
Richard P. Wolff, Ph.D.

Behavioral treatment for obsessive-compulsive disorder (OCD) in childhood is very new compared with the relatively recent but far more extensive behavioral work with adults. Despite the prominence and success of behavior modification with other childhood disorders in the past 20 years, childhood OCD received little behavioral attention due to its perceived rarity. However, a higher than expected prevalence rate in the general population directed new attention to behavioral treatment of childhood OCD. Since no standardized methods for behavioral treatment for childhood OCD are currently available, this chapter reviews behavioral treatment with adults, summarizes the published child behavioral reports, and, based on our clinical experience with these children, addresses special problems likely to be encountered in developing and implementing a behavioral program for this pediatric population.

Review of Behavior Treatment for Adults

Reports of behavioral treatment of obsessive-compulsive adults since the 1960s demonstrated the success of behavioral techniques in comparison to the more traditional psychotherapies (Foa et al. 1985; Murray 1986). Behavioral therapies showing varying degrees of effectiveness with OCD have included systematic desensitization (gradually acclimating the patient to the feared object/person); paradoxical intention (deliberately increasing the frequency or intensity of thought and/or behaviors); thought stopping (instructing the patient to "stop" the thought); and aversion procedures (increasing discomfort) (Foa et al. 1985). Relaxation techniques have proven to have little or no effect with OCD (Marks 1977). In vivo exposure combined with response prevention (forcing patients to remain in a feared situation and preventing them from carrying out the rituals) has become the adult behavioral treatment of choice since Meyer's (1966) successful treatment of two patients. Meyer hypothesized, combining exposure with prevention, the patient may discover that the feared consequences no longer take place, with the modification of expectations resulting in the cessation of ritualistic behaviors. In a study of 32 obsessive-compulsive patients in three treatment groups (in vivo exposure only, response prevention only, two procedures combined), patients showed greater changes with the combined treatments (Foa et al. 1984). Foa et al. (1985), in summarizing group studies of more than 200 obsessive-compulsive ritualizers treated with prolonged exposure and response prevention, found 51 percent of the patients were symptom-free or much improved at the end of treatment, 39 percent were moderately improved, and only 10 percent had no improvement. At follow-up, while the number of patients considered failures increased to 24 percent, this method of treatment was still rated as a success.

Foa and colleagues, combining these treatment techniques, have developed a comprehensive treatment program for adults that consists of three phases (Grayson et al. 1985) (Appendix 1). The first phase consists of gathering information about the patients' obsessive-compulsive behaviors, informing the patient about the treatment, and establishing a treatment plan. Imaginal flooding, in vivo exposure, and response prevention techniques are defined in relation to the patient's symptoms. The setting (home or hospital) and who will assist the patient with his or her assignments are decided. Patients are selected who manifest compulsive rituals, express a desire to get rid of them, and can identify and report a set of stimuli, thoughts, or objects that precede emission of, or urges to, emit the compulsive rituals (Foa and Tillmans 1980).

The information-gathering phase, which includes functional analysis of problem behaviors, is actually the most important task. Additional guidelines are available (Baer and Minichiello 1986; Emmelkamp 1982; Hersen and Bellack 1981; Steketee and Foa 1985) for probing for degree and severity of symptoms. Emmelkamp (1982) suggested the therapist question the functional relationship between problem areas as well as within a problem area to formulate a hypothesis of why a patient "is as he is" and not just focus on the obsessive symptoms that may be the end result of a complex behavioral chain. Since cause and effect are difficult to determine, the therapist can test different hypotheses from the developmental history before deciding on the treatment strategy. Obtaining information concerning antecedents and modifying variables is important for deciding on symptom focus and for avoiding a treatment failure.

Research treatment phases have consisted of 10 to 15 treatment sessions scheduled every weekday with a minimum of three sessions per week (massed sessions show greater improvement than spaced sessions). In the beginning of the session, the patient's mood, urge to ritualize, and prior homework are discussed. Flooding in imagination concerning objects, thoughts, or situations that provoke fear are discussed. In vivo exposure is then introduced based on a hierarchy of exposing the patient to moderate anxiety (40 to 50 based on a 0 to 100 Subjective Units of Discomfort, or SUDS, scale) and increasing over time, with exposure lasting for 90 minutes. Response prevention is continuous during this period to eliminate experiencing any anxiety relief. All nonessential washing and cleaning is eliminated, with gradual introduction of what is considered normal routine.

The third phase is a maintenance regime to prevent returning to former behavior and to continue exposure to previously avoided situations. Social skills and new patterns of behaviors may need to be learned or reestablished. Weekly sessions for a few weeks to months may be necessary.

Treatment failures with adults have been attributed to their lack of emotional processing (failure to activate the fear sufficiently during treatment or disconfirming information unavailable) (Foa and Kozak 1986). Patient characteristics of the latter group include cognitive avoidance (pretending to be elsewhere), absence of short-term habituation, depression, and overvalued ideation (fears are realistic vs. being silly). Obviously, some characteristics such as diagnosing depression and labeling realistic fears can be identified in the assessment phase whereas the others involve actual participation in the treatment process. The degree of family/spouse overinvolvement and need to keep the patient dependent can also affect outcome.

Reports of Behavioral Treatment with Children

We could locate only 20 studies published since 1967 of behavioral treatment of obsessive children (Table 1).

A total of 43 patients (26 males) 8 to 18 years of age received some

Table 1. Reported studies of behavioral treatment of obsessive-compulsive children

	No. of Patients	Age	Sex	Symptoms	Treatment	Follow-up	Comments
Weiner 1967	1	15	M	rituals with washing, dressing, reading, writing, placing objects, thoughts that something terrible will happen	positive response for rituals	7 months	symptom-free
Mills et al. 1973	1	15	M	morning and evening rituals, checking, putting things in order	response prevention: hospital and home		at home rituals returned after 2 months; parents used response prevention succesfully
Fine 1973	2	11	M	evening rituals, touching peers on behind, getting parents to repeat questions	extinction, response prevention, family therapy	1 year	minimal rituals
		9	M	evening rituals, dress certain order, think pleasant thoughts	family therapy, firm responses		minimal rituals
Campbell 1973	1	12	M	persistent thoughts about sister's death	thought stopping	3 years	symptom-free

Hallam 1974	1	15	F	persistent questions, washing and cleaning bathtub	extinction, social-skills training	14 months	questions eliminated; washing rituals remain
Freidman and Silvers 1977	1	18	M	counting numbers & steps, 6 steps before going thru doorway; sit down & stand up in certain way	paradoxical intention; thought stopping; positive reinforcement	2½ years	symptom-free
Ong and Leng 1979	1	13	F	contamination & dirt, lice, germs in hair, books, house; rituals: hand washing, baths; avoid: doorknobs, furniture, pets, food	implosion, modeling; response prevention; positive reinforcement	2 years	mild relapse; good response to further work
Harbin 1979	1	16	F	worry will fail school, redo homework; unpleasant thoughts	ordeal	8 months	symptom-free
Stanley 1980	1	8	F	morning and evening rituals, checks toys, ritual song	response prevention, family involved	1 year	symptom-free
Green 1980	1	15	M	touches objects, checks, cup just right, reenters doorways, fears terrible things may happen	relaxation, satiation, response prevention	6 months	minimal thoughts; rituals hardly ever

Table 1. Reported studies of behavioral treatment of obsessive-compulsive children *(continued)*

	No. of Patients	Age	Sex	Symptoms	Treatment	Follow-up	Comments
Queiroz et al. 1981	2	9	M	fears punishment, people; picks up trash & keeps it; shower rituals	positive reinforcement; in vivo desensitization	18 months	adequate behavior
		12	F	repeats gestures, questions; opens/ closes doors	family involvement	1 year	symptom-free
Hafner et al. 1981	1	16	M	fears contamination from sister; rituals: thumps floor, refuses to swallow	in vivo desensitization; family therapy	1 year	symptom-free
Phillips and Wolpe 1981	1	12	M	needs parent in sight; kicks things; does things 3 times; moves head, arms; calls Dad repeatedly; fears parents will die	in vivo desensitization; rewards, parent training	2 years	symptom-free
Clark et al. 1982	1	13	M	obsessional slowness; 6–8 hours to dress; checks taps, doors	response prevention; model, prompt, PACE, shape		gains not maintained with fading procedures

Bolton et al. 1983	15	12 –18	8 M 7 F	cleaning, checking, rumination	response prevention, family, drug, individual therapy	9 months to 4 years	13 cases followed: 7 symptom-free 3 mild 1 still severe 2 episodic
Dalton 1983	1	9	M	hand washing, checking behind doors, daydreaming	ignore, positive reinforcement, family therapy	1 year	symptom-free
Ownby 1983	1	13	M	hand washing, brushing teeth, showering 1 hour after school; fears germs, contamination	thought stopping	18 months	symptom reduction maintained
Zikis 1983	1	11	F	does things twice (one hand then the other); tics; keeps eyes open at night	in vivo exposure; response prevention	1 year	symptom-free
Apter et al. 1984	8	10 –16	5 M 3 F	cleaning, checking, rumination, washing most common; thoughts of sex, aggression	response prevention; in vivo exposure; drug & psychotherapy	2½ years	7 of 8 much improved; (4 symptom-free); 1 improved
Kolko 1984	1	16	F	avoidance behavior; thoughts of separation & death; checking and cleaning	in vivo exposure; paradoxical intention	9 months	almost symptom-free maintained

form of behavioral treatment. Sixteen are presented as single case reports, with the remaining reports presenting two to 15 cases.

Diagnosis of OCD was typically based on detailed behavioral description of the obsessive symptomatology in the present with some onset history. The presenting symptoms included: washing, checking, counting, touching, bedtime and morning rituals, fears (dirt, contamination, harm befalling self or family), persistent questions, and obsessional slowness. As seen in Chapter 2, these symptoms are typical of our clinical population. However, there is rarely reference to standardized definitions so that certain essential features of the DSM-III (American Psychiatric Association 1980) definition (e.g., the subject's view of the problem as rational or irrational) are not described and are not discussed. This distinction is important for differential diagnosis with thought disorders as well as for establishing the child's motivation to participate in treatment.

Classic single-subject protocols with treatment preplanning and a standardized method to measure effects were presented in five cases. Obsessive symptoms were observed for a period of time to establish a stable behavioral baseline, then treatment was implemented. For instance, Mills et al. (1973) videotaped evening rituals of a 15-year-old male inpatient, before and after response prevention, using nursing staff as therapists. Both Kolko (1984) and Green (1980) used a baseline treatment design but included follow-up measures as part of their methodology. Clark et al. (1982) used a more complicated multiple baseline design for treating a case of obsessional slowness, which consisted of modifying daily living activities one at a time with prompting/pacing/shaping techniques. Queiroz et al. (1981) presented extensive and useful behavioral analyses and descriptive clinical casework, giving a flavor of how complex design, assessment, and implementation of behavioral treatment can be. Several studies planned a specific behavioral strategy but implemented them without baseline observations or established treatment time course. In general, the behavioral component was presented as a segment of the total treatment, a multimodal approach. The extreme nondesign was Harbin's (1979), describing his unorthodox "ordeal" treatment for compulsive worries about failing school and compulsive homework behaviors as "trial and error." He first focused on the family and mother. Next his patient detailed frequency and type of rituals (uncontrolled thoughts while doing homework resulting in temper tantrums and beating on her body). Treatment consisted of a half hour of exercises at midnight if any "abnormal" behaviors had been present, with a reduction in frequency of behavior.

Measures for assessing baseline behavior and treatment/follow-up effects for obsessions, anxiety, and fear ranged from standardized self-report questionnaires (Maudsley Obsessive-Compulsive Inventory, Lynfield Obsessive-Compulsive Questionnaire, Fear Survey Schedule) to therapist global report of improvement. Patients evaluated at pre- and posttest (Green 1980; Kolko 1984), systematically demonstrated improvement with their symptoms. Phillips and Wolpe (1981) and Ong and Leng (1979), however, collected data only during the assessment phase and left the reader wondering about the outcome comparisons, particularly in the Ong and Leng study where ward staff collected extensive multiple baseline data for a hospitalized 13-year-old girl. Since observable rituals lend themselves to quantification and may not fit readily into a standardized scale, many ratings were based on therapist, staff, parent, or self-report global ratings of improvement. Green (1980) devised a self-rating scale of 0 to 9 (hardly ever to nearly all the time) for a 15-year-old patient who touched objects, checked, and had to place his cup just right. Behavioral diaries and charts were assigned to parents and patients for frequency and severity of symptoms and were reported as part of the global ratings. Naturalistic ratings ranged from Mills et al. (1973) using videotape to observe evening rituals to Friedman and Silvers (1977) subjectively assessing severity of obsessive behavior and depressive feelings, as well as using retrospective chart reviews and "personal communications."

Behavioral treatment for most of these 20 reports was one part of a multimodal approach. At times it was the major component, and at other times secondary to family therapy and other procedures. Single case studies composed the majority of reports and were not designed to specifically test the effect of a single behavioral procedure. Response prevention was the predominant treatment reported in nine studies, but was typically used together with other treatment techniques.

Response prevention was used with 11 of 15 obsessive adolescents in a retrospective report (Bolton et al. 1983). The general procedure was a progression of therapies with initial outpatient self-monitoring and concurrent parent engagement. If success was not attained, then inpatient self-monitoring was instituted with external controls applied by the staff to ensure compliance with the treatment. Graded exposure was used in three of the cases, flooding in one. Additional treatment included clomipramine (six cases), and a psychotherapeutic relationship in "most" cases. Improvement occurred in 87 percent of the adolescents after hospitalizations of 1 week to 2 years.

Ong and Leng (1979) employed response prevention along with several other interventions to successfully eliminate washing and cleanliness rituals in a 13-year-old girl. For 1 hour after "contamination," she was prevented from washing by being locked in her room or restrained on her bed. However, continual monitoring could not be provided, and the ward contained several water faucets, preventing determination of the rate of free responding. Concurrently, treatment was provided by in vivo participant modeling, positive reinforcement of other behaviors, drug treatment (diazepam 2.5 mg TID × 4 weeks), and family interventions. The girl improved, but it is not possible to single out the effect of any treatment.

Mills et al. (1973) at first used nursing staff, then later used the parents to prevent bedtime rituals. Stanley (1980) used the parents exclusively as therapists in the home for bedtime and song rituals.

The most successful approach with adults, response prevention combined with in vivo exposure, was only reported in two studies. Apter et al. (1984) reported complete failure of response prevention and in vivo exposure in all eight cases of hospitalized adolescents with OCD. Their procedure was to "enjoin" the subjects from performing the rituals and to ask them to think of something else in place of the obsessional thought. "When possible" a student nurse or other staff member was assigned to watch the patients and encourage them not to engage in the rituals, a procedure that does not comply with the usual and customary form. In view of this rather vague approach, it is perhaps not surprising that the adolescents did not cooperate, and the results were unsuccessful.

In contrast, Zikis (1983) successfully developed a treatment program for an 11-year-old girl using in vivo exposure and response prevention applied by the parents. The presenting problems were seven separate rituals, which were eliminated within 1 week, and tics, which disappeared 2 weeks later. Total time with the therapist was only 1 hour, which is in contrast with the time usually suggested, and no replications have been reported.

Positive reinforcement, which focused on reinforcing positive behavior, was the next favored treatment in four cases. Queiroz et al. (1981) gave points for adequate behavior. They also trained the parents to give social reinforcements for appropriate behavior. The therapist gave suggestions to the patient for positive, alternative responses to build up a repertoire of interactive behaviors and to allow the objectionable rituals to phase out.

In vivo desensitization was employed in three cases and as one of six elements of a treatment package to eliminate separation and rituals in a 12-year-old boy (Phillips and Wolpe 1981). Within 4 months of treatment, gains were noted, and treatment of 88 sessions eventually proved successful.

While the above techniques are more appropriate for overt rituals, thought stopping appears to be the likely treatment for rumination, and has been applied exclusively and as a treatment component. Campbell (1973) treated a 12-year-old boy who was experiencing negative thoughts relating to the recent and violent death of his sister. The usual procedure was modified to eliminate the disruptive stimulus "STOP!" when the thought occurred. Rather, the subject was to evoke the thought, disrupt it by loudly counting backward from 10, and then think of a pleasant scene. After 1 week the frequency had decreased 80 percent, was eliminated at 4 weeks, and revealed no relapse at 3-year follow-up.

Thought stopping was included in a multimodal approach in the inpatient treatment of an 18-year-old male with a severe counting compulsion (Friedman and Silvers 1977). During 13 weeks of inpatient treatment, he experienced insight-oriented individual psychotherapy (2 hours/week), family therapy (1 hour/week), group therapy, milieu therapy, and behavior therapy. Behavior therapy focused on thought stopping. Reinforcement was provided by other patients and the nursing staff. He also was asked to record the antecedent-behavior-consequences of each occurrence of a thought. The authors considered the response to this treatment program to be exceptionally good, and the changes were maintained at a 2½-year follow-up.

Finally, thought stopping in the usual form was applied by Ownby (1983) to eliminate excessive hand washing in a 13-year-old boy. The child imitated the therapist by imagining a pleasure scene immediately after saying "stop" to himself.

Most reports addressed the associated familial overinvolvement with the child's rituals in the overall treatment plan. Only three reports failed to mention the family interactive patterns or didn't use family members as therapists. Frequently, marital stress was present; often, one parent, usually the mother, had become overprotective toward the child while the other parent had withdrawn. While complaints centered around the control of the obsessive behaviors, Hafner et al. (1981) questioned the family's having a vested interest in preserving the pathology. Therapy consisted of sessions with the child and parents as a family unit to establish an alliance and/or having the parents cooperate as therapists for the child. Parents participated by performing behavioral observations and reports, response prevention of behaviors such as checking and washing, or refusing to answer repetitive questions. Outcomes were measured with family improvement as well as the child's success.

Successful outcomes were self-reported with the exception of two studies. Apter et al. (1984) attributed patients' failures to respond to in vivo exposure and response prevention to low staff-to-patient ratio, inexperience with behavioral treatment, and, most important from our point of view, secretive and resistant patient behavior. In Clark et al.'s (1982) single case of obsessional slowness, treatment produced an immediate response rate that did not maintain during treatment withdrawal. Speculatively, the slowness may have served to keep the patient dependent on his family, avoiding social situations.

Follow-up investigation, from 5 months to 4 years, was presented for 17 reports. Good maintenance with minimal to absent symptoms was found. Ong and Leng (1979) reported a mild relapse of handwashing rituals when one patient assisted her aunt in her hair salon. Further treatment helped her to respond rapidly.

The lack of prospective ongoing behavioral treatment studies with obsessive-compulsive children is striking in view of the early onset of the disorder and particularly the degree of sophistication and success of treatment in adults. During follow-up interviews of our former obsessive adolescents, we found many had designed their own "do-it-yourself" behavior treatment by purposely exposing themselves to fearful situations and contaminated objects rather than attempting to inhibit their responses. One boy forced himself through doorways without the prescribed counting rituals despite discomfort and fear of harm; another boy forced himself to read homework sentences only once, then go on despite his "need" to repeat (see Chapter 2).

Considerations for Future Studies of Behavioral Treatment of Childhood OCD

Many aspects of adult behavioral treatment can be extended directly with children. The same diagnostic inclusion criteria (overt rituals, desire to be rid of them, ability to report symptoms and cooperate with a treatment plan) would similarly apply. However, age and developmental stage of the child are major differential issues. Although we have had children as young as 8 viewing their behavior as senseless and reporting changes over time, older children tend to be better reporters. Having younger children read a rating scale aloud and tell the examiner what a word or item means is useful in assessing their self-report ability. A second major consideration is that the child is not acting as a self-agent and is brought in by parents or guardians. The child may see his or her own symptoms differently than the parent and the question to address is what is the parent's agenda for bringing the child to treatment. Parents may be overreacting to the child's behavior and/or looking indirectly for treatment for themselves. While family cooperation is important with adults, children are dependent for everyday needs, support, and transportation on significant adults.

The psychopharmacological treatment of childhood OCD (described in Chapter 13) exemplifies how behavioral assessment has already been used with childhood OCD. The week-long baseline assessment phase typically includes standardized OCD measures and extensive interviewing to delineate and quantify the various obsessive-compulsive behaviors and patterns. Behavioral emphasis differs in that the behavioral symptoms with the antecedents, consequences, fear cues, and avoidance patterns are the focus rather than global severity. Gaining the child's cooperation and willingness to collaborate with the therapist is especially important during this phase because of the initial stress of treatment implementation and need to tolerate initial anxiety for reward of longer-term gains. Explaining the rationale for treatment, than deciding and formulating the hierarchy of stressful situations together with patients, lessens their fear of the unknown and allows children to gain mastery in the situation. For instance, a child who fears contamination from germs rates the most feared items (dogs, dirt, door handles) with the therapist, deciding together on the degrees of exposure (which item, at what time) and the possible consequences. Asking the child to rate his or her subjective degree of distress with the SUDS rating of 0 to 100 (see Chapter 4) establishes the pace for treatment. One child said holding a can of oil was a 50 but having it on his hands was a zillion. Certainly the therapist's ingenuity is tested in devising individualized treatment plans for special symptoms. The key to successful cooperation is *no surprises!* Children need to know the worst feelings that can happen and that they will survive. The therapist is ultimately in charge of the treatment in order to push the discomfort levels, despite the patient's resistance, and gain results.

Treatment time will differ from more traditional protocols, with 90 minutes to 2 hours needed for imaginal and in vivo exposure. The therapist may guide the child through a feared scene verbally, then may model touching a feared object before the child does so. Items may be brought into the clinic and the child may be taken into the community (restaurants, muddy streams, stores), wherever the fear can be effectively confronted. The goal is to induce anxiety and have it be tolerated, until it gradually diminishes within the session. Patients are often surprised that what was a dreaded fear alone can be tolerated with the therapist. The boy, earlier mentioned with the fear of car oil, gingerly poured car oil on his hands, grimaced, then began to rub designs on his palms. By the next session, he rubbed it on his arms and face saying "no problem." The number and frequency of treatment sessions needed will depend on the rate of disappearance of rituals;

three to five sessions a week are recommended to maximize effects. Clinical dialogue and session strategies are presented elsewhere (Chapter 12; Foa and Tillmans 1980; Grayson et al. 1985; Steketee and Foa 1985).

Both hospital and home can be successful treatment settings. The obvious advantages to the hospital are the degree of environmental control, the availability of personnel to carry out the treatment plan, and the ability to use standardized ratings. The home setting may be more useful, however, for some behaviors; for example, checkers may feel more pressure to check at home than when in the hospital. In addition, hospital programs must be concerned about the ability to generalize to the home setting. Decisions about the appropriate setting are based first on the type and severity of the symptoms, degree of parental cooperation, ability of the child to separate from parents, transportation, and school situation.

Training the parents as co-therapists can keep the child at home in addition to educating the parents to develop new interactive behaviors with the child. Parents may be overinvolved in helping a sick child, inadvertently encouraging the child's inappropriate behaviors. One mother, functioning as her child's co-therapist, was delighted to learn she could set limits because she had become intimidated by her child's behavior. Removing the child from the home environment without investigating family interactive patterns may place the child at risk for relapse. Companions can be trained to go into the home to help with response prevention and guidance during the treatment period.

In commonsense terms, behavioral treatment is so widely used with children that it seems easy to put these techniques into practice. However, a lack of understanding the principles and techniques can doom a behavioral program to failure. Most of our patients have had vigorous "home remedies" applied without success. Adults often comment that they have tried the same techniques on themselves but were unsuccessful alone. The therapist is a powerful tool in planning out appropriate strategies, minimizing error and maximizing the child's potential. While the child may show improvement, the new learning may need to be reinforced.

Failure to adequately inform the parents and patient of the treatment plan and consequences (increased initial anxiety and fear) can also signal failure. Anticipating what can happen, even if unpleasant, and knowing others have managed the treatment successfully, can relieve some anxiety and midnight calls. Having a packet ready with therapy directions, daily direction and note-taking charts, symptoms, and rating scales can be useful.

Teachers, who typically participate in behavior management for other childhood disorders, should be involved only if the obsessive behaviors affect school. Usually children do not want teachers and peers to know about their difficulties, and it helps them not to "use" their behavior.

Maintenance strategies need to be planned to prevent relapse. As the children give up their behaviors, more time is now available and their lack of appropriate social skills may become apparent. Whether appropriate interpersonal behavior became lost from the isolation or was never learned, social-skills training may be needed to reintegrate interactions with others. Parents will need to relearn how to redirect their own lives when their lives no longer revolve around the child. Typically, one parent only is involved with the child to the exclusion of the other parent. The therapist must anticipate possible needs of the parents to reintegrate their lives once the child has improved. In addition, improvement can happen so rapidly that parents may worry about relapse into old behavior. Discussing the uncertainties of establishing new ways of behavior and interactions will provide and encourage this newer yet healthier existence.

References

Apter A, Bernhout E, Tyano S: Severe obsessive compulsive disorder in adolescence: a report of eight cases. J Adolescence 7:349–358, 1984

American Psychiatric Association: Diagnostic and Statistical Manual of Mental Disorders, 3rd ed (DSM-III). Washington, DC, American Psychiatric Association, 1980

Baer L, Minichiello WE: Behavior therapy for obsessive compulsive disorder. In Obsessive-Compulsive Disorders: Theory and Management. Edited by Jenike MA, Baer L, Minichiello WE. Littleton, MA, PSG Publishing, 1986, pp 45–75

Bolton D, Collins S, Steinberg D: The treatment of obsessive-compulsive disorder in adolescence: a report of fifteen cases. Br J Psychiatry 142:456–464, 1983

Campbell LM: A variation of thought-stopping in a twelve-year-old boy: a case report. J Behav Ther Exp Psychiatry 4:69–70, 1973

Clark DA, Sugrim I, Bolton D: Primary obsessional slowness: a nursing programme with a 13-year-old male adolescent. Behav Res Ther 20:289–292, 1982

Dalton P: Family treatment of an obsessive compulsive child: a case report. Fam Process 22:99–108, 1983

Emmelkamp PM: Phobia and Obsessive Compulsive Disorders: Theory, Research, and Practice. New York, Plenum, 1982

Fine S: Family therapy and a behavioral approach to childhood obsessive compulsive neurosis. Arch Gen Psychiatry 28:695–697, 1973

Foa EB, Kozak MJ: Emotional processing of fear: exposure to corrective information. Psychol Bull 99:20–35, 1986

Foa EB, Tillmans A: The treatment of obsessive-compulsive neurosis, in Handbook of Behavioral Interventions: A Clinical Guide. Edited by Goldstein A, Foa EB. New York, Wiley, 1980, pp 416–500

Foa EB, Steketee GS, Grayson JB, et al: Deliberate exposure and blocking of obsessive compulsive rituals: immediate and longterm effects. Behavior Therapy 15:450–472, 1984

Foa EB, Steketee GS, Ozarow BJ: Behavior therapy with obsessive compulsives: from theory to treatment, in Obsessive Compulsive Disorder: Psychological and Pharmacological Treatment. Edited by Mavissakalian M. New York, Plenum, 1985

Friedman CTH, Silvers FM: A multimodality approach to inpatient treatment of obsessive compulsive disorder. Am J Psychother 31:456–465, 1977

Grayson JB, Foa EB, Steketee GS: Obsessive compulsive disorder, in Handbook of Clinical Behavior Therapy with Adults. Edited by Hersen M, Bellack AS. New York, Plenum, 1985

Green D: A behavioral approach to the treatment of obsessional rituals: an adolescent case study. J Adolesc 3:297–306, 1980

Hafner RJ, Gilchrist P, Bowling J, et al: The treatment of obsessional neurosis in a family setting. Aust NZ J Psychiatry 15:145–151, 1981

Hallam RS: Extinction of ruminations: a case study. Behavior Therapy 5:565–568, 1974

Harbin HT: Cure by ordeal: treatment of an obsessive compulsive neurotic. International Journal of Family Therapy 1(4):324–332, 1979

Hersen M, Bellack AS (eds): Behavioral Assessment: A Practical Handbook. New York, Pergamon Press, 1981

Kolko DJ: Paradoxical instruction in the elimination of avoidance behavior in an agoraphobic girl. J Behav Ther Exp Psychiatry 15:51–57, 1984

Marks D: Recent results of behavioral treatments of phobias and obsessions. J Int Med Res 5:16–21, 1977

Meyer V: Modification of expectations in cases with obsessional rituals. Behav Res Ther 4:270–280, 1966

Mills HL, Agras WS, Barlow DH, et al: Compulsive rituals treated by response prevention: an experimental analysis. Arch Gen Psychiatry 28:524–529, 1973

Murray JB: Successful treatment of obsessive compulsive disorders. Genetic, Social and General Psychology Monographs 112:173–199, 1986

Ong SBY, Leng YK: The treatment of an obsessive compulsive girl in the context of Malaysian Chinese culture. Aust NZ J Psychiatry 13:255–259, 1979

Ownby RL: A cognitive behavioral intervention for compulsive handwashing with a thirteen-year-old boy. Psychology in the Schools 20:219–222, 1983

Phillips D, Wolpe S: Multiple behavioral techniques in severe separation anxiety of a twelve-year-old. J Behav Ther Exp Psychiatry 12:329–332, 1981

Queiroz LOS, Motta MA, Madi MBBP, et al: A functional analysis of obsessive compulsive problems with related therapeutic procedures. Behav Res Ther 19:377–388, 1981

Stanley L: Treatment of ritualistic behavior in an eight-year-old girl by response prevention: a case report. J Child Psychol Psychiatry 21:85–90, 1980

Steketee G, Foa EB: Obsessive compulsive disorder, in Clinical Handbook of Psychological Disorders. Edited by Barlow D. New York, Guilford Press, 1985

Weiner IB: Behavioral therapy in obsessive compulsive neurosis: treatment of an adolescent boy. Psychotherapy: Theory, Research, and Practice 4:27–29, 1967

Zikis P: Treatment of an 11-year-old obsessive compulsive ritualizer and Tiqueur girl with in vivo exposure and response prevention. Behavior Psychotherapy 11:75-81, 1983

Appendix 1
Guidelines for Planning a Treatment Program
(Published with permission of J. Grayson)

I. Information Gathering
  1. Obsessions
    a. External Cues
       Specifically elicit information about objects or situations
       that provoke high anxiety or discomfort (e.g., urine, pesti-
       cides, locking a door).
    b. Internal Cues
       1) Inquire about thoughts, images, or impulses that pro-
          voke anxiety, shame, or disgust (e.g., images of Christ's
          penis, numbers, impulses to stab one's child).
       2) Inquire about bodily sensations that disturb the patient
          (e.g., tachycardia, pains, swallowing).
    c. Consequences of External and Internal Cues
       1) Elicit information about possible harm that can be
          caused by the external object or situation (e.g., disease
          from touching a contaminated object, burglary if a door
          is not properly locked).
       2) Elicit fears about harm caused by internal cues
          a) From thoughts, images, or impulses (e.g., "God will
             punish me. I may actually stab my child").
          b) From bodily sensations (e.g., "I'll lose control").
          c) From the long-term experience of high anxiety (e.g.,
             "This anxiety will never go away and I'll always be
             upset").
          d) Strength of belief system—Assess the degree to
             which the patient believes that the feared conse-
             quences may actually occur. What is the objective
             probability that confrontation with feared cues will
             actually result in psychological or physical harm?
  2. Avoidance Patterns
    a. Passive Avoidance
       Gather a list of all situations or objects that are avoided
       (e.g., using public bathrooms, stepping on brown spots on
       the sidewalk, carrying one's child on a concrete floor, driv-
       ing). Attend to subtle avoidance practices (e.g., touching
       doorknobs on the least used surface, driving at times of
       least traffic).
    b. Rituals
       List all ritualistic behaviors including washing, cleaning,
       checking, repeating an action, ordering objects, requesting

reassurance, and cognitive ritual (e.g., praying, neutralizing thoughts, good numbers). Many patients exhibit more than one type of compulsion. Pay attention to subtle rituals such as the use of wipes or lotion to decontaminate hands. Wiping is a short version of a washing ritual.

   c. Relationship between Avoidance Behaviors and Fear Cues
Ascertain the functional relationship between the fear cues and the avoidance associated with it.

3. History of the Main Complaint
   a. Events associated with onset.
   b. Fluctuations in the course of symptoms and events associated with remission and recurrence of symptoms.
   c. Prior coping with symptoms, prior treatment efforts, and resultant effects.

4. Mood State
   a. Depression
Assess the level of depression by clinical interviews and inventory (e.g., Beck Depression Inventory or Hamilton Depression Rating). Consider antidepressant medication or cognitive therapy for depressed ratings prior to behavioral treatment.
   b. Anxiety
Consider ameliorating procedures such as anxiolytic drugs. If used, fade their use near the end of treatment.

5. General History
Include information about relationship with parents, siblings, and peers; educational achievements; employment history; dating history; sexual experiences; marital relationship; and medical history.

II. Treatment Program
1. Decision to Hospitalize
   a. During intensive treatment the patient is likely to be temporarily under high stress.
   b. Hospitalization should be considered for those who live alone or are in a stressful familial relationship.

2. The Use of Prolonged Exposure
   a. In vivo exposure for external objects or situations that evoke high levels of anxiety.
   b. Imaginal Exposure
     1) When in vivo exposure is practically impossible.
     2) When the feared catastrophes constitute a major component of the patient's fear model. In these cases imaginal exposure is used in combination with in vivo exposure.
   c. Suggestions for Exposure Treatment

1) All designated exposure items are arranged hierarchically according to the SUDs (Subjective Units of Discomfort) levels they evoke and are presented in ascending order beginning midway. That is, if the top item evokes 100 SUDs, exposure commences with items at a 50-SUD level; if the top item evokes 80 SUDs, a 40-SUD item is presented first.
2) A given item should be presented until the anxiety level provoked is reduced by half.
3) An exposure item should be repeated until it evokes no more than minimal anxiety.
4) Frequent sessions should be implemented preferably three or more times per week.
5) Ideally, the intensive treatment program should be terminated when the most feared item has been confronted and provokes only mild anxiety. If substantial gains are not evident after 15 sessions, continuation of intensive treatment should be questioned.
6) Regularly scheduled follow-up sessions are recommended to consolidate treatment gains.
7) For motivated patients, detailed instructions for self-exposure may be sufficient. If the relationship between spouses or family members is good, they can be actively involved in the treatment program.

III. Homework

A total of 4 hours of exposure homework is assigned. For patients whose treatment includes imaginal exposure, a tape of that day's fantasy exposure is made for later replay at home; an additional 3 hours in vivo exposure is also assigned.

IV. Response Prevention

a. Washers are usually permitted one 10-minute shower every fifth day and no hand washing except under unusual circumstances during the first 2 weeks of treatment. Thereafter, to facilitate learning of normal washing, the therapist may permit one 10-minute shower per day and 30-second hand washings after bathroom use, before meals, and when hands are visibly dirty or greasy.

b. Checkers are allowed one brief check of items that are normally checked after use (e.g., stove, door locks) and no checking of items that are not typically checked by most people.

c. Supervisors at home or in the hospital should not use force to prevent ritualizing but report infractions to the therapist.

Chapter 12

Case Study: Cognitive-Behavioral Analysis and Treatment of An Adolescent with Severe Multiform Obsessive-Compulsive Disorder

Charles S. Mansueto, Ph.D.

The significant successes of learning-based interventions in obsessive-compulsive disorder (OCD) continue to be substantiated in a steadily growing number of controlled studies. Foa et al. (1983) have asserted that "the treatment of choice for obsessive-compulsives is a combination of deliberate exposure and response prevention" (p. 287). While it has been noted that no systematic investigation of the efficacy of behavior procedures in child and adolescent populations has yet been conducted (Wolff and Rapoport 1986; see Chapter 11), the marked similarity between manifestations of OCD in children and adolescents and of OCD in adults suggests that some variant of exposure and response prevention is the treatment of choice for younger patients.

Applying published guidelines for exposure and response-prevention-based therapy in actual clinical practice is another matter. Published descriptions of behavior therapy for OCD rarely convey the problems encountered when conducting this type of treatment in actual clinical settings where patients often present complex, multiform, and ill-defined difficulties.

Within the ranks of behavior therapists, a commonly heard discussion addresses the significant discrepancies between "what is reported" and "what we actually do." Behavioral treatment of OCD can provide a striking illustration of such discrepancies. For example, a behavioral assessment described as taking 2 or 3 hours in literature accounts may be incomplete well after the treatment has formally begun. Likewise, other issues critical for successful behavioral treatment such as conceptualization of the problem, the choice of behaviors targeted for change, the selection of the intervention strategy, the determination of therapeutic goals, the orientation of the patient for treatment, and maximization of patient motivation are usually addressed superficially or not dealt with at all in published accounts. These components of therapy involve complex processes that do not lend themselves to analysis or reporting within the neat and efficient format of research reports nor to methodical elucidation in "cookbook style" therapy manuals. When the therapist confronts such critical but complex treatment issues in obsessive-compulsive patients who are commonly held to be a particularly challenging population, the therapist's knowledge, talents, and capabilities are likely to be "put to the test."

Work with younger patients offers an interesting mix of difficulties and opportunities. On the positive side, the fact that one-third to one-half of obsessive-compulsive individuals develop their disorder before age 15 (Rapoport 1986) suggests that early detection and successful treatment can minimize suffering in those patients by short-circuiting the evolutionary course of the disorder. Also, it seems reasonable to speculate that younger patients are more "treatable" during the relatively early stages of the disorder rather than after years of living with obsessive-compulsive functioning (although this is as yet unproven). Finally, because the disorder is relatively "fresh" in younger patients, it is likely that much can be learned by investigating the etiology and evolution of OCD in patients where the passage of years has not yet rendered retrospective analysis a futile effort.

It is in the spirit of the above considerations that this case study is presented. Unlike most reported case studies, it describes treatment still in progress. Although there may be empirical or scientific shortcomings to this approach, I have attempted to chronicle the complexities involved in the clinical application of behavior therapy to an adolescent obsessive-compulsive patient whose problem clearly does not lend itself to therapy "by the book." In addition, for purposes of instruction and clarification, the conceptualization of the problem within a cognitive behavioral framework is presented in more detail than is typically found in the behavioral literature. While the retrospective analysis of cause and course of psychiatric disorders is always a highly speculative process, the many unanswered questions regarding the origins and evolutions of OCD would seem to justify an additional descriptive study as a potentially useful adjunct to experimental studies.

As yet, the most comprehensive theory of OCD, besides psychoanalytic theory, is the cognitive behavioral theory of Rachman (Rachman 1978; Rachman and Hodgson 1980). The fundamental assumption in this view is that obsessive cognitions trigger conditioned anxiety in these patients, and that the compulsive ritual serves to remove or reduce the anxiety, thus serving as an escape or avoidance mechanism. The ritual behavior is thereby maintained and strengthened through the mechanism of negative reinforcement.

The strength of this conceptualization is that it provides an explanation of why obsessions and compulsions, once established, might be maintained. Rachman and Hodgson (1980) acknowledged that questions remain concerning certain etiological matters:

> Our account leaves several points unexplained. For example, it provides little enlightenment about silly insignificant obsessions such as number sequences, nonsensical phrases, and the like. Also, it does not tell why, of all the possible themes, certain ideas or images or impulses become repetitive—the selectivity of obsessions is unexplained. (pp. 274–275)

Sumners and Gournay (1986) described the case of a 20-year-old man whose obsessive-compulsive symptoms seemed to develop in a clear evolutionary process. Furthermore, the authors provided evidence that the obsessions and compulsions in the patient evolved from useful psychological strategies but became "mere flotsam" as the functional utility evolved into functional autonomy. The authors questioned whether the evolution of the disorder as presented in that case had wider relevance, since their patient had significant anomalies that were atypical of patients with OCD in general. Specifically, the patient had an array of physical defects, most notably severe visual handicaps.

In the present case, evolutionary characteristics of the developing disorder are examined in a patient with severe and complex symptoms that are much more typical of those seen in obsessive-compulsive patients. As presented, it provides an illustration of ongoing behavioral-based treatment of an adolescent with crippling obsessions and compulsive symptoms that formed a complex pattern of maladaptive response. The treatment strategy ultimately involved an active and direct attack on the symptoms. Passive avoidance constituted a major portion of the debilitating symptoms, and the many specific forms this took were targeted for exposure treatment. The obsessional system would be addressed by a cognitive restructuring treatment in which a learning-based conceptualization of the problem was provided to replace the existing, idiosyncratic, religious/moral conceptualization that impeded adaptive functioning and threatened treatment. Approaches to the modification of active rituals that constituted a smaller but significant and resistant component of the problem are also described.

This account provides a "close-up" view of the factors that led to the adoption of an evolving treatment strategy as the complexity of the problem unfolded in a young client with a fascinating history and a complex obsessional matrix. It is hoped that this will provide the reader with a unique perspective on the complexities that may be encountered in behavioral treatment of such cases.

Secondarily, this detailed view into the evolution of obsessive-compulsive functioning is presented in the hope that the clinical record, which provides a speculative account of the origins and development of the disorder in this one young patient, will have implications for the broader efforts underway to answer some of the puzzling questions that remain about the disorder.

The Case of Daniel

Daniel is a 19-year-old college student, the youngest child and only son of four children born to parents from an affluent suburban community. His infancy and childhood had been unremarkable; he was seen by family and friends as a bright, thoughtful, and friendly child, who had grown into a "good kid" and "B" student. He remained popular throughout grade and middle school. A short-lived preoccupation with "germs" near the end of sixth grade troubled his parents enough to have Daniel seen by a psychologist, but the problem seemed to pass and no one was particularly alarmed by it. However, by the end of middle school and his first year of high school, those close to him saw unmistakable indications that Daniel's problems again warranted professional attention. This time, however, therapy did not halt his steady deterioration into webs of obsessive-compulsive functioning.

Presenting Complaints: His Parents' View

Daniel was described by his parents as having a 6-year history of obsessive-compulsive problems, which had not improved much since diagnosis despite 3 years of psychotherapy with three different therapists and current pharmacological treatment with imipramine. He had managed to complete high school despite the many difficulties caused by his disorder, but he was now failing all his courses during his first semester at the local college in which he was enrolled full-time. During this time he was living at home.

His parents consulted me after a co-worker, in whom his father had confided, had described how her mother, a patient I had treated for a long-standing washing compulsion, had benefited dramatically from behavior therapy. Daniel, though still under treatment with an eminent psychiatrist, seemed to be getting worse. With the encouragement of his psychiatrist, Daniel agreed that behavior therapy should be explored.

According to his parents, Daniel was "preoccupied" and "behaved oddly," though the specific ways in which his problems manifested themselves had taken a variety of forms over the years. They thought that the earliest sign of the problem occurred in sixth grade. Daniel became concerned about germs and would "blow germs away" when someone sneezed, coughed, or was known to be ill, and would wash his hands frequently. With the help of a psychologist, the problem was "talked through" and overcome during the school year. His life from seventh through ninth grade was relatively uneventful.

It was during the 10th grade in high school, that the most severe problems began to develop. Daniel's adjustment to his new school was made more difficult by two factors: the death of his grandfather of cancer a month before school opened, and his fear of certain "rough kids" in school. In late fall he again became preoccupied with fears of germs. To prevent potential illness, he would wash his hands up to 30 times each day, scrutinize all silverware, dishes, and glasses for specks of dirt or food, and wash all money he received from any source. In addition, Daniel's parents noted that piles of clothes, books, papers, etc., accumulated on the floor and furniture of his room, and that he was unwilling to move them. As that school year progressed, Daniel decided to "become kosher" although his family did not closely follow the practices of their Jewish religion, and he severely limited the varieties of food he was willing to eat.

Greatly disturbed by all of this, his parents had him examined at Children's Hospital in Washington, D.C., where he was diagnosed as having OCD and was referred to a psychiatrist for treatment. After 6 months of "verbal psychotherapy," Daniel, his parents, and the psychiatrist agreed that no progress had been made and a second psychiatrist began treatment. Daniel seemed to "open up" to this person more and confided that much of his problem stemmed from chronic fears that he was "doing something wrong." His rituals, he said, were attempts to ward off punishment by God for the wrongs he had done.

The psychiatrist proposed to work with Daniel to help with these concerns, while his assistant would use behavioral techniques to eliminate the washing rituals and fears of contamination. Within a week, after systematic exposure to dirty hands, varieties of food, unwashed money, and the like, Daniel seemed "cured" of his problem. His hand washing was returned to appropriate levels, his diet was greatly expanded in variety (although he remained kosher for a while thereafter), and he would handle and use unwashed money. For a while, at least, Daniel seemed "almost normal" to his hopeful parents. But it was not long before his problems reappeared, escalated to alarming proportions, and took even more bizarre turns.

His parents were mystified and upset by some of Daniel's behavior over the summer before 11th grade. While walking he would incorporate "silly steps" into his movement. He refused to watch most of his favorite TV shows and wouldn't go to movies, or almost anywhere else, with friends. He would repeatedly walk in and out of rooms in a "very odd" manner. He would return to places he had just left to see if he had, as he would say, "done everything right." He would be found doing bizarre things, like washing the family car wearing only a bath towel. Worst of all from his parents' perspective was that Daniel, who had always been an open and communicative child, seemed to be "turning inward," refusing to explain his behavior, and appeared to be emotionally distancing himself from his parents.

Daniel's psychiatrist understood the general basis of his disorder—a fear that he "had displeased God by doing things wrong"—and that, in Daniel's mind, the probability of being punished by God was somehow lessened by performing these rituals. He described Daniel to his parents as a "classic example of an obsessive compulsive." Through his relationship with the boy, the therapist explored the dynamics of the disorder, provided emotional support, and urged Daniel to try to be normal by resisting his impulses.

But Daniel did not resist, and although he survived his final 2 years of high school, disaster was just in the offing. His academic work began to suffer. Where his writing was once fluent and logical, it began to seem childlike. By the end of 12th grade his sentences were stilted and primitive; his papers were almost incomprehensible, with words and phrases endlessly crossed out and rewritten. But he somehow passed his 12th-grade courses and graduated from high school. By this time, however, no sphere of his life was untouched by his disorder. His efforts at dating were doomed to failure by his noticeable bizarreness. He maintained some friendships, but it became necessary for his closer friends to tolerate his "weirdness"; to their credit, a few stuck by him.

On the basis of his previously strong academic record, Daniel was admitted to a local college to which he would commute from home in the fall. The summer prior to college seemed quieter. His parents became used to the many manifestations of Daniel's disorder and were hopeful that he would either "grow out of it," respond to his psychotherapy, or benefit from the imipramine that he would begin taking in late summer. By November their hopes were dashed. Daniel seemed stranger than ever, making unusual repetitive movements with head, arms, and legs; walking in and out of rooms of his house in "mechanical ways"; and still refusing to give any explanations. He was failing every one of his courses and had yet to receive anything but an F on any paper or test. It was time to try something new, and because Daniel was reluctant to try any other medication, he agreed to try behavior therapy.

Daniel's View of the Problem: Developing a Phenomenological Perspective

The phenomenological perspective here implies a perspective by which the world is seen through the patient's eyes. This is an essential component of a complete behavioral analysis of OCD.

Daniel was responsive and personable from the outset. He impressed me as a pleasant-looking, polite, and well-spoken young man. I presumed him to be of average to above average intelligence. As we spoke, I observed him to occasionally make subtle but "strange" movements of his hands, legs, and head. His eyes seemed to dart about as we spoke. I told Daniel that he could tell me as little or as much as he wished about his problem at this session, but that if I were to help him, he would have to eventually tell me *everything*. I offered to answer any questions he might wish to ask, and this made sense to him. He asked me if I knew where OCDs come from. I explained that while I certainly didn't know enough about his particular problem, I was confident that given enough information to work with, I would be able to understand his problem well enough to explain it to him. He would not only know enough about where it came from, I explained, but more importantly, he would understand what he must do to overcome it. Daniel was provided with a much more extensive education in learning principles and their application than is typical. However, all patients, even younger children, benefit from some degree of understanding of the mechanisms that maintain the disorder and those that constitute the basis for their therapy

He seemed interested and wanted to know more. I said it would be necessary for him to provide me with more information about the specifics of the problem so that I wouldn't have to speak in generalities. Daniel began his account by informing me that there would be many things he would be unable to tell me now, but that he would try to find ways of telling me these things in the future. I accepted that.

As Daniel began to tell his story, he described how hundreds of times each day he would "get a feeling" that he had "done something wrong," that is, "to displease God." To avoid possible punishment for these "wrongdoings" at God's hands, he would punish himself in some way, thus reducing his concern about some more awful punishment occurring at some later time. Additionally, he would avoid any actions or thoughts that had accompanied these feelings, and this led to the development of a complex system of "rules" that, in Daniel's mind, placed prohibitions or limitations on his behavior and thinking processes in virtually every situation of his life. His account was absorbing as he described the multitude of things he must do, or could not do, or must do in certain ways or in a certain order; of thoughts he could not think; of memories and information he could not retrieve; of things he could not say or must say in certain ways; or of using or not using certain words. He described a system that was so complex, so convoluted, so pervasive, that I wondered how he was able to function at all within the rigid requirements of his unforgiving system.

Daniel asked, "Did I give you enough to get you started?" And we both had a good laugh over the intended humor in his question. [Humor is a particularly useful element in therapy with obsessive-compulsive patients and its judicious use (never making "fun of" the patient, but instead encouraging a mutual appreciation of some of the "absurd" aspects of the disorder), can greatly relieve some of the difficult moments that behavioral treatment can involve.] As he left my office (with some self-monitoring forms in hand), I marveled at the spirit of this young man that enabled him to go on despite the oppressive weight of his unrelenting system. He would need to rally all that spirit if he was to regain his ability to function in this world.

The second session began with Daniel handing me his self-monitoring forms. The homework had required him to monitor three specific aspects of his problem during a 24-hour period: (a) repeating something; (b) stopping himself from doing something he wished to do; and (c) walking out of and back into a room. He would note the time of the occurrence, the activity or thought that evoked the ritual, his subjective distress (0–100), and the number of minutes spent on the ritual.

The page was literally covered with tiny notations, many crossed out and rewritten: back and front, in margins, between lines, wherever a coded entry could fit in. Minute by minute, hour by hour ritualizing had occurred: while walking, sitting, writing, eating, watching TV, brushing teeth, washing, attempting homework, driving, going to sleep, sleeping (he ritualized in his dreams). The record sheet was virtually unintelligible, but at least we had something of a baseline to work with. [Monitoring always constitutes an essential part of the continuous evaluation of treatment effectiveness in behavioral treatment. Self-monitoring is always necessarily involved, even with young checkers or ruminators.]

Just sorting through the myriad of prohibitions was a daunting task. Daniel listed hundreds. We organized them into things he couldn't eat or drink, places he couldn't go, things he couldn't use, clothes he couldn't wear, activities he couldn't be involved in, things he couldn't think about or talk about, things he couldn't buy, things he couldn't write down or say. No mundane aspect of everyday life seemed too insignificant to go unregulated in Daniel's private world. Even when there was no outright prohibition, he had developed special ways things had to be done, usually involving the "order" in which activities were carried out, or which seemingly entailed the meaningless repetition of insignificant movements. For example, just getting to a class was a major accomplishment in that every step—getting out of bed, washing, eating, getting dressed and out of the house, driving to the campus, parking the car, walking to the building, getting through the door and into a seat—was punctuated by endless occurrences of a sense of wrongdoing that, in turn, led to thousands of instances of hesitating, terminating, repeating, and ordering. Even making it to class only meant that Daniel might be prevented from listening to certain information, taking notes, sometimes even opening his notebook. Any behavior or thought, at any given moment, could trigger the sense of wrongdoing that permeated Daniel's consciousness, and led to avoiding actions and thoughts, being preoccupied about following rules, and "doing the right things."

"What would happen if you simply did things like everyone else did them?" I asked. Daniel said that while his thinking "usually doesn't go that far anymore," he firmly believed that punishment by God was inevitable if he did not follow the dictates of his beliefs and feelings. It was for this reason that no amount of exhortation by parents, friends, or therapists had been able to dissuade him from his unique way of going about things. [Some assessment of the patient's belief in the inevitability of catastrophic consequences should they fail to yield to their urges to avoid or ritualize is necessary, in light of the research of Foa (1979), which identified the presence of a "strong conviction that their fears were realistic" as a notable impediment to therapeutic success. Depression was also noted as a factor in treatment failures but this was not a problem in Daniel's case (his initial score on the Beck Depression Inventory (Beck et al. 1979) was 8, and is currently 3. If significant depression is present, the use of antidepressant medication or cognitive behavioral techniques should be considered prior to the beginning of treatment for OCD.] He acknowledged that he, in fact, was suffering from OCD because "everyone says that." However, in his own mind it was necessary that he avoid and ritualize in what had become his customary manner. He was convinced that his beliefs and feelings were the only valid guides to what he must do.

But I had made a commitment to provide Daniel with a perspective on his problems that involved no supernatural forces, no mysterious and unpredictable internal signals of wrongdoing. Instead, there would be a new scheme—one based on principles of conditioning and learning, and one that I hoped would motivate Daniel to cooperate in the demanding exposure phase of therapy, in which he would be required to face his fears and relinquish any short-term comfort he derived from his rituals in favor of the prospect of a life free from the constraints he had imposed on himself.

We embarked on a cooperative fact-finding mission into the early manifestations of the problem. While the history-taking and information-gathering proceeded over the next 2 weeks, Daniel's academic predicaments went from dismal to hopeless. A letter to his academic dean produced an administrative withdrawal and a promise of readmission for the spring semester contingent on my assurance that his academic potential was vastly improved by then. Spring semester was 2 months away.

I was very pleased with the relationship that was developing between us. Daniel wanted badly to believe the explanations I gave him for the development of his current patterns of thinking, feeling, and behaving. He knew that we were inexorably moving toward a direct confrontation with his fears and rituals. He listened intently as I described to him mechanisms of classical conditioning, negative reinforcement, habituation, and the like, interweaving learning-based explanations with elements of his own history, attempting to construct a mutually acceptable scheme that would explain how Daniel went from a fully functioning "happy kid" to an incapacitated, preoccupied, dysfunctional adolescent, all in just a few years, and under the watchful eyes of loving parents and skilled therapists. [The degree of attention given to the historical factors in this case was greater than that which is typically given. This seemed warranted in the present case because, fully accounting for the origins and development of the course of Daniel's problem in learning-theory terms, it became crucial for his acceptance of this alternative interpretation of his disorder.]

In four sessions, we finished our account and Daniel was pleased. He asked that we commit it to a "chart" so he could keep it with him and study it. It made sense to him; it was logical and scientific and explained the twists and turns his problems took in the course of the evolution of his disorder.

Historical Assessment and Cognitive-Behavioral Analysis

Daniel recalled his childhood as a happy one, filled with friends and relatives, free of problems. His parents were described as loving, supportive, and "easygoing" but he acknowledged that they both were "finicky about cleanliness and germs" and that his mother was an "emotional person who was easily upset." He also acknowledged some "minor" difficulties during childhood that had passed quickly (like fearing toilets would overflow if he flushed them), but he dismissed these as childhood "silliness." He mentioned the "germ problem" and its quick resolution during sixth grade, but he did not think it was particularly significant.

His previously tranquil homelife erupted into a series of crises during his middle school years. One of his older sisters began to use drugs and had gotten into some trouble with the school authorities. Daniel remembered much yelling and arguments in the family—often between his father and mother—about how to handle his sister, and he worried about the possible breakup of his home. Friction within the home "had his nerves on edge" and he would pray to God that things would get back to normal. Concurrent with these events was the slow and painful death of his paternal grandfather, whom Daniel loved and was very close to. It was with these factors as a backdrop that we identified an important series of incidents that were to be the first entries on Daniel's "chart" because they figured so significantly in the early manifestations of the disorder. [I would not argue that the present interpretation is elegant or even complete. It is simply, I think, a reasonable one that derives from widely accepted psychological principles of learning. The learning-theory-oriented reader can, no doubt, see numerous possibilities for "beefing up" the interpretation.

Phase I: Anxiety Conditioning

Daniel recalled the first occurrence of "that feeling" during December of 10th grade, as he sat in the synagogue at the long and emotional funeral service for his grandfather. He remembered it was hot and he was not feeling very well. It crossed his mind that he really didn't want to be there, when he suddenly felt a strong "twinge" of guilt; he thought to himself that it was wrong to think that; it was "against religion" to think about being elsewhere at a time like that, and that God must disapprove! As he sat there, he wondered how he could make amends but realized that he couldn't undo the thoughts that had already passed. He worried that God would punish him for having such thoughts during a holy service. His fear and discomfort mounted and went unabated until he left the service. It had been a very disquieting experience that would stay with him for a long time.

Shortly after that, another episode strengthened the link in Daniel's mind between the fear of punishment by God and his sense of personal wrongdoing. While masturbating late one night in his room, the TV happened to be on in the background. Much to his horror he suddenly became aware that the TV was tuned in to a religious program and that he had, in his view, "been masturbating in the presence of religion and God." Daniel was overwhelmed by strong feelings of guilt and the belief that what he had done was "wrong and against God" and that he "deserved to be punished." Worse yet, during other masturbatory episodes he was unable to keep his mind free of intrusive thoughts about God, or of occasional sacrilegious images involving his masturbating before holy objects. [That anxiety-provoking images or thoughts occur, and sometimes increase in frequency, is a theoretical paradox. Sumners and Gournay (1986) suggested that the "paradoxical enhancement by punishment effect" described by Gray (1971) has implications for this phenomenon.] These incidents drove him to even greater heights of unrest. He feared punishment, and every thought about God or religion triggered strong and lingering feelings of anxiety and guilt. Daniel began to worry a great deal more than he ever had before. This prompted him to search for ways to alleviate these powerful feelings. He decided that what he might do was to "prove himself to God" to escape the almost certain punishment that was forthcoming.

In the cognitive-behavioral view that Daniel was to adopt, anxiety became conditioned to certain cues associated with wrongdoing, and the prospect of God's punishment for these "transgressions." Critical conditioning incidents occurred at a time in his life when he was emotionally vulnerable to such conditioning. It was in the next phase of the evolution of the disorder that Daniel began to include specific attempts to escape and avoid these powerful conditioned responses that had generalized to many cues associated with religion or God (e.g., driving past a church, hearing someone say "Goddamn," seeing things that looked like a cross, even crossing "ts" as he wrote).

Phase II: The Emergence of Self-Punishment and Rules

As Daniel continued his efforts to cope with the strongly conditioned anxiety, he became more preoccupied with a concern to do what is "right." Unfortunately, as hard as he would try, he could not always control what he thought about or, being an otherwise healthy adolescent, what he would do. More and more he worried that he must take steps to prevent God from punishing him. He hit on the solution of punishing himself and in this way "proving" himself to God so that God would not see the need to punish him later. It was during this phase that he began to deprive himself of pleasurable activities. For example, he would not drink Coke or Pepsi, or watch his favorite TV shows, or go out to movies or go bowling. He would not eat certain candy or chew certain gum or even think about certain pleasurable memories. Daniel would also choose to do many things the "hard way" as opposed to the convenient way as another means of "proving himself to God." He would only go to certain stores, the ones that were inconveniently located; he would take long routes to places instead of short ones; he would eat only kosher foods. Finally to punish himself, he would allow himself to appear "foolish" in front of friends and strangers. He would walk in "silly steps," he would dress inappropriately, he would say ridiculous things, all without explanations.

These efforts were to provide him relief from his fear of punishment by God, but there were several problems with Daniel's strategy. First, it came at an obvious cost in terms of embarrassment in front of those who observed and questioned his behavior. (He obviously could not reveal the "shameful" reasons for all of this self-punishment.) Second, the relief was always temporary, and it seemed that more and more was required to regain the relief that he had experienced with these efforts early on. Finally, there was a "fatal flaw" in the system (discussed later) that would show up in a later phase of the problem. But for now the system was holding together, just barely. As a matter of fact, Daniel was unable to keep to his self-imposed "rules of punishment" to the degree that he felt he should. He began to cut corners to "cheat" a bit here and there, to let up on the requirement of constant vigilance. One night while watching an episode of the TV show "Hill Street Blues," a pivotal incident occurred. A character in the story died of AIDS and was revealed to be a homosexual. What an awful punishment! A thought flashed through Daniel's mind: if he were to be stricken with AIDS, the disease would be bad enough, but the humiliation of having family, friends, and acquaintances thinking he was gay would be the worst punishment by God that he could imagine, and so Daniel became a "washer" during the last few months of 10th grade.

In many ways this was easier for him to do than to follow so many difficult rules. In fact, his preoccupation with cleanliness served to distract him from thoughts that in many ways were more disturbing. It was not long to be, however, because a competent co-therapist using standard behavioral techniques quickly "broke him" of his contamination fears and washing rituals within a few sessions and then, as Daniel put it, his problems "really got bad."

These incidents were also represented on Daniel's chart. He understood the relationship between the arousal of anxiety by conditioned fear cues and his efforts to alleviate his distress through his discovery of a variety of techniques that would enable him to regain a sense of comfort. In this way he came to understand the ways in which his avoidance and escape from anxiety and worry, through self-punishment and through the imposition and following of self-imposed rules, served to reinforce his rule making and compliance with those rules. This, in turn, would maintain and strengthen his growing tendency to extend the self-imposed restrictions on his behavior. When the following of rules led to the greater immediate discomfort of punishment by ridicule from others, he temporarily found refuge in a similar but more controllable system in which fear of AIDS preempted more diffuse and complicated concerns. The effectiveness of the behavioral treatment for Daniel's washing compulsion soon deprived him of the "simpler" means he had found to deal with his problems by narrowing his focus to a distractive fear of contracting AIDS. Having accepted all of this as a "reasonable" alternative explanation for what he had experienced—one certainly worth considering—Daniel went on to explain from his perspective, why "things really got bad" after that.

Phase III: The Diminution of "Crystalized Obsessions"

Certain occurrences during the summer before 11th grade made it even more difficult for Daniel to maintain even a modicum of control over his difficulties. One problem was that, in his words, "the rituals went inside my head." While his parents and therapists were comforted by the fact that he was no longer washing and thus appeared more "normal," he was actually struggling to develop another way to relieve the greatly troublesome feelings that were triggered by so many different thoughts, actions, and situations. It was as if curing him of washing and contamination fears also eliminated the tunnel vision that had temporarily blocked out the bigger problems. Now Daniel's eyes were wide open and he could again see the full magnitude of the problem, and it was worse than before. Because now, with the passage of time, it became impossible to be certain that he could ever remember, much less comply with, the hundreds of "commitments to God" he had made. He had to cope with the likelihood that at any given moment he was, in fact, breaking a promise to God he had made earlier that year. A lie to God, a promise made in good faith but now broken, certainly had to warrant severe punishment, but Daniel was no longer willing to allow his thinking to go that far. Thoughts of God and potential punishment were replaced by anxiety in a generalized form—the feeling that was now cued by almost any kind of movement or thought—a dreadful sense that he was "doing something wrong." The intrusive feeling that he had, in fact, violated one of the hundreds, if not thousands, of self-imposed rules, had now generalized to any moment of self-consciousness in which he might question whether he was in compliance with previously made rules. Known rules were still adhered to, but a larger problem had emerged: hundreds of instances were now occurring daily in which self-conscious scrutinizing of ongoing behavior and thoughts would trigger anxiety responses "automatically," that is, with no identifiable cognitive antecedent. These occurrences led more often than not to the termination of the sequence of behavior (or thinking) that was underway. This avoidance brought some quick relief from the anxiety and from the consequent thought "I must be doing something wrong," but at a cost. From that moment on, that particular behavior or thought would exist in the future as a new prohibition, adding hundreds of new rules to those that already existed and increasing the probability that there was, in fact, a "rule" governing any given behavior or thought no matter how trivial or mundane. This was the "fatal flaw" in Daniel's system alluded to earlier. Adding rules was comforting, following rules was comforting, but so many rules were added that it was impossible to keep track of them all. Anxiety, doubt, and confusion became pervasive. The very mechanisms that had been developed to ensure a degree of comfort were now ensuring a great deal of discomfort. Daniel's thinking had evolved further and further away from "crystalized" ruminations about specific acts of wrongdoing that violated religious and moral principles. The fear of being punished by God had become a multitude of individual anxiety responses that had a life apart from specific thoughts about a punitive deity. Instead, there were vague and persuasive feelings of anxiety and doubt, and the search was now for relief from discomfort by mechanisms that were no longer logically linked with any moral or religious principles.

Phase IV: The Emergence of "Pure" Rituals

The identification and analysis of a fourth phase in the evolution of Daniel's disorder brought the situation to the state it was in during much of his last year of high school, and to the time he came to me for help. Although there were some elements of this final manifestation throughout each previous phase, it was the emergence of chronic, pervasive, and "pure" rituals (i.e., rituals that lacked "meaning") as a prominent feature of the symptom picture that distinguished this latest phase. Daniel's avoidance of "prohibited" or "wrong" behaviors was not providing satisfactory relief from his anxieties, and doubt as to whether he, on any given occasion, had done something in violation of his self-imposed rules, was becoming the order of the day. His efforts at monitoring his every thought and action required great concentration and exhausting effort. It was as if he had to keep an eternally vigilant "third eye" to process every moment and render a judgment as to whether it was appropriate to continue. Of course, he had to remain in contact with his external environment as well, and the task proved impossible. Inevitably he would "lose track" of what he had just done or thought and this loss of concentration triggered immediate anxiety and the concurring cognition that he had done something wrong. Since he had no way of knowing what it was, or what rule had been violated, he sought to repeat the sequence of behavior in the hope of ascertaining the wrongdoing. In fact, since there was no wrongdoing to be discovered, he would settle for (i.e., be comforted by) repeating the action, (e.g., rereading a sentence, getting up from a chair, moving his arm) without a loss of concentration. Thus he gained assurance that he had done as much as possible to protect against violating any rule.

Each repetition, usually of a movement but sometimes of a thought, resulted in a temporary respite from the emotional and cognitive dilemma. Daniel came to understand that this temporary solution (i.e., ritualistic repetition with its resulting restoration of comfort) was actually the mechanism by which this tendency to repeat actions was maintained and strengthened. He discovered over time that the repetition could and would take a variety of forms. If he were writing and the feeling came, words, phrases, or even whole lines had to be crossed out and rewritten, often with entirely different words (so much for neat, legible, and well-developed compositions). If the "feeling" occurred during conversation, Daniel had to go back to what he had said last and say it again before he could go on. (His conversational skills went, as one might imagine, downhill.)

If he were doing nothing notable when the feeling came, he would repeat whatever movement he could determine that he had last made. In the company of others, he would try to disguise these maneuvers by making them subtle enough to go undetected. The trouble was that if they were too subtle, they felt "inadequately done" and did not provide a satisfactory measure of relief. Therefore, the failed subtle maneuvers would often be followed by more apparent ones (e.g., getting up and leaving the room and returning after a short time). There was no way to keep such a staggering array of comfort-producing devices from people who were with him for long. Daniel's system was in shambles and he knew it.

He felt hope, however. With this new "learning-based" explanation, his problem was, for the first time, understandable to him without God, sin, religion, and the inevitability of divine intervention as explanatory concepts. In their place were principles like classically conditioned anxiety, generalization, reinforcement, escape, avoidance, and, best of all, the principles that held the possibility of successful treatment: extinction, habituation, counter-conditioning, and the like. Daniel wanted very much to "buy" this view. Did he? Well, yes and no.

Daniel carried his charts back and forth to therapy as he would a talisman. He consulted them frequently and would review them at bedtime. We would fit incidents, old and new, into the scheme, sometimes modifying the charts until they seemed "right." In a short time, Daniel was describing his problems of daily life in language that would warm the hearts of behaviorists everywhere. Yes, he believed that there was great promise in this new conceptualization. For the first time he felt his problem was really understood by someone else, and it made sense to him as well. He seemed more relaxed, his parents said, and spoke hopefully about therapy "really working this time." He began to confide in me more, providing me with background information that he had never disclosed before, such as romantic disappointments, sexual insecurities, and embarrassing moments, eventually providing me with the details of the larger phenomenological context from which his problems had emerged. None of these revelations struck me as clinically significant, but his openness was very encouraging.

But no, he could not yet fully discount his beliefs regarding the fundamental validity of his own views about the "true nature" of his difficulties although his confidence in this view was weakened. (The probability of being punished by God if he broke rules was now about 50 percent he thought.) Moreover, he had discovered a "Catch-22" in this new view that deeply troubled him. If he had, in fact, made numerous promises to God for any reason whatsoever, was it not, in fact, a sin to violate those holy commitments? And does God not punish those who have broken their vows to Him? I, of course, argued no and mustered up as many religious and ethical arguments as I could to support my conclusions. But Daniel was quick to point out that I was a psychologist, and not a Jewish one at that, and therefore my opinions on theological and religious matters did not carry much weight.

I realized he had a point here, and so I quickly decided to implement one more measure to prepare Daniel for the exposure phase of therapy that was to begin shortly. I employed a little known behavioral intervention known as "a visit with the rabbi."

It was during our meeting with a sympathetic and scholarly rabbi from a synagogue other than the one Daniel attended that Daniel and I learned of Hebrew sages of old and their encounters with obsessive-compulsive functioning (see Chapter 18). In fact, during the Middle Ages, a religious ceremony had been developed to address an ancient problem that proved to be an uncanny match to Daniel's circumstances. The rabbi scheduled the religious ceremony for one morning later that week. At that ceremony, I looked on as Daniel, standing before three rabbis who stood in judgment, read from a translation of an ancient text and asked release from

> every vow or oath or prohibition or restriction ... even a prohibition to derive enjoyment that I imposed upon myself ... that escaped my mouth or that I vowed in my heart ... both regarding vows that are known to me and those that I have already forgotten. ... it is impossible to specify them because there are so many. ...

So Daniel was released and the ceremony also had provisions for proactive release from any future vows, declaring them all "totally null and void, without effect and without validity." It was time, we agreed, "to get on with the treatment."

The Course of Treatment

Of course treatment had long since been underway. I had met with Daniel 12 times up to this point, usually Wednesday and Saturday of each week. By "treatment" was meant the exposure phase that constituted the behavioral core of my intervention. For this to be successful, it was necessary that Daniel systematically violate every existing rule that could be identified. This would address and, I hoped, alleviate the phobic avoidance component of his disorder. He was well aware that this was to be a crucial element of treatment, one that was aimed at dismantling the incapacitating system of prohibitions that Daniel had developed over the years. "Where to begin?" and "How to proceed?" were questions of no trivial importance in that we were dealing with a formidable system. It was clear to both of us that all of our preparation for this moment, including the religious ceremony, and a later "booster session" with the rabbi, increased Daniel's motivation and provided a degree of confidence that would support his direct confrontation with the seemingly endless array of forbidden actions and thoughts.

It was not to be an easy task for Daniel, however. His thinking about what all this meant may have been modified, but the anxiety conditioned to the behavior of rule breaking would not dissolve so easily. [Here is a situation where changing cognitions did not eliminate strongly conditioned anxiety responses. As in many instances, cognitive changes set the stage for, but are not sufficient for, the alleviation of conditioned maladaptive responses. Behavioral treatment is required.] It would take a great deal of courage and stamina for him to "stare down the dragon" as he went about the mission of doing exactly that which his deeply entrenched emotions told him he must not do.

He would do what was necessary, however, because his recent experiences provided him with a cognitive framework that made his problem less intimidating: learning may have been at the root of his disorder but learning principles were now going to be working *for* him. If Daniel's problem were only "habits" of thoughts, feelings, and actions, if even those rules that were based on actual promises made to God were invalidated, if the weight of his religion were thrown behind these therapeutic efforts, then he could face his greatest fears.

While there is no clear point that overvalued ideas become "appropriately" valued, or even acceptably valued, ideas, I was pleased that Daniel now rated the probability that he would be punished by God if he broke his rules as less than 30 percent. He now seemed willing to tackle the rules head on, and I felt satisfied that he would have a fighting chance.

Because much of the rule breaking would eventually be done by Daniel alone as "homework" assignments, he carried a card in his wallet on which were listed four guidelines that we gleaned from the religious ceremony, or from a subsequent meeting with the rabbi. Daniel consulted these when confronted with a difficult choice or a "weak moment." These were:

1. It is proper to enjoy God-given gifts of life, and improper to deny oneself life's everyday pleasures (or the full use of one's faculties).
2. No thought is inherently evil or sinful in that we don't have complete control of our thoughts and also because thoughts serve to discharge tensions.
3. Self-imposed vows, promises, rules, etc. are invalid and unacceptable unless they are grounded in accepted religious principles and/or practices and even then are valid only if they are reasonable ones (i.e., ones that we can be expected to follow).
4. We are urged to refrain from engaging in "self-conceived false religious practices," and rituals should be viewed in this way when they are done for religious purposes.

I warned Daniel in advance that while we hoped many taboos and rituals would "evaporate" before systematic exposure to them, he should be prepared for the fact that many of these involved long-standing and well-practiced responses. So it could very well be an arduous task to win back the lost ground. He understood this better than I did.

The sheer magnitude of the task required a carefully prepared plan of attack. I chose to work first on the avoidance because success here would provide immediate payoff in the form of increased adaptive functioning in Daniel's daily life. In the process we would gather information about the effect "violating the taboos" had on the frequency and intensity of the "pure" rituals. If the hoped-for improvements in daily function could be achieved, we would then focus on the rituals.

Daniel agreed that he would try to add no new rituals as rules were broken. It was now December, 8 weeks into therapy with Daniel, and he was totally withdrawn from imipramine. After a day or two of headaches, he seemed fine; his score on the Beck Depression Inventory was stable between 5 and 8. It was interesting to note that during the previous month, our somewhat crude measures of frequency and intensity of obsessions and rituals indicated a gradual worsening of his disorder. This was corroborated by general agreement (parents and Daniel) that he was "as bad as he had ever been" during the information-gathering phase. This suggested that so called nonspecific factors in therapy were contributing little or nothing to his improvement. In fact, his ability to function in the academic sphere came to a virtual halt: papers and tests earned only F's and were so awful that the concern of several instructors for Daniel's state of mind was expressed in comments on his papers. Just getting to class became almost impossible because of difficulties in getting out of the house, driving, parking the car, walking to the building, going through doors, sitting down, and so on. Moreover, he was being bombarded almost constantly with "spontaneous feelings" that led to the ritualistic repeating, walking in and out, and so on.

From the standpoint of therapeutic strategy, this was not a bad thing because it made Daniel eager to "get on with the therapy." It was at this point that my letter resulted in his administrative withdrawal from college for the semester. I freed up my schedule so we could spend part of therapy time out of the office.

The assault on the rules began with some imaginal work in my office. The in-office setting was one that did not have a significant history of taboos and rituals. In fact, the office and my presence had become "countercues" for obsessive-compulsive symptoms, I learned, when it became apparent that it was not easy to produce the "feelings" that occurred so frequently in all other settings. This would limit the possibilities for in vivo exposure in the office.

To impose some organization on the exposure phase, we developed broad "categories" of rules based on what items or activities they governed. The categories were food and drink, dressing and grooming, household chores, driving places, walking places, writing things, remembering things, talking about things, playing the guitar, reading, taking notes, going to various places, and so on.

Within these categories were lists of specific, previously taboo activities. These were arranged in a rough hierarchical fashion, using a 0–100 scale as an indicator of how much anxiety Daniel anticipated in the performance of the activity. All ranged from 60 to the maximum 100, and we would approach them from the least to the most.

It was apparent from the first session of office work that this would be a fruitful approach. Beginning with certain memories that were "wrong" to think of (there was no apparent rhyme or reason as to why some memories were OK to remember and others were not), Daniel privately dredged up memories that generated moderate levels of anxiety. It got easier and easier for him to think of these as he went on to more anxiety-provoking memories, and these too were thought of until they could be recalled without significant anxiety. Next he imagined telling me those memories; then he *did* tell me. Soon memories began to flow, and he was able to write about them without any crossing out. He managed fine and was impressed because it seemed to be getting easier as he did this. Soon he promised he would be able to tell me every "forbidden memory," and he did. And these, it turned out, were rather unremarkable in content—not traumatic or "Freudian" by any stretch of the imagination. Most likely they represented contents of consciousness that had, by a stroke of randomness, occupied the forefront of Daniel's awareness during one of the many occurrences of an intrusive feeling of wrongdoing.

Homework consisted, as it usually did, of practicing what we had done in my office (i.e., violations of existing rules) in his natural environment. He noted that it was harder to do these things without my presence, but he mostly managed, and made notes of things that hung him up. We later would accomplish these things either in the office or, when it was necessary, with my accompanying him "in vivo." Soon momentum began to build, and the rules came "crashing down." Many hard ones were accomplished with help but soon Daniel was "breaking through" even very difficult ones on his own.

His life began freeing up in substantial ways. He began to act and feel more normal. The records he kept for me showed a drastic reduction in rulebound behavior. There was, however, little if any noticeable change in measures of the "spontaneous feelings" or subtle repeating rituals. These apparently would have to be dealt with later with another therapeutic strategy. Daniel said that he was enjoying life more but that the detailed record keeping was becoming a burden for him. For that reason, and because I discovered that up this point there had been close agreement between the "frequency, intensity, and time spent ritualizing" records and a 0 to 100 "Global Measure of Improvement" scale I had been obtaining each week (0 = "the problem is as bad as it has ever been" to 100 = "I feel totally cured"), the former was temporarily discontinued. Over the weeks I watched as the global scores inched higher and higher. The scores were a bit over 50 when the college's spring semester began. At that time, Saturday sessions were scheduled for work in settings that had a history of triggering particularly strong negative feelings (e.g., certain stores, roads, eating places); these too were rapidly yielding to our attack. The Saturday before spring semester classes began, I accompanied Daniel as he drove to campus along "forbidden" roads, parked in various "taboo" spaces in different "prohibited" parking lots, walked to buildings along "unacceptable" pathways, and went through "verboten" doors—all with very little difficulty.

Spring semester was a very different experience for Daniel. By the end of May, after 4 months of therapy, he had passed every test, attended every class, turned in every paper, and earned grades of B or C in every course. By summer vacation there was a virtual absence of any self-imposed rules. The picture had improved greatly. He was now functioning more capably than he had been for years, but his global self-rating score of 70 indicated that, for Daniel, the fight was not over yet. During the spring semester he had gotten a taste of what freedom from OCD could be like. He had had some very good days, but he also experienced some trying moments as well. For one thing, we had discovered that it was necessary to exercise his newly gained freedom from rules because if a previously rule-governed behavior was neglected as Daniel put it, "the rule creeps back into place." While the few occurrences of these returning rules were relatively easy to overcome by exposure tactics, Daniel found these slips frustrating and unnerving. On the positive side, this served to revitalize Daniel's commitment to therapy, thus helping to counter any wariness or complacency that could threaten further progress.

A more worrisome factor to us both was that we had not yet found a satisfactory solution to the problem of the spontaneous feelings (we called them "false alarms" by then) and for the sometimes subtle, but often disruptive, repeating rituals that would follow them. Daniel had learned to function effectively despite these intrusive feelings and thoughts that he had "done something wrong." But the sheer frequency of the false alarms—up to 150 per day—and the fact that Daniel still felt compelled to repeat *something* following each feeling meant that a solution had to be found. Although most of the repeating rituals involved subtle movements (e.g., the twitch of a finger, a sidelong glance, or a tap of the foot), some, particularly those following occurrences of very strong feelings, prompted Daniel to exit the room and return after a brief time with a comforting sense of "starting fresh." Daniel said these feelings, and the behaviors they triggered, made him feel abnormal, distracted him, and exhausted him emotionally. This aspect of the problem caused me concern not only because it troubled Daniel, but because it seemed to me to be the emotional "core" of the problem; an element present at the genesis of Daniel's disorder and possibly the motivational force for the establishment of the complex structure of rules that had required such an extraordinary investment of time and effort to dismantle.

So Daniel and I agreed that our twice weekly, hour-long sessions during June would focus on the quest for an effective strategy to resolve the "false alarm" problem. We knew what would *not* work because we had tried a few things already.

"Trying harder to resist" didn't work, but then it never had. Relaxation exercises that we tried had no effect on this aspect of the problem either. One strategy looked promising for about 2 weeks but did not hold up well in the long run. In that effort, Daniel self-monitored and recorded the spontaneous feelings and urges to ritualize for increasingly longer intervals during the day. However, he did not ritualize during those intervals. Because he was unable to prevent himself from ritualizing entirely (the discomfort was too strong he said), he was allowed to perform the accumulated rituals "en masse" during the hour before bedtime. The learning-theory-oriented reader will note that, from a theoretical standpoint, this approach had much to recommend it. Indeed, I was pleased with the "elegant simplicity" of this strategy. However, I reluctantly abandoned this approach four sessions later, strongly influenced by an exhausted and angry Daniel who vehemently stated "It's not working and I won't do this anymore." Fortunately I had several alternative strategies to fall back on.

Twice weekly sessions with a "therapeutic companion" were added to our plans. [Therapeutic companions are persons in my employ who work with the patient in vivo. These are typically BA or MA level psychology students who oversee therapy in the patient's "natural environment." Often a close bond forms between patient and companion, which facilitates the companion's role as a model, facilitator, guide, and "cheerleader."] The companion was to accompany Daniel for prolonged periods in his home and to places he frequently visited in order to provide support and direction while he totally refrained from ritualizing for ever-increasing amounts of time.

Within a few sessions with his companion we were hopeful: Daniel would go for hours experiencing fewer and fewer "false alarms" and each was diminishing in strength. He was able to resist, under these conditions, and he was convinced that he was ready to tackle one of the "biggies." By this he meant he would totally abstain from any ritualization within one of the remaining categories of false-alarm-triggered rituals. By this time a number of categories had already been overcome: "crossing things out" (when writing); "repeating things" (when talking); "looking away" (while looking at someone or something). These categories had been reduced from frequencies of up to 100 per day to zero. The remaining categories consisted of "walking in and out" of rooms, which occurred 25 to 30 times each day; and repeating movements, which were occurring 60 to 70 times each day. These were the "biggies." Of the two, "walking in and out" was the more disruptive of ongoing behavior, was more noticeably "strange" to other people, wasted more energy, and had a greater negative impact on his self-esteem. Being freed of that ritual would lift a giant weight from Daniel's shoulders. For these reasons, we chose that category as the one to go.

And go it did; but not without a fight. While the companion was with him, he resisted totally; when she left, he walked in and out. So I put together a 3-minute "endless" tape on which was recorded some upbeat guitar music superimposed over which were statements like: "Walking in and out is a false religious practice"; "Walking in and out interferes with life's activities"; "When you feel an urge to walk in and out, it's an opportunity to make a healthy choice"; "Walking in and out has no ethical or religious basis." Daniel agreed to listen to it over and over on his Walkman tape player during all sorts of activities. He said it was corny, but he stopped walking in and out. To this day, he will not acknowledge that the tape had anything to do with it, but insists he was just ready to stop. Maybe he was.

Things began to happen quickly then. Daniel said "It's getting easier and easier." In early July Daniel took a much-needed vacation from therapy to spend a week at the ocean with a friend and his friend's parents. He was back a week later. He had had a "great" time and had "felt normal" and did "all the normal things" (foremost among these was meeting girls, it turned out). The prior "taste" of normality was just a nibble; he was feasting now and loving it. But he felt confused. He didn't know if he could trust his feelings. He said he felt "too good."

The rest of the summer went much like that for Daniel, and he was learning to trust his feelings. His friendships blossomed; he dated and had a bad case of "puppy love" that I wasn't sure he'd survive until I remembered that we all survive. He survived. He got a job that he liked and did well at, even managing to save some money. He found an apartment with a college buddy and moved out of his parents' home in the late summer. Daniel was at a time in his life in which separating from his family and establishing independence was a "healthy" step. For this reason I chose not to involve the family much in the therapy, other than to to invite them in for occasional "updates." [If Daniel had been younger, it is very likely that the whole family would have been asked to meet with my co-worker, who functions as a behavioral family therapist. This is to ensure that the breaking of maladaptive habits and the substitution of adaptive functioning is being supported by other family members.] Daniel returned to school for the fall semester with a fresh outlook. The 6 weeks since he has returned to college have gone extremely well. He has been active in campus activities and has found a social "niche." He has developed excellent study habits, is earning all A's and B's now, and is genuinely enjoying his classes. He is busy with the day-to-day concerns and activities of the typical 19-year-old college student.

He is not "cured" yet or I would not have described this as a "case in progress." I still meet with Daniel 1 or 2 hours each week. He continues to complain of "very minor" false alarms occurring a few times each day, and he is wary of them. He said, "I can see I have to be careful of these things" because he remembered how his great difficulties were built on just a few troubling incidents. It bothers him that he has occasional lapses where he repeats a subtle movement or behavior almost reflexively, and has voiced the fleeting worry about whether the problem could "come back." But he seems to understand that his therapy has not masked, suppressed, camouflaged, or otherwise driven his problem "undercover." Rather, his treacherously debilitating obsessive-compulsive cognitive, affective, and motoric habits have been virtually eliminated, and in their place are the healthy, adaptive habits that have made the world for Daniel a different place.

Perhaps Daniel said it best in statements he made during the past few sessions:

> I've had a good time these past months . . . great . . . terrific . . . compared with the way it was last year . . . and it hasn't been up and down. . . . Rules just haven't been a problem. . . . I'm not really concerned about it now. . . . I feel confident that I'm a lot stronger. . . . It's been good and continuous. . . . I'm in the routine of life now as opposed to an obsessive-compulsive daily routine. . . . I feel relaxed, my attitude is

good . . . everything is really good. . . . Hours go by, maybe days where I
can't remember any specific [obsessive-compulsive] incidents . . . every
ritual [category] is "dropping down" further and further and I can't
think of any rules or rituals that have taken anything out of my
day. . . . I'm really happy with this.

And of the future, Daniel said:

I'm not really worried about it. . . . I feel like any problems that might
come up can be solved pretty easily. . . . There's comfort in knowing we
can go the distance with the problem. . . . These methods are
reliable. . . . I feel that we can take care of whatever's left when it's
time. . . . I trust these methods.

Conclusion

Daniel's is not the kind of case that behavior therapists hope will walk
through their doors. Like all patients, some are easier than others, and
from the first it was clear that Daniel was not going to be easy. It can
be relatively simple to design a behavioral program for some cases, a
relatively circumscribed washing compulsion, for example. Daniel responded well when he was a "washer." Behavior therapy has a strong
literature for OCD, and a casual reading of treatment accounts in the
literature can give the impression that OCD is a unified disorder that is
responsive to a well-defined treatment "package." Just "flood" them
with the things they fear, and "prevent them from ritualizing." Anyone who has worked with more than a few patients with OCD knows
how complicated it can be to translate this simple formula into an
effective therapeutic procedure. Cases such as the one presented here,
where the obsessions are pervasive and where the patient is particularly resistant to therapeutic procedures, are unlikely to benefit significantly from "cookbook-style" treatment. It is hoped that the reporting of this case will provide an opportunity for a view into the
process of outpatient, clinical behavior therapy for OCD where the
case is, I think, a challenging one by any standards. This report has
highlighted the clinical art that surrounds therapeutic technique and
often determines the outcome of therapy.

Perhaps the reader questions whether or not the preceding has
indeed been a description of behavior therapy. It is my contention that
published descriptions of behavioral interventions may encourage the
impression that behavior therapy is a limited "bag of tricks." Rather, I
see it as a wonderfully diverse approach to treatment that has, as
guideposts, empirically derived psychological principles. If the appli-

cation of these principles as presented here seems inelegant or intuitive, it is because that is the way it often is. This is not "seat-of-the-pants" therapy, I would argue, because each step is monitored for effectiveness and is integrated into an overall therapeutic strategy that relies on behavioral principles for its inspiration and direction. The research literature of behavior therapy sets clearly defined but narrow parameters for the conduct of therapy. The clinical practice of behavior therapy, of necessity, goes beyond the boundaries set by research. This is not a weakness but rather it is the source from which the field is enriched and broadened. As techniques derived from research enrich clinical practice, so does clinical practice enrich research by raising new questions that can and should be addressed through research endeavors.

Daniel's case, as reported, suggests that his rituals, while apparently "meaningless" to close observers, actually comprised an elaborate system of evolving habits, derived from a complex and changing cognitive system. The genesis of both could be traced to specific experiences in which principles of learning served as explanatory mechanisms. This exercise in no way denies nor does it confirm the role of biological factors operating in OCD. Instead, the emphasis here is on the contribution of psychological principles as they are applied to the analysis and treatment of the disorder in one individual. Here, behaviors that served adaptive psychological ends in early phases of the disorder evolved into nonadaptive rituals that seriously impeded normal functioning. A cognitive system struggling to understand and cope with conflicting beliefs and feelings metamorphosed into an elaborate obsessional system characterized by a diffuse, ill-defined, and pervasive sense of doubt, worry, and foreboding. Both were fueled by emotions that did not remain linked to the incidents that aroused them but that instead spread, virtually unchecked, to influence every aspect of life. Whether the internal logic and gradual evolution of Daniel's case has implications for a broader understanding of OCD is now open to speculation.

References

Beck AT, Rush AJ, Shaw BS, et al: Cognitive Therapy of Depression: A Treatment Manual. New York, Guilford Press, 1979

Foa EB: Failure in treating obsessive compulsives. Behav Res Ther 16:169–179, 1979

Foa EB, Grayson JB, Steketee GS, et al: Success and failure in the behavioral treatment of obsessive-compulsives. J Consult Clin Psychol 51:287–297, 1983

Gray JA: The Psychology of Fear and Stress. New York, McGraw-Hill, 1971

Rachman SJ: Fear and Courage. New York, Freeman, 1978

Rachman SJ, Hodgson R: Obsessions and Compulsions. Englewood Cliffs, NJ, Prentice-Hall, 1980

Rapoport JL: Annotation: childhood obsessive compulsive disorder. J Child Psychol Psychiatry 27:289–295, 1986

Sumners D, Gournay K: Obsessive compulsive neurosis: a speculative account of an unusual case. Behavioral Psychotherapy 14:162–170, 1986

Wolff R, Rapoport JL: Behavioral treatment of childhood obsessive-compulsive disorder. Behavior Modification 12:252–266, 1988

Chapter 13

Drug Treatment of Obsessive-Compulsive Disorder

Henrietta L. Leonard, M.D.

Until recently, there was little research on drug treatment of obsessive-compulsive disorder (OCD) at any age, and even fewer studies with children. Because so few controlled pediatric studies have been completed, we present a brief overview of drug treatment of OCD in adults, and then focus on the experience of children and adolescents. A number of more detailed reviews have been written on the general subject of psychopharmacology of OCD and these should be consulted for more details in treatment of adults (Klein et al. 1985; Zohar and Insel 1987).

Studies with anxiolytics, antipsychotics, nonselective antidepressants, and the more selective serotonin reuptake blockers are reviewed here. Of the latter group, only clomipramine (CMI) has been examined extensively. The two controlled studies with adolescents will be discussed in greatest detail. It is ironic that with the increased recognition of the syndrome and early reports of efficacy of clomipramine (Lopez-Ibor 1966), there is now as much known about drug treatment of adolescent OCD as there is for depression and anxiety in this age group. Even with limited data, there is cause for optimism.

Anxiolytics

Waxman (1977) compared diazepam and CMI in 41 patients with phobias and obsessional disorders and found CMI "useful" in their treatment. However, the diagnosis of OCD was not clear, and conclusions were hard to draw from the information presented. Burrell et al. (1974) reported bromazepam to be useful in an open trial of 220 patients with obsessional symptoms. In general, the open trials have had mixed results (Ananth 1976), and there are major unresolved issues. Anxiety may exacerbate the obsessions and the rituals, and anxiolytics may improve OCD only via their anxiolytic action. Whether OCD is an anxiety disorder or not remains debatable. At the very least, further work is needed before the usefulness of anxiolytics for OCD can be established.

Alprazolam has been reported in several individual cases (Hardy 1987; Ketter et al. 1986; Tesar and Jenike 1984; Tollefson 1985). Tesar and Jenike, for example, reported its efficacy in one patient with OCD with generalized anxiety and a history of panic attacks. On the (generous) dosage of 12 mg/day, his obsessive thoughts became infrequent. Tollefson reported a moderate to marked improvement in four obsessive-compulsive patients in an open trial of alprazolam, ranging from 1.25 mg to 6 mg/day. Two of the four cases had a panic component. Ketter et al. and Hardy reported improvement in adult patients on much smaller doses of 1 to 3 mg/day.

Antipsychotics

There are no clinical controlled trials of antipsychotics used for the treatment of OCD. Ananth (1976) obtained equivocal results with haloperidol. In general, antipsychotics are not felt to be efficacious.

Antidepressants

Antidepressants other than clomipramine and serotonin reuptake blockers are not consistently helpful in OCD. Only one controlled study of an antidepressant, which was not a serotonin reuptake blocker, could be found. Foa et al. (1987) treated 37 obsessive-compulsive patients with imipramine or placebo for 6 weeks. Imipramine and placebo were not different in their effect on obsessive-compulsive symptoms. Imipramine reduced depression in highly depressed patients with OCD, but did not affect obsessive-compulsive symptoms in these or less depressed patients. Case reports of individual improvement for trazodone (Lydiard 1986; Prasad 1985), doxepin (Ananth et al. 1975), tranylcypromine (Jenike 1981), phenelzine (Isberg 1981), and L-tryptophan (a serotonin precursor) suggest occasional usefulness. But there is no systematic evidence to support any consistent efficacy of antidepressants other than potent serotonin reuptake blockers.

Serotonin Reuptake Blockers

The three serotonin reuptake blockers studied to date for OCD are CMI, fluoxetine, and fluvoxamine (Figure 1).

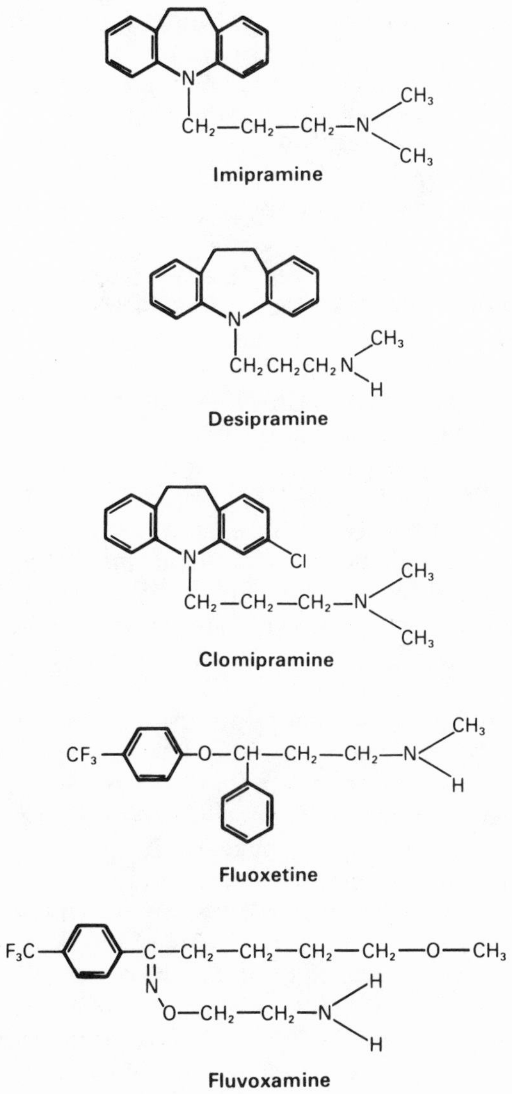

Imipramine

Desipramine

Clomipramine

Fluoxetine

Fluvoxamine

Figure 1. Chemical structures of imipramine, desipramine, clomipramine, fluoxetine, and fluvoxamine.

Clomipramine

Pharmacology of Clomipramine

Clomipramine hydrochloride ("Anafranil SR 75") is a relatively selective and potent inhibitor of active serotonin uptake in the brain. It also blocks histamine H_2 receptors, cholinergic, and alpha$_1$ noradrenergic receptors. Its antidopaminergic properties are weak.

Clomipramine is almost completely absorbed following oral dosage. Metabolism takes place primarily in the liver. The plasma half-life of CMI itself is 24 hours, but desmethylclomipramine, CMI's major metabolite, has a much longer half-life. Metabolism can be induced by cigarette smoking and reduced by phenothiazines through competitive inhibition.

Since 1976 there have been nine controlled trials of CMI in adult patients (Table 1) and two in children and adolescents with OCD (Table 2). Of the controlled drug trials comparing CMI to placebo, CMI is superior in nine of the nine studies (Yaryura-Tobias et al. 1976; Thoren et al. 1980; Marks et al. 1980; Montgomery 1980; Insel et al. 1983, 1985; Mavissakalian et al. 1985; Flament et al. 1985; Leonard et al. 1988). Four of the six controlled studies comparing CMI to a standard antidepressant found CMI superior. Clomipramine was significantly better than clorgyline (Insel et al. 1983), imipramine (Volavka et al. 1985), desipramine and zimelidine (Insel et al. 1985), and desipramine (Leonard et al. 1988). In the other two studies comparing CMI to another antidepressant, CMI seemed promising but did not differ significantly from the comparison drug. Thoren et al. (1980) found a 42 percent decrease of obsessive-compulsive symptoms on CMI and only 21 percent on nortriptyline, but the latter treatment was not significantly different from either CMI or placebo. However, when CMI was given as an open trial to the eight nortriptyline subjects (only one of whom had responded), four of eight responded. Ananth et al. (1981) found significant improvement in obsessive-compulsive, depressive, and anxiety symptoms on CMI and not amitriptyline. However, no significant difference was seen when the two active medications were compared directly. They conclude that CMI is more efficacious than amitriptyline, although statistical comparison was not significant.

Mavissakalian et al. (1985) suggested that the antiobsessive effect of CMI is at least partially independent of its antidepressant effect. They reported that depression, but not obsessive-compulsive symptoms, improved in the placebo group and that CMI was equally effective in the high and low depressed patients with OCD. Eight of the nine controlled studies showed that improvement in OCD symptoms was independent of pretreatment depression (Thoren et al. 1980; Montgomery 1980; Ananth 1976; Ananth et al. 1975, 1981; Insel 1983;

Table 1. Drug treatment of obsessive-compulsive disorder (OCD): controlled trials with clomipramine (CMI) in adult patients

Author	Sample and Diagnosis	Dosage (mg)	Design	Results and Comments
Yaryura-Tobias et al. 1976	OCD $N = 18$ age 18–65 yr	100–300	4 mo double-blind placebo given for 2 wk either 4th or 6th wk	5 of 18 dropouts. Significant decrease of OC sx at termination. OC sx worse 1 wk after placebo when compared to wk prior to placebo. Limitations: small N, short placebo phase not allowing for carry-over effect.
	OCD & schizophrenia $N = 18$ age 18–65 yr	25–300	8-wk open trial, antipsychotics given ad lib	4 of 10 dropouts. Decreased OC sx at wk 4.
Thoren et al. 1980	OCD (RDC) 24 patients age 19–61 yr	CMI to 150 NOR to 150	6-wk trial, double-blind CMI vs. NOR vs placebo	CMI: 42% decrease OC sx. NOR: 21% decerase OC sx. Placebo: 7% decrease OC sx. CMI was superior to placebo.
			parallel groups placebo $N = 8$ CMI $N = 8$ NOR $N = 8$	NOR did not differ significantly from CMI or placebo. Limitations: small N, short duration, low dosage.
Marks et al. 1980	OCD (Ritualizers) $N = 40$ age 15–18 yr	CMI to 225 day (mean dosage 183 for 10 wk, 145 thereafter)	2×2 design CMI vs placebo exposure vs relaxation 36 wk	CMI superior to placebo. CMI effect only seen in depressed patients. Exposure improved rituals. CMI enhanced compliance with exposure and with relaxation.
Montgomery 1980	OCD (RDC) $N = 14$	CMI to 75	double-blind crossover design CMI vs. placebo 4 wk each	CMI superior to placebo at wk 4. No improvement in depression. Limitations: low dosage, short duration, crossover design carry-over effect, behavior therapy concurrent.

Table 1. *(continued)*

Author	Sample and Diagnosis	Dosage (mg)	Design	Results and Comments
Ananth et al. 1981	OCD $N = 20$ age 22–56 yr	75–300 133 CMI (mean) 197 AMI (mean)	4-wk double-blind CMI vs. AMI	CMI improved OC sx, depression, & anxiety. Improvement in the AMI group was not significant. However, no significant difference between the two drugs. Improvement of OC independent depression. Limitations: small N, short duration, low dosage.
Insel et al. 1983	OCD (DSM-III) $N = 13$ age 19–57 yr (mean = 32)	CMI to 300 (mean 236) clorgyline to 30	24-wk double-blind crossover CMI vs clorgyline (MAOI)	CMI superior to clorgyline & placebo for OC sx, anxiety, & depression. Antiobsession independent of baseline depression. Limitations: small N (10 completed crossover)
Volavka et al. 1985	OCD (DSM-III) $N = 23$ CMI: 11 age 21–54 yr (mean = 31) IMI: 12 age 19–42 yr (mean = 28.7)	CMI & IMI to 300 (275 at 12 wk) (IMI mean 262 at 12 wk)	12-wk double-blind parallel design no placebo CMI vs IMI	CMI superior to IMI on OC sx & depression. CMI response independent of initial severity of depression. Limitations: No placebo, small N. IMI patients sicker at baseline.
Mavissakalian et al. 1985	OCD (DSM-III) $N = 12$ (CMI = 7; placebo = 5) age 20–58 yr (mean = 36)	CMI 150–300 (mean 229)	12 wk double-blind CMI vs placebo parallel	CMI superior to placebo for OC sc. 43% response (3/7) on CMI. No response to placebo. Limitation: small N
Insel et al. 1985	OCD (DSM-III) CMI $N = 9$ DMI $N = 8$ Zimel $N = 5$ age 20–55 yr	DMI 275 (mean) Zimel 280 (mean) CMI 258 (mean)	placebo-controlled double-blind crossover (5 wk each active medication)	CMI superior to both DMI & Zimel for OC sx. No difference between Zimel & DMI. Limitations: 9 of original 16 patients completed CMI (full study). CMI trial limited to DMI & Zimel nonresponders.

Note. OC sx = obsessive-compulsive symptoms; RDC = Research Diagnostic Criteria; NOR = nortriptyline; AMI = amitriptyline; DSM-III =*Diagnostic and Statistical Manual of Mental Disorders*, 3rd edition (American Psychiatric Association 1980); IMI = imipramine; CMI = clomipramine; Zimel = zimelidine; DMI = desmethylimipramine.

Table 2. Drug treatment of obsessive-compulsive disorder (OCD): controlled trials with clomipramine (CMI) in children and adolescents

Author	Sample and Diagnosis	Dosage (mg)	Design	Results and Comments
Flament et al. 1985	OCD (DSM-III) $N = 19$ age 19–18 yr (mean 14.5)	CMI 100–200 141 (mean)	10-wk double-blind crossover of CMI vs placebo (5 wk each)	CMI significantly better than placebo in relieving OC sx. No correlation between plasma CMI levels & treatment response. Limitations: Crossover design, small N, short duration.
Leonard et al. 1988	OCD (DSM-III) $N = 32$ age 10.9 yr	CMI to 300 157 (mean)	12-wk double-blind crossover 5 wk each active med CMI vs DMI 2-wk initial placebo single-blind trial	CMI superior to DMI. OC sx ameloriation independent of depression.

Note. DSM-III = *Diagnostic and Statistical Manual of Mental Disorders*, 3rd edition (American Psychiatric Association 1980); OC sx = obsessive-compulsive symptoms; CMI = clomipramine; DMI = desmethylimipramine.

Volavka et al. 1985; Mavissakalian 1985), including pediatric studies (Flament et al. 1985; Leonard et al. 1988).

In summary, controlled trials make a strong case for CMI's antiobsessional effect. Even these studies, however, suffer the shortcomings of limited treatment duration, low dosages, and relatively small sample size.

Clinical Experience with Drug Treatment of Childhood Obsessive-Compulsive Disorder

Flament and her colleagues (Flament et al. 1985; Flament et al. 1987) published the first controlled study of the pharmacological treatment of childhood OCD. For the most part, results parallel those seen with adults. Clomipramine was significantly superior to placebo in a 5-week double-blind crossover study utilizing a mean daily dose of 141 mg. All but one of the 19 children had received prior treatment; 15 had previous medications, of whom 10 had received a tricyclic antidepressant other than CMI. Only one child (who had received lithium) had shown any hint of prior drug response. This suggested a specificity of effect, more conclusively demonstrated by Leonard et al. (1988) also for an adolescent population.

For these trials, clinical ratings were adapted from those used with adults or used unchanged. It was extremely important, however, to include parental weekly ratings for this predominantly outpatient population because of the child's secretiveness.

Of these adolescents, 75 percent had a moderate to marked improvement, whereas 16 percent were unchanged. In general, response pattern (usually no improvement until week 3 of treatment, although occasionally sooner), side effects, and plasma concentration were similar to that seen for adults. Plasma concentration of the desmethyl metabolite were 2.6 times greater than those of CMI. A wide variability between patients' plasma levels relative to oral doses occurred, as had been noticed in other studies (Stein et al. 1980), and levels did not correlate with response. Thus while there is not complete agreement on this point, in my impression plasma concentration is not useful.

Clomipramine-Desipramine Comparison in Children With OCD

In order to compare CMI with a standard (and available) tricylic antidepressant as well as to ensure a true double-blind study by using a comparison drug with similar side effects, a double-blind crossover study was carried out with CMI and desmethylimipramine (DMI), a selective noradrenergic reuptake inhibitor (Leonard et al. 1988) (Table 2).

The first 32 (22 males) children and adolescents with severe OCD have completed this ongoing study (Table 3). Following a 1-week diagnostic evaluation, the outpatient drug treatment trial consisted of an initial 2-week single-blind placebo phase. Any subject with a 20 percent improvement on a global OCD scale would be excluded. The double-blind crossover phase consisted of two consecutive 5-week

Table 3. Characteristics of 32 children and adolescents with obsessive-compulsive disorder (OCD) participating in the clomipramine (CMI)–
desipramine (DMI) comparison study

Characteristics	Mean ± SD	Range
Age (years)	13.91 ± 2.7	8–19
Age of onset (years)	10.94 ± 2.8	5–16
Duration (years)	3.00 ± 2.4	1–9
Hamilton Depression scores	8.00 ± 4.8	1–20
IQ score		
Verbal	111.8 ± 12.8	84–136
Performance	103.1 ± 12.9	78–131
Full-scale	108.4 ± 11.8	83–129
CMI dose (mg)	157.5 ± 54.4	68–250
DMI dose (mg)	161.7 ± 52.7	75–250

treatment periods with doses of CMI or DMI targeting 3 mg/kg. Depression, anxiety, obsessive-compulsive symptoms, and side effects were rated weekly as in the Flament et al. (1985) study.

Clomipramine was superior to DMI in ameliorating obsessive-compulsive symptoms at 5 weeks of treatment. In fact, DMI did not seem more effective than had the placebo been in the Flament et al. (1985) study, producing little or no improvement from baseline. Clinical improvement could be seen as early as week 3. As shown in Figure 2,

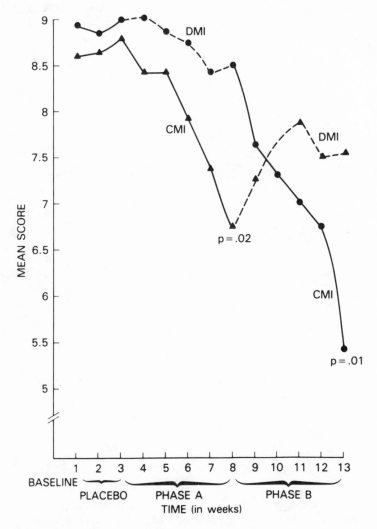

Figure 2. Global OCD scores for children and adolescents during clomipramine (CMI) and desipramine (DMI) crossover study ($N = 32$).

relapse on crossover to DMI was seen quickly, usually after 2 weeks when DMI followed CMI.

Figure 3 shows collapsed data for the controlled trial in which ratings of obsessive-compulsive symptoms are pooled for DMI and CMI regardless of order. As can be seen, there is improvement on CMI, which differed significantly from DMI at weeks 4 and 5 of treatment. There was a mild decrease in depressive symptoms in Phase A on both drugs; however, depression ratings *increased* during Phase B if DMI was given second. This appeared to be secondary to demoralization of these obsessive-compulsive patients as their obsessive-compulsive symptoms returned on DMI, following improvement on CMI during the first phase.

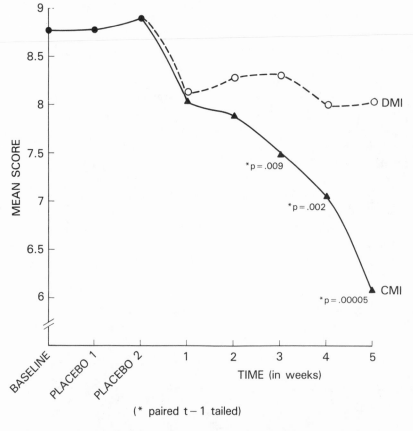

Figure 3. Global OCD scale collapsed scores for children and adolescents during clomipramine (CMI) and desipramine (DMI) crossover study ($N = 32$).

In general, both drugs were well tolerated, with no nausea, vomiting, or seizures. Side effects were similar for CMI and DMI, although CMI produced slightly more insomnia, sweating, tremor, and drowsiness. Even our youngest patients (ages 6 to 8) tolerated the medication well with few complaints. Those patients with coexisting attention deficit disorder experienced improvement in their concentration, as has been documented with other tricyclics. My clinical impression was that the children and adolescents experienced fewer side effects than do adults on CMI. Withdrawal from CMI was more difficult than from DMI, with patients on CMI needing to be tapered more slowly.

Clomipramine responders were continued on CMI at a dose of 3 mg/kg. Currently, a trial of 12 weeks is considered adequate to see if long-term maintenance is indicated. Three child patients went from a partial to a complete response to CMI after 500 to 1,000 mg L-tryptophan (QHS) was added to their maintenance dosage. Lithium augmentation has not been tried in the children, although it has been successful in several of our adult patients.

Prediction of Response

There are no agreed on predictors. Thoren et al. (1980) found that patients who responded to CMI had a higher pretreatment concentration of cerebrospinal fluid (CSF) 5-hydroxyindole acetic acid (5-HIAA) and homovanillic acid (HVA) than did nonresponders. Clinical improvement was correlated with a decrease in CSF 5-HIAA.

In children, Flament et al. (1985) found that drug response in the CMI–placebo comparison could not be predicted from any baseline clinical measure, including computed tomography (CT) scan measure of ventricular brain ratio, electroencephalogram (EEG), dexamethasone suppression test, neuropsychological or psycholinguistic measures, age, IQ, mode or age of onset, duration, or severity of illness. Males responded better than females ($p = .05$), and there was a trend for ritualizers as compared to pure obsessionals to do better ($p = .08$). There was one biochemical predictor. Clinical response to CMI *did* correlate significantly with pretreatment platelet serotonin concentration ($p < .001$). A high pretreatment level of platelet serotonin was a strong predictor of a favorable clinical outcome. In the CMI–DMI comparison, the findings were similar: age, sex, severity, duration, coexisting depression, and constellation of obsessive-compulsive symptoms did not predict response.

The literature is mixed as to whether clinical response to CMI correlates with CMI plasma concentration. Insel et al. (1983) found that CMI improvement correlated with plasma level, whereas Thoren et al. (1980) found a *negative* correlation. No correlation was found by Flament et al. (1985) or Flament and Rapoport (1987) between clinical response of her adolescent sample and plasma level of parent or metabolite compound. Thus it seems unlikely that plasma concentration correlates with response. All agree, however, that relatively low values may be efficacious.

Mechanism of Action of Clomipramine

Speculations about the mechanism of action of CMI are based on pre-clinical and clinical studies. Agren et al. (1987) found that CMI did not significantly change the pre- and posttreatment level of HVA, but significantly and dramatically decreased 5-HIAA and 3-methoxy-4-hydroxyphenylglycol (MHPG). Nortriptyline decreased HVA ($p = 0.05$), decreased 5-HIAA ($p = .001$), and decreased MHPG ($p = .0001$). Desipramine did not significantly change HVA (trend for decrease), but did significantly lower 5-HIAA and MHPG ($p < .01$ and $p < .0001$ for 5-HIAA and MHPG, respectively). These changes showing effects of other tricyclics on 5-HIAA therefore do not explain the differential clinical response of obsessive-compulsive patients to CMI and not to DMI and nortriptyline.

However, when comparing the effect of CMI, nortriptyline, and DMI on the HVA–5-HIAA angle, a measure Agren et al. (1987) derived using polar coordinates rather than simple ratio, a dramatic difference is seen between CMI and the others. Clomipramine significantly increased the HVA–5-HIAA angle ($p = .0001$), whereas nortriptyline and DMI had no effect on this measure.

The serotonergic action of CMI appears most likely to be a necessary condition for antiobsessional effect in light of the similar efficacy of other serotonin reuptake blockers (see discussion below). However, Murphy et al. (1985) reinvoked the "shotgun effect," reminding one that different known biochemical target sites of the tricyclics might contribute in differing proportions to their known therapeutic effects in differing disorders. Sites to be kept in mind are muscarinic, beta-adrenergic, alpha-adrenergic, histaminic, serotonergic receptors, and imipramine binding sites.

Despite the serotonergic action appearing a likely candidate, other effects of CMI should be noted. Clomipramine, for example, has a potent antiparasitic effect on protozoan membranes (Zilberstein and Dwyer 1984) and Ca^{++} channel opening (Insel et al. 1985). Its anti-Leishmania and antiphosphorylation effects remain interesting, although unclear if in any way related to clinical efficacy.

In any case, the focus in antidepressant research has moved from a simplistic notion of monoaminergic specificity to conceptualizing the interaction between the more monoamine neuronal systems. Any simplistic notion of dopaminergic overactivity in this disorder is contradicted by the lack of efficacy of antipsychotics in the treatment of OCD. Interestingly, high-dose stimulant medication in an attention deficit disorder population has caused children to become more obsessive-compulsive (Koizumi 1985), and the increased dopaminergic activity may exacerbate obsessive-compulsive symptoms.

Other Serotonin Reuptake Blockers

Zimelidine, a relatively selective bicyclic serotonin (5-HT) reuptake blocker has been useful in one controlled study (Prasad 1984), but not in another (Insel et al. 1985). In any case, zimelidine has since been removed from the market because of a Guillain-Barré-like syndrome associated with its use.

Fluvoxamine, a unicyclic antidepressant, is a selective serotonin reuptake blocker with little or no effect on the noradrenergic system. Perse et al. (in press) found it to be safe and effective in 13 of 16 patients with OCD in a double-blind crossover study. Price et al. (1987) found significant improvement in 6 of 10 patients with OCD in a single-blind placebo-controlled study (Table 4).

Fluoxetine, a bicyclic chemically unrelated to fluvoxamine, is also a selective serotonin uptake inhibitor. Fluoxetine seemed effective for OCD in an open trial (Fontaine and Chouinard 1986) and a single-blind trial (Turner et al. 1985). This is of considerable practical interest because the drug is available in the United States as an antidepressant, while the other better-studied serotonin reuptake blockers are not yet approved. To date, however, fluoxetine has not been used in children.

Antiandrogens

Hormonal manipulation may be effective in the treatment of OCD. Several of the National Institute of Mental Health (NIMH) study sample patients have reported the onset or exacerbation of their OCD symptoms during puberty. In addition, female patients often experience an increase in thoughts and rituals immediately before their menses. Dr. Steven Rasmussen (personal communication, 1988) has collected a series of 20 OCD cases with postpartum onset. These anecdotal reports and speculations about the role of androgenic hormones in receptor formation and sensitivity make the single report of antiandrogen treatment particularly interesting.

Casas et al. (1986) reported a series of six female and one male adult outpatients with obsessive-compulsive symptomatology treated with cyproterone acetate, a potent antiandrogenic agent. The male

Table 4.   Drug treatment of obsessive-compulsive disorder (OCD): controlled trials of other serotonin reuptake blockers

Author	Sample and Diagnosis	Dosage (mg)	Design	Results and Comments
Price et al. 1987	OCD (DSM-III) $N = 10$ age 20–58 yr (mean 35)	fluvoxamine 50–300 274 (mean)	single-blind placebo controlled; placebo (initial 2 wk), then 4 wk fluvoxamine	Significant improvement in 6 of 10 patients. Limitations: did not distinguish between antiobsessional and antidepressant properties.
Perse et al. in press	OCD (DSM-III) $N = 16$ age 18–60 yr (mean 40)	fluvoxamine 50–300	20-wk double-blind crossover; fluvoxamine vs placebo 2-wk placebo, 8-wk placebo or fluvoxamine, 2-wk placebo, 8-wk fluvoxamine or placebo	Fluvoxamine sign better than placebo on OC sx. 13 of 16 improved on fluvoxamine; 9 of 13 showed major improvement.
Turner et al. 1985	OCD (DSM-III) $N = 10$ mean age 30 yr	fluoxetine 20–80	single-blind; placebo initial 2 wk, then fluoxetine next 10 wk	Significant improvement on 5 of 7 self-report obsessive-compulsive scales. Great variation in response (some marked improvement, others had little). The most anxious & depressed patients improved the most. Limitations: single blind, pilot study, small N (2 dropouts)

Note.   DSM-III = *Diagnostic and Statistical Manual of Mental Disorders*, 3rd edition (American Psychiatric Association 1980); OC sx = obsessive-compulsive symptoms.

was symptom-free during his brief antiandrogen trial; the four women with primary OCD were significantly better; the two women with obsessive-compulsive features secondary to psychosis and phobic disorder were unimproved. The trials were brief. The women were given cyclic courses to allow for monthly menses. All women reported that their symptoms returned during their "off" phase and that each reintroduction of cyproterone acetate was somewhat less effective than the previous month. All patients tolerated the medication well and requested that they no longer be cycled. None of the remissions, however, were permanent.

Because of the promising pilot results of Casas et al. (1986), I report ongoing open trials in some detail here for antiandrogen in my child and adolescent subjects. To date, two male patients who had failed CMI therapy trials have been given open trials of spironolactone (a peripheral antiandrogen, specifically antitesterosterone) and testolactone (an antiestrogen, also peripherally effective) (Dr. S. Swedo, personal communication, 1987). One 15-year-old adolescent was midpuberty (Tanner III) when his 10-week trial was initiated. He reported a moderate improvement in his symptoms with no side effects. Although his major ritual of exercising 1 to 2 hours per day was unchanged, he was washing significantly less (5 minutes instead of 1 hour) and was able to sleep in his room for the first time in 2 years.

The second case, an 8-year-old, prepubertal male, entered the antiandrogen trial with frequent, disturbing obsessions and touching rituals. After 1 week on the spironolactone and testolactone, he was symptom-free. His remission lasted approximately 6 months, with gradual recrudescence of obsessive-compulsive symptoms. He was then taken off the antiandrogens and started on a behavior modification program.

The limited success in our NIMH clinic and Casas et al.'s (1986) patients is encouraging. Clearly, antiandrogen treatment for OCD may prove to be a useful adjunct treatment, and a controlled trial should be undertaken.

Are Patients With OCD Different Biochemically at Pretreatment Compared to Controls?

Thoren et al. (1980) studied CSF 5-HIAA, MHPG, and HVA in controls and in patients with OCD pre- and posttreatment of 3 weeks of CMI. There was no difference in the baseline values of HVA, MHPG, and 5-HIAA in the normal controls and in the pretreated patients with OCD.

Peripheral measures of serotonergic and noradrenergic function were compared in 29 children and adolescents with OCD with age- and sex-matched controls (Flament and Rapaport 1987). The pretreatment of patients with OCD did not differ from the controls on measures of platelet serotonin and monoamine oxidase (MAO) activity, nor on plasma epinephrine and norepinephrine concentrations at rest and after orthostatic challenge procedure. Lower platelet serotonin concentration was found in the more severely symptomatic patients.

CSF monoamines were available for 26 adolescent subjects pretreatment. CSF and 5-HIAA correlated negatively with illness baseline severity. The most severely impaired patients had the lowest CSF 5-HIAA (Dr. S. Swedo, personal communications, 1987). This finding is consistent with the peripheral platelet serotonin lower concentration with a more severe illness. However, pretreatment CSF 5-HIAA did not predict drug response, unlike the earlier findings of Thoren et al. (1980) or those of Flament et al. (1987), in the peripheral system.

The "serotonergic hypothesis" of OCD is based primarily on drug response data. Clomipramine's main pharmacological effect in vitro is the selective inhibition of serotonin reuptake into presynaptic nerve terminals (Hamberger and Tuck 1973; Ross and Renyi 1975). Even its major metabolite, desmethylclomipramine, is a relatively potent serotonin reuptake inhibitor (Table 5).

In pediatric samples, as cited above, reduction of platelet serotonin correlated significantly with antiobsessional effect. Moreover, limited experience with lithium and L-tryptophan augmentation for obsessive-compulsive adolescents supports reports of others (Rasmussen 1984), that those agents with presumed increase in serotonergic function augment CMI response. It is beyond the scope of this chapter to review this subject in depth, but the interested reader is referred to other studies of selective agents that further support a serotonergic mechanism of drug action in OCD (e.g., Zohar and Insel, in press).

The short-term efficacy of serotonin uptake inhibitors in OCD leaves a number of important questions. The long-term efficacy of drug treatment, its relative usefulness in comparison with behavior treatment, and the usefulness of CMI (and other serotonin reuptake blockers) in other childhood disorders with stereotypies or repetitive behaviors remain open questions.

The 2- to 5-year prospective follow-up of the first 27 adolescent subjects seen in the NIMH childhood OCD project showed continued pathology in most of the sample (see Chapter 2). However, this group had not been followed actively during the interim period and only 12 subjects received the drug for more than a few months following the initial treatment study. There was no evidence, however, that good responders in the short-term trial had better long-term outcome than

Table 5. Comparative potencies of uptake inhibition of noradrenaline (NA), 5-hydroxytryptamine (5-HT), and dopamine (DA) into synaptosomes in rat brain

Drug	IC_{50} NA uptake (M)	IC 5-HT uptake (M)	IC_{50} DA uptake (M)
Clomipramine	6.8×10^{-6}	5.0×10^{-9}	7.0×10^{-6}
Desmethylclomipramine	2.5×10^{-7}	3.4×10^{-8}	5.3×10^{-6}
Imipramine	4.2×10^{-6}	2.8×10^{-8}	2.4×10^{-5}
Desmethylimipramine	8.5×10^{-6}	3.5×10^{-7}	1.0×10^{-5}

Note. Reproduced with permission from Benfield et al. 1980.

did nonresponders. A second prospective follow-up study is underway with more strenuous follow-up and greater avalability of drug and behavioral treatment as indicated.

More recent work at NIMH with females with trichotillomania (compulsive hair pulling) suggests a close relationship between this condition and OCD. Trichotillomanics are primarily females having childhood onset. For the most part these women do not have other symptoms of OCD. However, they do regard their habit as undesirable, but are unable to stop. Following an open trial, Swedo et al. (in preparation) conducted a double-blind comparison of CMI and DMI with eight trichotillomanic patients, with superiority for CMI in comparison to DMI. It may be that other uncontrollable behaviors (impulse disorder not otherwise classified in DSM-III-R) such as nail biting, kleptomania, or even some of the paraphilias such as cross-dressing (all of childhood onset) will also respond selectively to CMI.

Clomipramine has not been studied systematically in other childhood disorders involving repetitive or stereotyped behaviors except for a small treatment trial with unselected patients with Tourette's syndrome, for whom it was not effective (Caine et al. 1979). The question of CMI efficacy for the subgroup of patients with Tourette's syndrome with severe obsessive-compulsive symptoms remains unanswered.

In summary, CMI treatment of childhood OCD appears to be safe and effective. It seems likely that the other serotonin reuptake blockers would also be useful in a pediatric population, but these have not yet been tried. A number of important questions remain unanswered. This chapter is written only as a beginning of our understanding of the biochemistry and drug treatment of OCD.

References

Agren H, Potter WZ, Nordin C: Antidepressant drug action and CSF monoamine metabolites: new evidence for selective profiles on monoaminergic interactions. Presented at the Sixth Catecholamine Symposium, Jerusalem, 1987

American Psychiatric Association: Diagnostic and Statistical Manual of Mental Disorders, 3rd ed (DSM-III). Washington, DC, American Psychiatric Association, 1980

Ananth J: Treatment of obsessive compulsive neurosis: pharmacological approach. Psychosomatics 17:180–183, 1976

Ananth J, Solyom L, Solyom C, et al: Doxepin in the treatment of obsessive compulsive neurosis. Psychosomatics 16:185–187, 1975

Ananth J, Pecknold JC, Van Den Steen N, et al: Double blind comparative study of clomipramine and amitriptyline in obsessive neurosis. Prog Neuropsychopharmacol 5:257–262, 1981

Benfield DP, Harries CM, Luscombe DK: Some pharmacological aspects of desmethylclomipramine. Postgrad Med J 56:13–18, 1980

Burrell RH, Culpan R, Newton K, et al: Use of bromazepam in obsessional, phobic and related states. Curr Med Res Opin 2:430–436, 1974

Caine E, Polinsky R, Ebert M, et al: Trial of chlomipramine and desimipramine for Gilles de la Tourette Syndrome. Ann Neurol 5:305–307, 1979

Casas ME, Alvarez P, Duro C, et al: Antiandrogenic treatment of obsessive compulsive neurosis. Acta Psychiatr Scand 73:221–222, 1986

Flament MF, Rapoport JL: Biochemical changes during clomipramine treatment of childhood obsessive compulsive disorder. Arch Gen Psychiatry 44:219–225, 1987

Flament MF, Rapoport JL, Murphy DL, et al: Biochemical changes during clomipramine treatment of childhood obsessive compulsive disorder. Arch Gen Psychiatry 42:977–983, 1985

Foa EB, Steketee G, Kozak MJ, et al: Effects of imipramine on depression and obsessive-compulsive symptoms. Psychiatry Res 21:123–136, 1987

Fontaine R, Chouinard G: An open clinical trial of fluoxetine in the treatment of obsessive compulsive disorder. J Clin Psychopharmacol 6:98–101, 1986

Hamberger B, Tuck JR: Effect of tricyclic antidepressants on the uptake of noradrenaline and 5-hydroxytryptamine by rat brain slices incubated in buffer or human plasma. Eur J Clin Pharmacol 229–235, 1973

Hardy J: Obsessive compulsive disorder. Can J Psychiatry 31:290, 1987

Insel TR, Murphy DL, Cohen RM, et al: Obsessive compulsive disorder: a double blind trial of clomipramine and clorgyline. Arch Gen Psychiatry 40:605–612, 1983

Insel TR, Mueller EA, Alterman I, et al: Obsessive compulsive disorder and serotonin: is there a connection? Biol Psychiatry 20:1174–1188, 1985

Isberg RA: A comparison of phenelzine and imipramine in an obsessive compulsive patient. Am J Psychiatry 138:1250–1251, 1981

Jenike MA: Rapid response of severe obsessive compulsive disorder to tranylcypromine. Am J Psychiatry 138:1249–1250, 1981

Ketter T, Chun D, Lu F: Alprazolam in the treatment of compulsive symptoms. J Clin Psychopharmacol 6:59–60, 1986

Klein DF, Rabkin JG, Gorman JM: Etiological and pathophysiological inferences from the pharmacological treatment of anxiety, in Anxiety and the

Anxiety Disorder. Edited by Tuma AH, Maser J. Hillsdale, NJ, Lawrence Erlbaum Associates, 1985

Koizumi H: Obsessive compulsive symptoms following stimulants. Biol Psychiatry 20:1332–1337, 1985

Leonard HL, Swedo S, Rapoport JL, et al: Treatment of childhood obsessive compulsive disorder with clomipramine and desmethylimipramine: a double blind crossover comparison. Psychopharmacol Bull 24:93–95, 1988

Lopez-Ibor JJ: Ensayo clinico de la monochloripramine. Presented at the Fourth World Congress of Psychiatry, Madrid, 1966

Lydiard RB: Obsessive compulsive disorder successfully treated with trazodone. Psychosomatics 27:858–859, 1986

Marks M, Stern RS, Mawsen D, et al: Clomipramine and exposure for obsessive compulsive rituals. Br J Psychiatry 136:1–25, 1980

Mavissakalian M, Turner SM, Michelson L, et al: Tricyclic antidepressant in obsessive compulsive disorder: antiobsessional or antidepressant agents? II. Am J Psychiatry 142:572–576, 1985

Montgomery SA: Clomipramine in obsessional neurosis: a placebo controlled trial. Pharmaceutical Medicine 1:189–192, 1980

Murphy DL, Siever LJ, Insel TR: Therapeutic responses to tricyclic antidepressants and related drugs in non-affective disorder patient populations. Prog Neuropsychopharmacol Biol Psychiatry 9:9–13, 1985

Perse TZ, Greist JH, Jefferson JW, et al: Fluvoxamine treatment of obsessive compulsive disorder. Am J Psychiatry 144:1543–1548, 1987

Prasad A: A double blind study of imipramine versus zimelidine in treatment of obsessive compulsive neurosis. Pharmacopsychiatry 17:61–62, 1984

Prasad A: Efficacy of trazodone as an anti-obsessional agent. Pharmacol Biochem Behav 22:347–348, 1985

Price LH, Goodman WK, Charney DS, et al: Treatment of severe obsessive compulsive disorder with fluvoxamine. Am J Psychiatry 144:1059–1061, 1987

Rasmussen SA: Lithium and tryptophan augmentation in clomipramine-resistant obsessive compulsive disorder. Am J Psychiatry 141:1283–1285, 1984

Ross SB, Renyi AL: Tricyclic antidepressant agent: I: comparison of the inhibition of the uptake of ^{3}H-noradrenaline and ^{14}C-5-hydroxytryptamine in slices of the midbrain-hypothalamus region of the rat. Acta Pharmacol Toxicol (Copenh) 36:395–408, 1975

Stein RS, Marks IM, Mawson D, et al: Clomipramine and exposure for compulsive rituals: II: plasma levels, side effects and outcome. Br J Psychiatry 136:161–166, 1980

Tesar GE, Jenike MA: Alprazolam as treatment for a case of obsessive compulsive disorder. Am J Psychiatry 141:689–690, 1984

Thoren P, Asberg M, Cronholm B, et al: Clomipramine treatment of obsessive compulsive disorder: I: a controlled clinical trial. Arch Gen Psychiatry 37:1281–1285, 1980

Tollefson G: Alprazolam in the treatment of obsessive symptoms. J Clin Psychopharmacol 5:39–42, 1985

Turner SM, Jacob RG, Beidel DC, et al: Fluoxetine treatment of obsessive compulsive disorder. J Clin Psychopharmacol 5:207–212, 1985

Volavka J, Neziroglu F, Yaryura-Tobias JA: Clomipramine and imipramine in obsessive compulsive disorder. Psychiatry Res 14:83–91, 1985

Waxman D: A clinical trial of clomipramine and diazepam in the treatment of phobic and obsessional illness. J Int Med Res 5:99–109, 1977

Yaryura-Tobias JA, Neziroglu F, Bergman L: Clomipramine for obsessive compulsive neurosis: an organic approach. Current Therapeutic Research, Clinical and Experimental 20:541–548, 1976

Zilberstein D, Dwyer DM: Antidepressants cause lethal disruption of membrane function in the human protozoan parasite Leishmania. Science 226:977–979, 1984

Zohar J, Insel TR: Obsessive compulsive disorder: psychobiological approaches to diagnosis, treatment and pathophysiology. Biol Psychiatry 22:667–687, 1987

Zohar J, Insel TR: Drug treatment of obsessive compulsive disorder. Psychol Med, in press

Chapter 14

Families and
Obsessive-Compulsive Disorder

Marge Lenane, M.S.W.

In this chapter, I will summarize my clinical experience with more than 100 families with children who have obsessive-compulsive disorder (OCD). Although they have many reactions in common with families of children with any psychiatric disorder, there are unique features of OCD that particularly trouble those living with its victims. I am increasingly impressed with the high frequency of the disorder in the parents of obsessive-compulsive patients, and the special issues this raises for family therapy. Finally, experience has been gained in the usefulness of patient and family support groups as adjunct treatments for OCD.

Marcus (1977) described different ways that mothers and fathers react to their sick child.

> Typically, the mother is closer to the situation, is more aware of the youngster's disabilities, and feels more responsible. With less direct contact, fathers are confused and often analytical and quasi-objective in their judgments. While mutual support and recognition of the problem is vital, parents struggling by themselves often blame each other for contributing to the problem or argue over the best discipline technique, or in the early stages at least, over whether or not a problem even exists. Parents report stress and tension in the marriage and loss of effectiveness as marital partners. (p. 392)

While the child's pain causes the family sadness, even the most understanding parents can't see why their child can't "just" stop the odd behavior. Some of the family issues are encountered by any family with a psychiatrically disturbed child.

There is also stress from the lack of useful support from the community and extended family. Perhaps more stressful than the negative input from the general public is the criticism and lack of understanding of relatives outside the immediate family. Close enough to the situation to be aware of the problem but too far removed to have a real appreciation, these relatives, usually from good intentions, freely express opinions that contribute to the parents' feeling of guilt and inadequacy. Extended family members sometimes underestimate the significance of the problem, impose their own attitudes and experiences without accounting for the different circumstances, and are usually not available when needed (to follow up or take responsibility for their suggestions). It is usually difficult for the suffering family to reject out of hand this type of advice, especially if given by a respected person. Thus the mother or father feels some obligations to reply and to heed the opinions. Not surprisingly, conflicts arise and relationships are strained.

Specific family stressors from OCD are also engendered by the child's secretiveness and desire to involve the family in the compulsions and obsessions, and from the lack of familiarity of health professionals with this disorder.

Parents may become aware that their child may have OCD only months or years after the problem has begun. Spouses may share their concern and observe the child's behavior for a while before confronting the child; this occurred in about 70 percent of our cases.

Other parents are taken by surprise when their child tells them about his or her behavior and asks for help from the parent. In our series, about 30 percent brought the problem to the parents' attention and asked for help.

A major issue for parents is how to resist being drawn into the child's rituals or obsessive thoughts. A mother of a "checker," for example, began to go around the house nightly with the child, reassuring the child that appliances were turned off and that doors and windows were locked. When the child asked her to put her hand over the empty electrical outlet "just to make sure there are no plugs in it," the parent obliged. Eventually verbal reassurance stopped working, and the mother devised a checklist for checking all the appliances, doors, and windows. At 11 every night, parent and child made a tour of the house, checking off each item. The parent would then sign and date the checklist for the child to take to bed. Because the child would not go to bed until this ritual was performed, the parents stopped going out on weekends or made sure they were home before 11 p.m. Next, the 11 p.m. checking tour was not sufficient to quell the child's anxiety, so the parent would agree to be wakened at 2 a.m. to redo the checking tour. It is not unusual for parents of "washers" to do five times the ordinary amount of laundry or to purchase 10 bars of soap a week. Children with obsessive thoughts may engage parents in fruitless, repetitive discussions related to an obsessive thought, such as the following. Child: "Is the sky blue?" Parent: "Yes, I'm sure it's blue." Child: "Are you sure?" "Yes, I'm sure it's not greenish blue. It is really blue." These discussions can take hours.

We had become accustomed to working with parents who themselves have OCD. The pain of knowing that he had passed the disorder on to his son kept one father from acknowledging his son's illness. I suggested that there could be some benefits to his son in knowing they share the same disorder. He responded "How could I tell him? He looks up to me." I said I was certain that his son would still look up to him and would probably be reassured knowing he wasn't alone. Not surprisingly, the son already knew. Most obsessive-compulsive children of an obsessive-compulsive parent know, without being told, that the parent has OCD or some other problem. Their imagined fears are at least as bad as the reality, and, at least for children who are over 7, disclosure seems helpful. (See Chapter 9 for an illustration of this.)

A family therapist, therefore, assists families with an obsessive-compulsive parent by openly discussing the disorder and its impact on family life. Education about the disorder should be provided, and members given an opportunity to negotiate ways of dealing with the ramifications. Family therapy helped the Carrs from overindulging their 13-year-old son Michael. Mr. Carr had bad memories of his parents' intolerance for his own obsessive-compulsive rituals when he was Michael's age, and he was determined to be more understanding. Unfortunately, the father's extreme indulgence was not helpful. In family therapy, Mr. and Mrs. Carr achieved a balance between overindulgence and intolerance. Michael clearly benefited.

For spouses in a conflictual marriage, the knowledge that a spouse may have transmitted the disorder can be a powerful weapon. Mrs. Himmelhoch used their son's disorder to attack her husband about everything, from "bad genes" to his earning capacity. He couldn't deny his genetic contribution to his son, so Mr. Himmelhoch ended up accepting as valid the rest of his wife's accusations. When the Himmelhochs learned ways of improving their marital relationship, Mr. Himmelhoch's OCD stopped being used as a weapon against him. Some parents with OCD are wonderfully empathic and accepting with their child with OCD and at the same time are more likely than parents without the disorder to set appropriate limits. For example, when Joanie complained to her mother how her OCD would make it impossible for her to get a job, Mrs. Sharp made it clear to Joanie that her (Mrs. Sharp's) OCD hadn't stopped *her* from getting and keeping a job and she expected her daughter to do the same. Joanie got the job.

Other psychiatric disorders were common in parents. Of the parents in our study, 50 percent were given some psychiatric diagnosis. Almost 20 percent of fathers had OCD. Affective disorder, OCD, alcoholism, and general anxiety disorder appeared most often. The siblings of the child with OCD fared better. Only 20 percent of them received a psychiatric diagnosis. However, many of the siblings are quite young; they may, therefore, display more psychiatric problems as they get older.

It is particularly hard for parents of obsessive-compulsive children to accept that their child has serious problems, as so often these youngsters' previous development was normal. They had been regarded as "regular kids" with only the usual minor problems. Some were top basketball players or soccer stars, held class offices, and were voted "most popular" in their class. In addition, when the youngster has concealed the disorder for a long time, parents feel guilty that they hadn't recognized something was wrong. Parents see society as holding them responsible for their child's illness. Society, however, is not the only source of criticism.

Siblings

I am distressed by the impact OCD has on siblings. Siblings complain that they don't get enough attention, time, or love. "Family life is ruined!" they say. Parents, of course, are in the middle.

Normal rivalrous feelings may be exacerbated by the disproportionate time given to the ill sibling. But it is common for siblings to be burdened with caretaking responsibilities and put under pressure to develop a possibly unfair and unrealistic level of tolerance.

In the Hartog family, for example, 14-year-old Claudia's rituals involved daily 2-hour showers in front of her mother so that the mother could reassure Claudia that she had washed enough. When Mrs. Hartog was not free to do this, 15-year-old Daniel was told to take Mrs. Hartog's place, watching Claudia shower for 2 hours. Even though Mr. and Mrs. Hartog knew that Claudia's demands were unreasonable, they urged their son to oblige "just to keep peace." Brother is bewildered and resentful. A less stressful, but also bewildering, situation existed for the Markers. Nine-year-old Kelly Marker demanded that her 6-year-old brother wash his hands for 15 minutes in presurgery fashion before she would allow him to use her toys. Her parents told him to do it rather than face Kelly's tantrums.

Youngsters with OCD are often teased by their siblings, who seem to be both jealous and embarrassed. Just as the children with OCD are teased by their peers for their obsessive-compulsive behavior, so too the siblings are teased by their peers about their brother's or sister's behavior. The 13-year-old brother of one obsessive-compulsive patient denied knowing his brother and begged his parents to send the brother to another school so that he wouldn't be humiliated by the rituals (going back to his locker 20 times to make sure it was locked; repetitive touching of walls). The siblings of a 17-year-old OCD girl teased her cruelly in an attempt to make her "snap out of it."

Sibling support groups are not new; one, for siblings of chronically ill children, was formed in response to continued parental concern for these siblings (Schultz 1984). It was initiated also in recognition of the often-noted "emotional risk" siblings face growing up in a family stressed by chronic illness and in recognition of the limited support services available to them.

We have not yet started a sibling support group, but will be forming one shortly. The group will provide education about OCD and a chance to discuss their frustration, embarrassment, and resentment toward the child with OCD.

Even when the parents know that their child has a "problem" with OCD, professional diagnosis and treatment are still hard to obtain. We see months and years of delay as blind alleys are explored. (See Chapter 8 for a firsthand account of such frustration.)

Some of the parents wondered first whether their child was on drugs, and a drug screen was done. Friends and professionals were consulted; alternative ways of stopping the compulsions were tried. Reasoning, punishment, and, not infrequently, bribery was usually tried and didn't work.

Finding a knowledgeable mental health professional for OCD has been difficult, although the situation is improving. Many have never treated a case. It's not surprising that the pediatricians and school counselors, often the first to be consulted, do not make the diagnosis. More surprisingly, we see youngsters with severe primary OCD who have been evaluated by more than four psychologists and psychiatrists without receiving the proper diagnosis. One child had been evaluated by 18 therapists!

While the family struggles to locate treatment, depression is a common development.

Acts of violence are not uncommon among teenagers with OCD, and these acts are often related to the OCD itself. The children are not violent themselves. The diagnosis of conduct disorder, for example, was made in only 3 of the 63 cases seen as of June 1987. However, 4 of the last 25 children in our study have physically attacked a parent. Attacks ranged from just shoving and punching to pounding a parent's head into a pet food dish before putting the pet food on the parent's head. These physical fights begin inevitably after a parent interrupts a compulsive behavior pattern.

Fear of one's own child has forced several of these uncertain parents to "walk on eggs" around the child to avoid triggering these displays. One boy, age 14, broke the glass shower door with his fist when his father tried forcibly to remove him from the shower. His parents now avoid any interaction that could lead to confrontation regardless of whether it has to do with curfews, cursing at parents, physical fights with siblings, or failing grades at school. These children had not been aggressive previously but now were physically and verbally assaulting their parents.

Most youngsters with this disorder never physically assault family members. But where violence occurs, parents are at a loss how to stop it even though they realize that it is imperative that it be stopped. In such cases, this is a priority goal.

Education about OCD is an important part of family treatment. Our screening interviews include all the adults living in the home as well as noncustodial parents having at least monthly contact with the child. Siblings are evaluated at a later date. These inclusive screenings allow for on-site assessment of family functioning while providing a family education session. Relevant articles are mailed before the initial interview; families don't absorb all the information the first time, and there are many repetitions.

Self-Help Groups

Chesler et al. (1984) described how self-help groups are an important resource for parents of children with any serious and chronic illness.

They provide parents with medical information and identification with others in a like situation, various kinds of social and emotional support, and practical and material assistance. Although the parents sought support and help from a variety of sources and used a broad range of coping strategies, some found the support group to be a unique resource.

Parent support groups are useful in providing a nonthreatening environment in which parents can gain insight. Parents of anorexics, for example, went through a mourning period for their previously held images of well-functioning children and benefited from an arena in which they could talk about their feelings of helplessness, despair, failure, anger, and loss of confidence in their parenting abilities (Lewis and MacGuire 1985).

Self-help groups focus on a specific common problem. Their main mechanism for meeting affective and cognitive needs is interaction among peers, rather than professional influence. They bring together people who empathize, who help the individual to mobilize psychological resources and master emotional burdens, and who provide feedback about an individual's behavior.

We have not been troubled by the heterogeneity of our families. The common concern over their psychiatrically ill children is a unifying force in our quite heterogeneous family support group. Similarly, for a long-term weekly support group run at the Massachusetts Mental Health Center, Grinspoon et al. (1961) found parents' heterogeneity became superficial and unimportant as long as the focus was on the children or parenting.

Not all parents elect to attend the support group. Participants are more likely to have higher educational backgrounds and naturally to live geographically closer to the meeting site. Because our patients are overwhelmingly middle and upper middle class, we have not found a strong class difference between attendees and nonattendees. Personality traits influence participation, and participants are more likely to be open and revealing about issues in general and can reach out and accept support from friends, family, and even strangers during stress.

Not all parents benefit from parent support groups; some parents have a negative impact. Often parents in marginally satisfying marriages will work hard to put forth an image of marital solidarity. However, parents in highly conflicted marriages usually cannot manage that and consequently do not attend support group meetings or attend singly. Rose and Garfinkel (1980) found that parents in fragmented, irrevocably split families do not make good support group candidates due to conflict and decreased motivation.

When a parent tries to monopolize group time in an attempt to meet unmet emotional needs, we have been impressed with the group's ability to limit these attempts. Some support in the form of brief comments in the group setting or more lengthy private comments after the meeting is over can be offered.

Some parent support groups are totally self-directed; others involve varying degrees of professional leadership. Our parents group and young people's group have similar leadership. The leader opens and closes the meeting, summarizes themes, facilitates discussions, and provides a safe and permissive atmosphere. The responsibility for benefiting from the groups rests with the individual parents. Hausman (1974) identified three main categories of leader tasks: (a) helping members to contribute by facilitating discussion and creating a permissive atmosphere; (b) encouraging insight by finding meaning in remarks and clarifying feelings; and (c) preventing things from "getting out of hand" (controlling hostility). Newton's (1985) discussion of "Tough Love" parent groups identifies four major advantages of professional participation: (a) to provide training on specific topics to orient parents; (b) to provide access to more resources in the community; (c) to coordinate treatment with the family's therapist, if necessary; and (d) to increase the group's ability to confront apathy, calm anger, and curb overzealous action by some parents. We have found that, rather than foster dependence, good group leaders could reduce reliance on experts by emphasizing mutual dependence and sharing. I decline to answer parental questions that I think could be answered by other parents, saying, "I wonder whether another parent might know the answer to that, or may have an opinion about that."

I have found, as have leaders of other support groups, great consistency regarding group themes. These common themes include the stigma of mental illness, the impact on other family members, medication, and other treatment options. Our parents at the National Institutes of Health (NIH) study used the group as a way of checking out the "rightness" of their dealings with the obsessive-compulsive youngster. For example, Mr. Framer told the group how he left his son behind when the family went to church because his son had made the family late the previous four Sundays. Several parents applauded Mr. Framer's actions. Another parent asked Mr. Framer about how he had gotten the gumption to leave his son behind. After listening to Mr. Framer's explanation, the other father said, "I think I've been too easy on my child."

Our parents get support from learning that others lose their tempers, say things they've regretted, or have wished their children were out of their lives. Mrs. Solomon said, "I thought I was the worst mother alive until I learned I was responding normally to abnormal behavior." Mr. Fort added, "It was such a relief to learn about people sometimes wish their kids were dead. The group members accepted what I said and didn't make judgments."

In summary, the group process has served (a) to provide an experience in which parents could regain confidence in their problem-solving skills; (b) to provide an arena for decreasing guilt, since guilt is so interruptive and counterproductive to good parenting; (c) to reduce isolation by helping parents share the trauma of their experience; and (d) to receive back understanding, useful feedback, and comfort.

Our parents tended to reject, passively or actively, attempts at "insight" that does not seem to be a useful model for our families.

Parents are receptive to other parents' suggestions for dealing with misbehavior but have not found that looking at family dynamics, which could have contributed to the onset of the particular behavior, to be helpful.

The NIH Family Support Group

During a 1985–1986 follow-up study of former obsessive-compulsive patients, parents were asked for suggestions for our program. The change most frequently recommended was an opportunity to meet with parents of other children with OCD.

Mr. Boris talked of his feelings of isolation.

> The staff of NIH knew what OCD meant but no one else did. For example, when I tried to get some support from my own parents by explaining Ellen's problem to them, they told me I'd always spoiled her and what could I expect but to have a kid who refused to do as she was told! When my wife and I tried to tell the school that Ellen would be missing classes to be treated at NIH, the teachers acted like we'd caused Ellen's problems.

Others voiced similar experiences.

> I felt so alone. Other mothers were talking about their daughters' braces or going to dances while my thoughts were about Jeannie who washed her hands at least 100 times a day and spent more than 6 hours a day doing an hour's worth of homework. My worries were so unlike those of my friends and there was no one I could talk to who would understand.

At first we introduced parents in the clinic waiting room to each other. When possible, we scheduled inpatient admissions of similar youngsters for the same time. The feedback from parents and young people affirmed our belief that they had something to offer one another that no professional could give them: a sense of a shared struggle involving pain, frustration, hope, and sometimes, success.

In September 1986, letters were mailed to all families of young people who had been through the study and who lived within a reasonable distance of NIH. Parents were asked if they were interested in attending a planning meeting and, if so, which day of the week and times were best.

Early Sunday evening was the time most requested. Eight families attended the first meeting; they expressed considerable relief in finally meeting others whose children had OCD. The meeting started promptly at 5 p.m. and ended promptly at 7 p.m. In telephone contacts before the meeting, there were concerns about confidentiality and self-disclosure, so we addressed the issue of confidentiality first. Other rules were: (a) no one has to talk unless they want to talk; (b) a speaker should limit his or her comments to five minutes per issue; and (c) the group will make decisions with regard to frequency, date, and time of meetings. It was decided by mutual agreement that each person would give his or her name, their child's name and age, approximate date of study participation, and the child's main symptoms and present status. My leader tasks included (a) discouraging one-on-one contact with me by avoiding eye contact with the person who was speaking and by modeling eye contact with all group members at a time; (b) summarizing similarities or concerns; (c) suggesting that a questioner ask the group rather than me unless it referred to a research study issue; (d) discouraging side conversations; and (e) following up to see whether a questioner felt he or she had gotten an answer to a question.

Each parent contributed to the discussion. At the end, parents broke up into small groups to follow up on issues raised during the meeting. The feedback from parents at that first meeting about the value of the group was extremely positive.

The rule that no one has to talk until or unless they're ready to do so has relieved the parents who are shy and reticent and would never discuss their concerns with anyone. They have benefited from hearing more outgoing parents talk about how the disorder impacts on their lives. Some parents drive 6 hours each month to the support group. Other parents fly from out of state to attend.

Some results of group participation are quite concrete. Due in part to group feedback, one family followed through on their decision to have their 22-year-old son John move out of the home and into a halfway home. This positive move was not easy for John or his family. The group supported John's parents at the same time that they reinforced John's need for independence.

One single parent was helped to be more forceful in setting limits with his teenage daughter by hearing other parents talk about not letting their children use the disorder to get away with unacceptable behaviors. Another couple realized they had focused too much on their child and not enough on their relationship. Now they make a weekly date with each other.

Others have similarly reported how support-group parents of chronically mentally ill individuals set better limits, effected separations (adult children moved out), resumed activities as a couple, and increased family self-esteem (McLean et al. 1982).

The primary purpose for the NIH support group was neither research nor public relations. However, as several parents expressed interest in educating the public about OCD, they were eventually interviewed by the media, and their stories led to other referrals. Other parents became involved in the legal issues surrounding new drug approval.

The children also benefited from the parents support groups. We found that when parents vented their anger, they were less likely to verbally attack the patient. Acknowledgment of the sadness about the patient's handicap allows the family to then refocus on their child's assets. Reducing guilt decreases parents' tendencies to overprotect and infantalize. Families become less defensive.

At the first parents group meeting, several families requested a concurrent young peoples group.

Mr. Tomaselli described his son Tony's feelings of despair.

> At home Tony was hassled by his younger brother for clogging up toilets and monopolizing the bathroom. At school he was hassled by his peers for "weird" behavior, like pulling his socks on and off 10 times after gym and for going back to his locker 10 times to make sure it was "really" locked. In the neighborhood he was teased for retracing his steps and retouching everything 10 times. Tony told me that *no one* was as crazy as he felt he was and that no one else ever did the things he did. It really would have helped him if he could have talked with even one other kid with OCD.

We had planned to have the parents support group firmly established before starting a patient group but the need was pressing. Because a response to a questionnaire survey was positive, a patient group that met at the same time as the parents group was started and continues to meet. The adolescent groups were first led by a medical student with considerable group experience, then by a pediatrician with some adolescent group experience, and now by a Ph.D. candidate who has worked with the NIH project for 7 years. Participants are from 8 to 22 years of age. They all assume responsibility for running the meeting. The older ones have been very considerate of the younger ones, attempting to draw them out but also respecting their right to be silent. Here, too, the role of the leader is to provide a safe atmosphere, monitor the flow of the meetings, and summarize concerns. The issues discussed most frequently include medicines, dealing with peers in reference to the OCD, and coping strategies.

In the fall we plan to start a siblings group, again in response to parental requests, and anticipate that the primary focus will be educational.

Our parents support group, like other parents groups, identified three main goals for their group participation: (a) educating and updating about recent research, (b) helping in dealing with sibling needs, and (c) setting guidelines for handling obsessive-compulsive behavior. There were no other goals identified, and at least one of these three was voiced by every participant.

In line with the parents' requests, the author gave a presentation at the fourth parents meeting on options for parental response to OCD, the school's role, children's attempts to get parents to participate in the obsessions and compulsions, impact of OCD on siblings, and ways parents can reduce the negative impact. At the fifth parents meeting, a child psychiatrist with the study spoke about recent developments in the treatment of OCD and future research plans.

Parents tell us how the group now fills their need to discuss their children's problems with others having firsthand knowledge of the disorder. Parents give the group regular follow-up on issues raised in earlier sessions. In the last session, Mrs. Greco spoke with pride about her daughter Kim's regular attendance at school. The change in Kim's behavior was partially the result of group suggestions that the family had acted on. Mr. McCarthy joked that his son Kyle should thank the group for being allowed to get his license. (The group had told Mr. McCarthy he was being too protective of Kyle and that he "should loosen up on the boy.")

Lists of parents' names, addresses, and telephone numbers are mailed out to all persons who put their names on the group mailing list. Almost half of the parents have telephone contact between meetings. One mother allows herself one long distance call each week to a different parent. Attendance is very good; at present, the average attendance is 22 at the parent group and 10 at the young people's group.

In summary, the support groups have served an important function in decreasing stress in these families. While drugs and behavior modification are our major treatments, the family support groups will go a long way in preventing lasting harm to marriages and family life.

References

Chesler M, Barbarin O, Lebo-Stein J: Patterns of participation in a self-help group for parents of children with cancer. J Psychosocial Oncology 2:41–64, 1984

Grinspoon L, Courtney PH, Bergen HM: The usefulness of a structured parents' group in rehabilitation, in Mental Patients in Transition. Edited by Greenblatt M, Levinson DJ, Klerman GL. Springfield, IL, Charles C Thomas, 1961

Hausman M: Parents' groups: how group members perceive curative factors. Smith College Studies in Social Work 44:179–198, 1974

Lewis HL, MacGuire MP: Review of a group for parents of anorexics. Psychiatry Res 19:453–458, 1985

Marcus LM: Patterns of coping in families of psychotic children. Am J Orthopsychiatry 47:388–399, 1977

McLean CS, Greer K, Scott J, et al: Group treatment for parents of the adult mentally ill. Hosp Community Psychiatry 33:564–568, 1982

Newton B: Tough Love: help for parents with troubled teenagers—reorganizing the hierarchy in disorganized families. Pediatrics 76:691–694, 1985

Rose J, Garfinkel PE: A parents' group in the management of anorexia nervosa. Can J Psychiatry 25:228–233, 1980

Schultz SK: Use of a support group to aid parental coping with a chronically ill child. Paedovita 1:22–28, 1984

Section VI

Theory and Research

Chapter 15

An Epidemiological Study of Obsessive-Compulsive Disorder in Adolescence

Martine Flament, M.D.
Agnes Whitaker, M.D.
Judith L. Rapoport, M.D.
Mark Davies, M.P.H.
Carol Zaremba Berg, M.A.
David Shaffer, M.D.

Systematic studies have affirmed that from half (Pitres and Regis 1902) to one-third (Black 1974) of adult cases of obsessive-compulsive disorder (OCD) have had their onset by age 15. Moreover, unlike depression and schizophrenia, the disorder in childhood appears in virtually identical form to that seen in adults, as discussed elsewhere in this book (Chapter 2).

The clinical literature describing childhood OCD is meager, but all agree that the disorder presents itself rarely in clinical populations, with a reported incidence of 1 percent in child psychiatric inpatients (Judd 1965) and 0.2 percent of total clinical populations (Hollingsworth et al. 1980). However, recent data suggest that the disorder may be more common. Although no "pure" cases of OCD were described in the survey of more than 2,000 10- and 11-year-olds on the Isle of Wight (Rutter et al. 1970), a total of seven cases were seen with mixed obsessive and anxiety features, giving a prevalence of up to 0.3 percent, depending on how these cases were classified.

In the United States, the recent Epidemiologic Catchment Area (ECA) surveys of adult populations have estimated lifetime prevalence rates of 1 to 2 percent (Karno et al., in press; Robins et al. 1984). The ECA data indicated specifically that OCD is considerably more prevalent in adults than had generally been expected.

The National Institute of Mental Health (NIMH) study of children and adolescents received an unexpectedly large number of referrals from the Baltimore–Washington area alone. Within the first year, referrals totaled considerably more than 1 percent of the area inpatient populations for children and adolescents. About half of the severely impaired patients had never been in treatment and had never been in treatment and had appeared only in response to TV advertisements rather than the usual clinical referral.

Because of our increasing perplexity over the "true" incidence of OCD in adolescence, a two-stage epidemiologic study of a county-wide school population was carried out, the first such study of childhood and adolescent OCD. The study addressed several questions:

1. Is the Leyton Obsessional Interview—Child Version (LOI-CV) (Berg et al. 1986) a useful screening instrument for epidemiological purposes?
2. Are the characteristics of community-derived samples similar to those of referred cases, particularly with regard to demographic, intellectual, and associated medical characteristics?
3. What is the prevalence of OCD in an adolescent population?

The Survey

The general design of the study is described in detail elsewhere (Whitaker et al., in press). Briefly, the study population was the entire 9th- to 12th-grade enrollment in the eight high schools (six public, two independent) of a single semirural county, approximately 80 miles from New York City. This population consisted of 5,596 students, ages 12 to 22.

The study was carried out in two stages. Stage 1 was a population survey, using a self-report questionnaire composed of a variety of mental health screening instruments, and administered in the schools during Fall 1984. Stage 2 consisted of semistructured clinical interviews administered to a stratified sample of students. Strata were defined by scores from scales used to assess symptoms of obsessive-compulsive, depressive, panic, and eating disorder.

Stage 1: The Adolescent Health Behaviors Study

In October 1984, all students enrolled in the eight county high schools, were asked to complete a questionnaire regarding "health and behavior, including eating habits, in people your age." The questionnaire was administered in supervised classrooms, with 45 to 50 minutes' completion time. Absentees in six of the eight schools were given the questionnaire within 3 weeks of the survey date.

The questionnaire was a composite screening instrument designed for the study. To assess obsessive-compulsive pathology, we used a shortened form (20-item) of the LOI-CV (see Chapter 5). The LOI-CV asks for presence or absence of a number of preoccupations and behaviors (summed up in the "yes score") as well as, for each positive answer, a rating of interference in personal functioning (all added for the "interference score"). The LOI-CV assesses current symptomatology.

Along with the LOI-CV, the entire questionnaire included the Eating Symptoms Inventory (Whitaker et al., in press); the Eating Attitudes Test (Garner et al. 1982); the Beck Depression Inventory (Beck et al. 1961), whose time frame was extended to "the past few weeks"; items developed by the investigators to assess anxiety; and items from the Framingham and Tacoma scales for Type A behavior (Siegel et al. 1981). Other items elicited sociodemographic characteristics, school attendance and grades, and personal and family health.

Stage 2: Clinical Interviews

A semistructured clinical interview was designed for the study, using parts of existing standard diagnostic instruments to which were added questions specific to the areas of eating, obsessive-compulsive, and anxiety disorders.

Obsessive-compulsive pathology was assessed with the OCD section of the Diagnostic Interview for Children and Adolescents (DICA) (Herjanic and Campbell 1977), the Addendum for Compulsive Personality Disorder from the Interview Schedule for Children (Kovacs, unpublished), and a few additional questions regarding checking habits, tics, and extracurricular activities. The other sections of the interview included: the Eating Symptoms Interview (Whitaker et al., in press), the Columbia Clinical Interview (Shaffer et al., in preparation), and the Adolescent Panic Attack Interview (Kalikow, unpublished). From the DICA (Herjanic and Campbell 1977), demographic and sociofamilial information and psychosocial stressors were obtained. A mental status examination was conducted and a brief medical history was obtained. In addition, all students filled out the Achenbach Youth Self Report (Achenbach and Edelbrock 1979) and, in two schools, the Beck Depression Inventory (Beck et al. 1961) regarding the past few weeks. The clinician rated the child on the Children's Global Assessment Scale (GAS) (Shaffer et al. 1983), which assesses the child's most impaired level of general functioning on a continuum from 0 to 100.

The interviewers were 13 trained clinicians (5 child psychiatrists, 2 child psychiatry fellows, 3 psychologists, 2 social workers, and 1 registered nurse), all with extensive clinical experience with adolescents. Of those students positive on the obsessive-compulsive screen, 70 percent were interviewed by the NIMH team. Written consent for the interview had been obtained from each subject's parents. The interviews were conducted in the schools or occasionally at home on the parents' request, and were about 75 minutes in duration. All students were interviewed during Winter 1984 or Spring 1985.

Diagnosis

Based on the interviews, all cases were written up with brief clinical vignettes, and provisional multiaxial DSM-III (American Psychiatric Association 1980) diagnoses were given by the interviewer. The cases were then reviewed blind by other teams of clinicians, and differences were resolved by consensus.

The interviews allowed for current as well as lifetime diagnosis of OCD. For compulsive-personality disorder, we used the DSM-III criteria of constant (lifelong) patterns of rigidity, stubborness, indecisiveness, and preoccupation with details.

We were not prepared for the high frequency of a phenomenon we labeled "subclinical OCD," or "obsessional features" because it defied other classification. In numerous instances, we noted one or two obsessive or compulsive symptoms that had a definite date of onset and that did not appear developmentally continuous, or accountable by situation or personality, and that occurred in subjects who did not meet full criteria for OCD (or another disorder). One example is a 16-year-old girl with a 1-year history of washing the walls of her room for 3 hours each week; in this case there was not significant interference with her life, but the behavior had commenced quite suddenly and was regarded as undesirable by the girl and her family. Other instances were mild but senseless straightening or cleaning rituals, infrequent but ego-dystonic obsessive thoughts, and so on.

In other cases, clear obsessive-compulsive symptoms appeared to be part of the clinical picture of a psychiatric disorder other than OCD. All "interview" vignettes were typed in narrative form shortly after the interview was completed.

Using this diagnostic classification, a very high agreement for OCD, compulsive personality, or subclinical obsessive-compulsive "feature" was obtained between interviews: on 81 cases, reviewed independently by two clinicians, the kappa value was .85 ($p < .0001$).

Data Management and Statistical Analysis

All Stage 1 and Stage 2 data were computerized, and descriptive statistics were obtained for the population. Stage 2 sampling followed a stratified design.

Comparisons between different groups of students were obtained by chi-square test statistics, Yates corrected for discrete characteristics, and by analysis of variance for measures that were assumed to be approximately gaussian in distribution.

Results

Stage 1

From the 5,596 adolescents enrolled in the eight county high schools in October 1984, 5,108 (91 percent) returned valid questionnaires. Completion rates by school ranged from 81 to 97 percent. Students not represented in the survey results include 203 absentees who did not complete the questionnaire within 3 weeks of the survey (4 percent), 35 refusers (1 percent), 35 learning-disabled students who were considered unable to participate by the school administration (1 percent), 51 pranksters who gave responses that were inappropriate or humorous (1 percent), and 164 students not officially listed as absent but not present in class (3 percent). In addition to these students who did not complete or return the questionnaire, 557 subjects (10 percent) had 50 percent or more of the answers missing on the LOI-CV and were excluded from subsequent sampling on the basis of this screen. Thus the total number of students who completed the LOI-CV was 4,551, a valid completion rate of 81.3 percent.

The sociodemographic characteristics of the survey population of 5,108 have been described in detail elsewhere (Whitaker et al., submitted). Briefly, there were 2,564 boys (50.2 percent) and 2,544 girls (49.8 percent), evenly distributed (24 to 26 percent) across grades 9 through 12. They ranged in age from 12 to 22 years, the four major age groups being 14 years old (20 percent), 15 years old (25 percent), 16 years old (24 percent), and 17 years old (23 percent). The majority of the students were white (94 percent), 2 percent were black, and 4 percent were from other ethnic groups.

Most students were Catholic (43 percent) or Protestant (37 percent); 2 percent were Jewish, 9 percent were another religion, and 9 percent reported no religious affiliation. The distribution of the survey population on the Hollingshead-Redlich four-factor index of social status (Hollingshead and Redlich 1958) was class V, 5 percent; class IV, 15 percent; class III, 24 percent; class II, 37 percent; class I, 20 percent.

The frequency distribution of LOI-CV scores are shown in Figure 1 (see Chapter 5).

Stage 2 Sampling

We selected for Stage 2, subjects having the highest yes and interference scores. Cutoff scores were derived from our previous clinical study (Berg et al. 1986), with which the 20-item LOI-CV could have

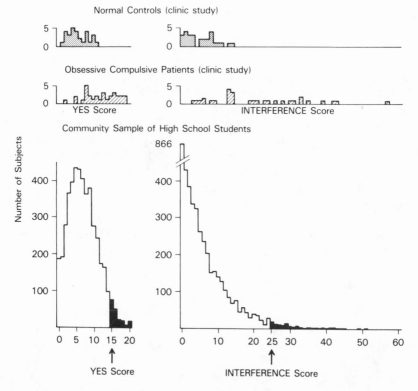

Figure 1. Frequency distribution of responses to the Leyton Obsessional Inventory—Child Version in a clinic study of 30 obsessive-compulsive patients, 28 normal controls, and a community sample of 4,551 unselected high school students.

best differentiated 30 obsessive-compulsive adolescents from 28 age- and sex-matched normal controls on the yes score ($p < .0001$) and the interference score ($p < .0001$).

These cutoff scores for Stage 2 sampling were chosen to be in the range suggestive of psychopathology and to yield a subsample of the population of appropriate size for clinical evaluation: 15 or more for the yes score and 25 or more for interference (Figure 1). These values were much above those obtained by any normal control in our previous study, but also above scores of more than half of the patients, a major methodologic problem in the identification of this disorder.

In our experience, the interference score had been the best indicator of psychopathology, but we were also interested in the possibility of selecting "healthy" or even "supernormal" individuals with noninterfering, ego-syntonic obsessional features. We therefore defined for Stage 2 clinical evaluation two distinct groups of subjects "positive" on the obsessive-compulsive screen. The first group, called the "High Yes/Low Interference" group (shortened to "High Yes") consisted of all subjects with a yes score of 15 or more but an interference score of 10 or less. The second group, termed here the "High Interference" group, included all the subjects with an interference score of 25 or more regardless of the yes score. It should be noted that subjects with a high yes score (≥ 15) but an interference score in the medium range (between 10 and 25) are not represented in this sampling design (i.e., are considered "negative" on the obsessive-compulsive screen).

As presented on Table 1, 35 subjects (10.7 percent) were selected from Stage 1 into the High Yes category, and 81 (1.6 percent) into the High Interference group. Thus the total number of students positive on either obsessive-compulsive screen was 116, 2.3 percent of the total

Table 1. Sampling and completion rate for Stage 2 clinical evaluation

Screening Status	No. of Subjects Selected	% of Population Studied	No. of Subjects Interviewed	% of Subjects Selected
High yes/low interference	35	0.7	26	74.3
High interference	81	1.6	67	82.7
Either positive obsessive- compulsive screen	116	2.3	93	80.2
"Other positive screens" control group	253	5.0	188	74.3
"Negative screens" control group	99	1.9	75	75.8
Total	468	9.2	356	76.1

population surveyed. Of this group, 49 scored positive only on the obsessive-compulsive screen, whereas 67 also scored positive on one or more of the other screens.

The other groups of subjects selected for clinical evaluation were a "negative screen" control group of 99 students (1.9 percent of the total population), randomly selected from subjects scoring negative on all Stage 1 screens, and "other positive screen" comparison groups consisting of subjects positive on one or more of the other screens (e.g., the depression screen, the eating disorders screen, and the panic disorder screen). Selection and evaluation of the latter groups are described elsewhere (Whitaker et al., in preparation). For this report, they provide a large "positive screen" comparison group of 253 subjects (5 percent) to contrast with the positive obsessive-compulsive screen samples. A total of 468 students was selected for Stage 2 clinical evaluation.

Stage 2 Completion

Diagnostic interviews were administered between January and August 1985 by the clinician team, which was blind to each subject's screening status. As shown in Table 1, the completion rate was 82.7 percent for the High Interference group and 74.3 percent for the High Yes group, overall 80.2 percent (either positive obsessive-compulsive screen), slightly higher than the 75.8 percent completion rate obtained in the negative screen control group and the 74.3 percent in the positive screen control group.

In the positive obsessive-compulsive screen samples, 84 of the students (90 percent) were interviewed in their school of attendance and 9 (10 percent) during home visits. The 23 subjects not interviewed included 16 who declined the interview, 2 who moved away and could not be located, and 5 who could not be identified from Stage 1.

Stage 2 Results

The psychiatric diagnoses given by the clinicans to subjects interviewed in Stage 2 are summarized in Table 2. In the positive obsessive-compulsive screen groups (combined), 14 subjects received a DSM-III diagnosis of OCD and 6 of compulsive personality disorder. Nine had what we termed "subclinical OCD" or "obsessional features": most frequently cleaning or straightening rituals, in other cases hand washing, "doing things a certain way," checking rituals, or obsessive thoughts. Eleven subjects reported some obsessive or compulsive symptoms associated with a disorder other than OCD—an anxiety

Table 2. Clinical diagnoses given to subjects in the four groups derived from a screening questionnaire of 5,108 high school students

Clinical Diagnosis (Stage 2)	Screening Status (Stage 1)				
	High Interference[a] (N = 67)	High Yes[a] (N = 26)	"Other Positive Screens" Controls (N = 188)	"Negative Screens" Controls (N = 75)	Total Interviewed (N = 356)
OCD	12	2	4[b]	0	18
Compulsive personality disorder	4	2	4[c]	1	11
Subclinical OCD	7	2	4	1	14
Other psychiatric disorders with obsessive-compulsive features	9	2	5	0	16
Other psychiatric disorders (no obsessive-compulsive symptoms)	12	2	46	9	69
No diagnosis	23	16	125	64	228

Note. First column indicates the current diagnosis only.

[a] Refers to the yes score and interference score on the Leyton Obsessional Inventory—Child Version.

[b] Two had onset of OCD since initial survey; one had yes = 20, interference missing; one had yes = 15, interference = 17.

[c] One had yes and interference missing.

disorder for 6 of them, major depression for 3, borderline intellectual functioning for 1, and atypical psychosis for 1.

Fourteen subjects who had scored positive on the obsessive-compulsive screen revealed no salient obsessive-compulsive symptoms during the interview but received a variety of other psychiatric diagnoses: depressive disorders (6 cases), anxiety disorders (5 cases), bulimia (2 cases), borderline intellectual functioning (2 cases), conduct disorder (1 case), and chronic motor tic disorder (1 case). Finally, 39 adolescents with either High Yes or High Interference on the LOI-CV received no psychiatric diagnosis.

In the negative screen control group, no one had a diagnosis of OCD and only one subject received a diagnosis of compulsive personality disorder. In the positive screen control group (subjects with posi-

Table 3. Clinical characteristics of 20 OCD cases identified in the epidemiological study of a high school student population (N = 5,108)

Age	Sex	Main Symptoms		Duration of Disorder (by age)	Other Disorders	LOI-CV Scores			Other Positive Screens
		Obsessions	Compulsions			GAS	Yes	Interference	
16	M	thoughts of mousetraps and flypaper	checking	13–current	overanxious disorder	70	17	51	depression, panic
18	M	thoughts of an accident		8–9 and 16–current	none	90	16	3	
15	M	fear of contamination	washing	13–current	ADD–residual type, history of 1 panic attack	70	18	40	
14	M		cleaning, checking things "just right"	12–current	ADD–residual type, compulsive personality disorder		16	36	depression
14	M	fear of contamination	cleaning, checking	9–current	none	81	15	17	eating
14	M		washing, straightening	7–current	none	72	14	27	
17	M		washing, cleaning, straightening, slowness	15–current	compulsive personality disorder	68	14	37	
16	F		hand washing, redoing papers	13–current	overanxious disorder, bulimia	50	14	30	eating, depression
16	M	fear of hurting other people	closing/opening drawers, straightening, checking	7–current	dysthymic disorder, history of 1 panic attack	80	15	0	
16	F		hand washing	15–current	bulimia, major depression	60	19	38	eating, depression, panic
16	M	thoughts of hurting other people	hand washing, checking	14–current	major depression, overanxious disorder, compulsive personality disorder	57	15	28	eating, depression

18	F	thoughts of hurting other people	hand washing, cleaning, straightening	18[b]–current	bulimia, major depression	50	8	6	eating
16	F	fear of contamination	hand washing, cleaning, straightening things "just right"	16[b]–current		50			depression
17	M		cleaning, checking, straightening	14–current	past separation anxiety disorder (age 3–12)	81	15	27	
16	F	fear of contamination	hand washing, avoiding touching, checking, straightening, rereading	15–current	none	65	20		eating, depression
17	F	thoughts of hurting self or others	washing, cleaning	13–current	2 past episodes of adjustment disorder with depressed mood	75	16	27	
17	F		hand washing, checking	13–current	phobia of strangers, history of 1 panic attack	61	9	25	
18	M	thoughts of getting hurt, fear of contamination	things "just right," cleaning	15–current	simple phobias (ladders; tarantulas)	75	16	31	
18	F	fear of contamination	hand washing	10–11	bulimia, major depression	9	13	16	eating, depression
15	F	fear of contamination	hand washing	13–13	overanxious disorder, atypical eating disorder, subclinical panic attacks	9	12	23	eating, depression, panic

Note. GAS = Children's Global Assessment Scale; LOI-CV = Leyton Obsessional Inventory—Child Version; ADD = attention deficit disorder.
[a] From initial survey questionnaire.
[b] Symptoms developed after the survey.

tive screen for other disorders), two adolescents had histories of OCD in the past and currently met criteria for other disorders (see Table 3), whereas four had a current diagnosis of OCD. Among those four, two had had onset of their disorder since the initial screening had taken place.

Three cases had had a yes score on screening of 20 (maximum score) but had not completed the inteference questions. The fourth case had a high yes score (15) but an interference score of 17 (too low to be selected in the High Interference group but too high for inclusion in the High Yes group).

Cases of Obsessive-Compulsive Disorder

Thus a total of 18 current cases of OCD were found among the 356 adolescents interviewed in Stage 2, 0.35 percent of the population surveyed in Stage 1 ($N = 5,108$). In addition, 2 subjects had histories of past episodes of OCD. From these data, we estimate a minimum figure of 0.35 percent for the point-prevalence rate of OCD in the adolescent population and a minimum figure of 0.40 percent for its lifetime prevalence rate.

The main clinical characteristics of these cases identified in the community survey are shown in Table 3. Of the 20, 11 were males. Their mean age was 16.2 years (range, 14 to 18), compared to a mean ($\pm$SD) age of 15.6 $\pm$ 1.4 years in the whole population. The onset age varied from 7 to 18 years (mean, 12.8), onset was most often gradual, but sudden in some cases. One boy had had an early episode of obsessions (age 8 to 9) followed by remission until age 16. Although duration of the disorder ranged from ½ to 7 years, only 4 subjects had ever been in treatment, 2 of whom for associated depression or anxiety. Only one boy had obsessions solely (intrusive thoughts of having a ski accident). All the other subjects had compulsive rituals, usually also related to obsessive thoughts (e.g., fear of contamination, fear of hurting self or others). Of those who feared hurting self or others, one specified fear of hurting parents, one fear of hurting neighbors, and another fear of hurting children. The most common rituals were washing and cleaning rituals, followed by compulsive checking and straightening. One boy had the compulsion to repeat his actions and another had primary obsessional slowness. As seen on Table 3, 15 of the 20 adolescents with OCD had one or more other lifetime concurrent psychiatric diagnosis (10, currently), most frequently major depressive disorder, bulimia, or overanxious disorder. Two would have also met criteria for compulsive personality disorder. Four students (1 male) had been in treatment at some time.

Demographics of Cases

OCD cases did not differ from the sample as a whole in terms of family constellation, social, race, religious affiliation, grade point average, medical history, or past head injury. More specifically, our cases were *not* more likely to be Catholic than Protestant (see Chapter 18), and their grades were not higher than average.

Our screening procedure had yielded very few false negative cases but a large number of false positives. Using a cutoff interference score of 25 or more (the High Interference group), the sensitivity of the instrument for OCD was 75 percent (12/16 cases), its specificity 84 percent, but its positive predictive value only 18 percent. Using a selection criterion of a yes score of 15 or more (High Interference and High Yes/Low Interference groups combined), the sensitivity increased to 100 percent, the specificity was 77 percent, and the predictive value 17 percent. Although the LOI-CV was not designed to identify compulsive personality disorder, the broader selection criterion (yes score $\geq$ 15) gave to the instrument a sensitivity for compulsive personality disorder of 55 percent. Moreover, its parent scale, the LOI, was not designed to discriminate between disorder and personality, and, in fact, was used for personality assessment (Cooper 1970). The obsessive-compulsive screen proved crucial for case finding; one of the other screens in this study identified only about half of the total cases of OCD.

Discussion

This is the first study of the frequency of OCD in an adolescent population. The minimal figure we obtained, of .35 percent of an unselected population, while much greater than any previous estimates, is probably still very minimal. There are four reasons why we believe the true rate to be much higher. First, the sample was school-based, and children with the most severe forms of the disorder would not be in school. Second, the 557 cases not completing the questionnaire would, based on our clinical experience, be likely to contain a higher than chance proportion of subjects with obsessive-compulsive symptomatology. Third, the 20-item screening LOI-CV used in this study, while the most successful instrument of its kind to date, would undoubtedly produce a number of false negative scores. The reason for this is that, again, in our clinical experience, up to 50 percent of referred patients with OCD have a few albeit severe symptoms, thus generating a relatively low yes score on which the interference score is based. Finally, the secretiveness and denial associated with the disorder would lead to under-reporting of both yes and particularly of interference items in the LOI-CV. Based on all of the considerations, the true prevalence is probably closer to .70 percent.

The subgroup of children termed "obsessional features" or "subclinical" OCD was particularly intriguing. These children did not meet criteria for obsessional personality nor did they, for the most part, show tendencies in this direction. Their symptoms appeared discreet, often with specific date of onset, and they adapted their lives around it without interference. However, the behavior appeared so discontinuous from their other patterns, and they were so aware of it when it began, that a de novo pathological process is postulated. Follow-up of this group will be most pertinent, and such a study is underway.

The equal male/female ratio in diagnosed cases differed from the male preponderance of clinical sample seen at the National Institutes of Health. This may reflect referral bias, or be related to differential severity, with female cases less often requiring clinical attention.

We identified 11 cases meeting criteria for compulsive personality disorder. While the diagnosis is not intended for subjects under 18, the interviewers had little doubt about the appropriateness of the diagnoses in these cases. Follow-up will shed light on the validity of compulsive-personality disorder in adolescence and on its relation to OCD.

These findings have major implications for mental health practice. Our prospective follow-up data indicate a poor prognosis for clinically referred adolescents with OCD (see Chapter 2). This unexpected high frequency of adolescent cases tells us that there may be as many as 200,000 children and adolescents in this country suffering from this disorder. With the recognition of effective treatments (Flament et al. 1985; Chapters 11–14), more aggressive case finding is indicated.

References

Achenbach T, Edelbrock C: The Child Behavior Profile: II: boys aged 12-16 and girls aged 6-11 and 12-16. J Consult Clin Psychol 47:223–233, 1979

American Psychiatric Association: Diagnostic and Statistical Manual of Mental Disorders, 3rd ed (DSM-III). Washington, DC, American Psychiatric Association, 1980

Beck A, Ward CH, Mendelson M, et al: The Beck Depression Inventory. Arch Gen Psychiatry 4:561–571, 1961

Berg CJ, Rapoport JL, Flament M: The Leyton Obsessional Inventory—Child Version. J Am Acad Child Psychiatry 25:84–91, 1986

Black A: The natural history of obsessional neurosis, in Obsessional States. Edited by Beech HR. London, Methuen, 1974

Cooper J: The Leyton Obsessional Inventory. Psychol Med 1:48–64, 1970

Flament M, Rapoport JL, Berg CJ, et al: Clomipramine treatment of childhood obsessive compulsive disorder: a double-blind controlled study. Arch Gen Psychiatry 42:977–983, 1985

Garner DM, Olmsted MP, Bohr Y, et al: The Eating Attitudes Test: psychometric features and clinical correlates. Psychol Med 10:647–656, 1982

Herjanic B, Campbell W: Differentiating psychiatrically disturbed children on the basis of a structured psychiatric interview. J Abnorm Child Psychol 5:127–135, 1977

Hollingshead A, Redlich F: Social Class and Mental Illness: A Community Survey. New York, John Wiley & Sons, 1958

Hollingsworth CE, Tanguay PE, Grossman L, et al: Long-term outcome of obsessive-compulsive disorder in childhood. J Am Acad Child Psychiatry 19:134–144, 1980

Judd LL: Obsessive compulsive neurosis in children. Arch Gen Psychiatry 12:136–143, 1965

Karno M, Golding J, Sorenson S, et al: The epidemiology of obsessive compulsive disorder in five U.S. communities. Arch Gen Psychiatry (in press)

Pitres A, Regis E: Les Obsessions et Les Impulsions. Paris, Doin, 1902

Robins LN, Helzer JE, Weissman MM, et al: Lifetime prevalence of specific psychiatric disorders in three sites. Arch Gen Psychiatry 41:949–958, 1984

Rutter M, Tizard J, Whitmore K: Education, Health and Behavior. London, Longmans, 1970

Shaffer D, Gould M, Brasic J, et al: The Children's Global Assessment Scale. Arch Gen Psychiatry 49:1228–1231, 1983

Siegel JM, Matthews KA, Leitch CJ: Validation of the Type A interview assessment of adolescents: a multidimensional approach. Psychosom Med 43:311–321, 1981

Whitaker A, Davies M, Shaffer D, et al: The struggle to be thin: a survey of anorectic and bulimic symptoms in a nonreferred adolescent population. Psychol Med (in press)

Chapter 16

Rituals and Releasers: An Ethological Model of Obsessive-Compulsive Disorder

Susan E. Swedo, M.D.

Ethology, founded by Whitman and Heinroth in the late 1800s and brought to recognition by Lorenz in the 1930s, is devoted to the investigation and comparison of animal behaviors. Konrad Lorenz dubbed himself and other ethologists as "starers-at-animals," which unassumingly summarizes the ethologist's role of naturalistic observation without interpretation (Lorenz 1970a, 1970b).

Ethologists scrutinize the similarities and differences in behavior across genus and species, trace the development of behavior by phylogenetic and ontogenetic studies, and attempt to assign meaning and function to consistently observed behaviors (Hess 1965).

Neuroethologists pursue the relationships between behavior and brain locus and neurochemical changes, and examine effects of hormones and neurotransmitters on observed behaviors. We have turned to these disciplines for possible models of the seemingly useless ritualized behaviors of the obsessive-compulsive patient. For many, obsessional rituals are well executed but misplaced or mis-timed "normal" human behaviors, and most bear some similarity to functional animal behaviors. For example, besieged obsessive-compulsive washers spend hours scrubbing their hands in a meticulous, stylized manner, while rats stressed with adrenocorticotropic hormone (ACTH) repeti-

269

tively scrub face, paws, and anogenital region in a predictable, invari-
ate pattern. Similarly, obsessive patients with hoarding rituals collect
mounds of materials that are then carefully arranged, much as a
mother bird collects materials for a nest or a chipmunk squirrels away
foodstuffs.

Lorenz (1937) discriminated two criteria that best defined the
concept of "inherited drives of fixed behavior." These were that the
pattern occurs in nearly all members of a species and that animals
reared in isolation would still exhibit the pattern. In addition to the
ethologically meaningful content of the rituals (grooming, protection
from danger), the uniformity of behaviors in obsessive-compulsive
disorder (OCD) and their emergence in childhood in patients having no
models whatsoever first brought an ethological model to mind.

In this review, analogies between specific animal behaviors and
common compulsive rituals are considered (i.e., grooming and washing, nesting and ordering, hoarding by animals and obsessive patients,
stereotypies and repeating rituals, and courtship dances and repetitive movement sequences). To link this with other biological analogies
to OCD (see Chapter 19), mediating mechanisms are discussed, based
on neuroethological data and preliminary clinical studies.

Ethology is the study of behavior or "patterns in time" (Eibl-
Eibesfeldt 1970). The investigations of behavior deal with sequences
that are not always completely visible. To compare interobserver findings, the observation of behavior has been divided into four categories:
(a) the manner in which an organism becomes sensitive to certain
physical, biotic, and social factors as key stimuli; (b) the means by
which these stimuli are presented and integrated into the brain; (c)
what changes in the organism's internal state are affected by the
environmental stimuli; and (d) how the internal milieu's changes influence the interaction of the organism with its environment (Ingle and
Crews 1985).

Ethologists primarily study the natural stimuli that elicit biologically important behaviors, the spatiotemporal structure of ensuing
action patterns, and the motivational, developmental, and physiological conditions that determine which response is likely to be elicited by
a given stimulus (Ingle and Crews 1985).

Definition of Terms

Innate or instinctual response patterns can be thought of in terms of a
complex reflex arc in which external and internal stimuli are received
and integrated to result in an efferent response. Ethologists generally
agree with this simplification, but point out that not all responses are
due to an afferent signal. In some instances, the response is spontane-

ous; in others, the expressed behavior is the result of disinhibition of an inner constant state by removal of an inhibitory control. For example, removal of the supra- and subesophageal ganglia in the praying mantis disinhibits the mating and locomotor behaviors, which then occur continuously. Normally, releasing stimuli are required for expression, and the two behaviors are mutually exclusive (Eibl-Eibesfeld 1970).

The basic unit for ethological observations is the fixed-action pattern, an inborn, internally coordinated sequence, that merely requires a releasing stimulus for actualization. Innate behavior patterns may be fully functional at the time of hatching or birth, such as the pecking, scratching, and drinking of the newly hatched chick. A young duckling will dive, feed below the water's surface, and oil its feathers, whether or not models are available. Other inborn behavior patterns, such as courting and mothering, require maturity for expression but are still innately determined.

Fixed-action patterns, once initiated, continue to completion whether appropriate or not. For example, a dog's turning in circles before lying down was historically necessary to trample the grass in preparation for a bed, but the modern dog performs this circling whether sleeping outdoors or on a thin living room rug. Similarly squirrels, even those living in wire mesh cages, when given excess food search for a vertical structure, deposit the nuts, push them into a corner, and make covering and tamping-down movements. The entire sequence is preprogrammed and "runs," once released, from start to finish, independent of what is happening around them.

Fixed-action patterns such as these are usually accompanied by orienting movements or taxis that, although inborn, are dependent on external stimuli. For example, the egg-rolling movements of the graylag goose consist of a fixed-action pattern—the pulling in of the egg (which continues even if the egg is removed), orienting movements (taxis), and lateral balancing movements of the neck—which *cease* when the egg is removed (Lorenz 1970b). Fixed-action patterns are like the engine of a car, which, once started, will continue; taxis are like the steering, requiring continued external stimulation.

Initiating stimuli can be innate or learned. Innate-releasing mechanisms (IRMs) become effective without any explicit learning. For example, a frog's tongue thrusting at moving forms is an innate prey-catching behavior, but experience and learning are required to limit the thrusting motions toward small, rapidly moving objects, which are usually insects and food.

An animal's responsivity to key stimuli requires the appropriate state or drive. The state or drive, in turn, is influenced by internal and external factors. Other reactions can compete; for example, flight can overcome hunger, satiety, and hormonal influences.

Thirst and hunger are other examples of drive states that can define a response. For example, a thirsty cat reacts to water but not food. Internal as well as external milieu influence drive states. Sex hormones produce an aroused state that promotes the fixed-action pattern of courting and mating if the appropriate releasing stimulus (an eligible partner) is present.

Figure 1 summarizes this ethological definition of behavior. The *automaticity* of the fixed-action pattern is of major importance for our obsessive-compulsive perspective (i.e., the way the fixed-action pattern continues once it starts even when the behavior is inappropriate).

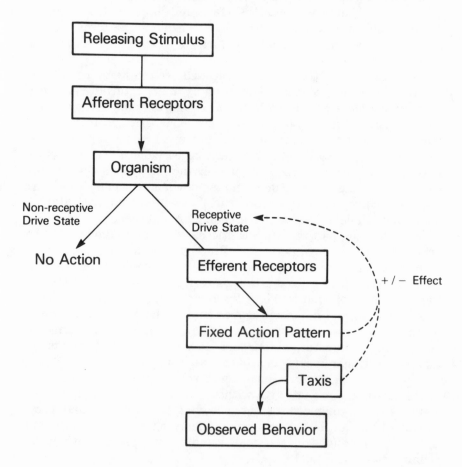

Figure 1. An ethological model of behavior.

Ethology: A Possible Model for Obsessive-Compulsive Disorder

Obsessive-compulsive rituals can be viewed as inappropriately released fixed-action patterns. Our work with more than 200 children and adults has led us increasingly to view OCD in this fashion. For example, obsessive patients, who check and recheck that the coffee pot is unplugged, all seem to perform each checking pattern in an identical fashion. Their behavior is perfect in form, but after the first check, it is ineffectual and inappropriate. To follow an ethological model, one must, of course, ask: what is the releasing stimulus in OCD? Is it internal (e.g., chemical) or external (e.g., environmental stress). How does it effect the release of the ritualized fixed-action pattern?

The washing of an obsessive-compulsive washer, our most typical behavior (see Chapter 2), is highly ritualized and specific. One young man, like dozens of others, spends hours in the shower, first stroking the right side of his head eight times, applying shampoo, then stroking another eight times, rinsing for eight counts, and finally stroking a last eight times. He repeats this entire routine for the top, the left side, and the back (in that order) before proceeding with his face, neck, and the rest of his body in similar fashion. Another patient, an elaborate hand washer, details every aspect from the "right" way to turn on the water, to the "correct" method for rehanging the towel with its edges exactly even. Stereotypies are "the persistent repetition of senseless acts or words" (Dorland's Medical Dictionary 1974), and these no-longer-useful ritualized behaviors *are* stereotypies.

Grooming

Grooming is a species-characteristic movement pattern with definable components; much is known about the biology of animal grooming but little about that of humans. Grooming serves a role in body surface care (Swenson and Randall 1978), temperature regulation (through evaporation of saliva) (Hainsworth 1967), social interaction (male saliva changes body odor and influences sexual behavior of the female partner rat) (Wiepkema 1979), and as a displacement response to conflict and frustration (Spruijt and Gispen 1983).

Self-grooming is less prevalent in primates than in other mammals. In monkeys, for example, grooming is primarily a social function. Ritualized grooming behaviors have become greeting expressions in many species. The lemur greets others with a movement that is used to comb the fur, accompanied by rhythmic calls and licking of the air (Eibl-Eibesfeldt 1970). Presentation of the head or other body part for symbolic grooming is a signal of submission and can defuse a threatening attack.

A few but quite intriguing human grooming studies have been carried out. Brief grooming behaviors are a regular portion of human greeting rituals (Kendon and Ferber 1973). Tapes of adults greeting each other at a birthday party reveal occasional grooming specific to the individual:

> CB usually strokes his beard, drawing the palm of the hand downward toward the tip. RC was observed either to touch the right side of her glasses or she would place the tips of the fingers of her right hand on the left side of her head, and draw the hand over her hair in an apparent hair adjustment movement. (Kendon and Ferber 1973, p. 637)

Adolescents meeting for a band concert exhibited considerably more grooming behavior. Seventy percent of the grooming occurred during the initiation or termination of an interaction, less than 10 percent when the teenager was alone. Self-grooming behaviors also can become stylized and integrated into the greeting ritual, such as stroking the beard or smoothing locks of hair (Michael and Crook 1973).

Self-grooming during stress and conflict seems irrelevant and unnecessary, but has been viewed as a *displacement activity* or as a reaction to the autonomic stimulation of the skin resulting from the stress reaction. The rat's grooming behavior is cephalocaudad in sequence, with face washing preceding body grooming, which, in turn, precedes anogenital grooming. The order in which the grooming is performed recapitulates the ontogeny of development of the component behaviors (Richmond and Sachs 1980). The pattern of rat grooming is presented schematically in Figure 2.

Novelty and conflict situations, both strong releasers of ACTH, induce grooming behavior. There is also strong direct evidence for ACTH involvement in grooming (Gispen and Isaacson 1981).

Intracerebral ventricular and intracranial injections of ACTH elicit a dose-dependent grooming response that is identical to that of saline-injected rats exposed to novel situations (except that ACTH-induced rats groom for longer periods). One microgram of ACTH injected into the lateral ventricle of a rat causes it to groom for 90 percent of the subsequent hour (Dunn and Vigle 1985) in a fashion indistinguishable from naturally occurring grooming (Gispen and Isaacson 1981; Zwiers et al. 1981). An intact hypothalamo-pituitary-adrenal system is not necessary for the expression of grooming behavior (Jolles et al. 1979), but ACTH-antibodies, which bind to an inactive ACTH, do prevent novelty-induced grooming (Dunn et al 1979). Thus ACTH mediates the external key stimulus and acts as the internal

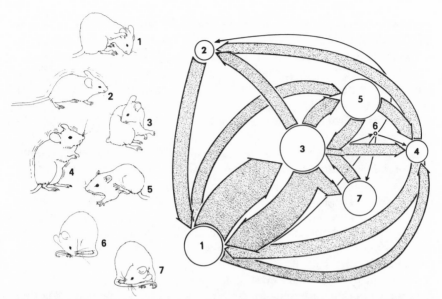

Figure 2.   Grooming behavior in the rat after ACTH administration. Element durations and transition frequencies were transformed to relative values for proper structure comparison. Area of the circles represents the log of element duration. Width of the arrows denotes square root of transition number. Direction of arrow indicates direction of transition: 1 face washing; 2 body shake; 3 body grooming; 4 vibration; 5 scratching; 6 tail sniffing; 7 anogenital grooming. (From Richmond and Sachs 1980.)

stimulus key to activate the grooming fixed-action response in a wide variety of conditions sharing in common only ACTH release.

Grooming is clearly a fixed-action pattern, as is shown by the ACTH trials as well as by experiments with mice (Fentress 1973). Adult house mice whose forelimbs were amputated at birth, for example, display patterns of facial grooming identical to those of normal litter mates. The absence of peripheral feedback did not alter the grooming behavior.

Other peptides, such as vasopressin, substance P, prolactin, and corticotropin releasing factor (CRF), while less potent than ACTH, also induce grooming behavior. However, the grooming induced by these peptides is not identical to novelty-induced grooming, as there is more scratching. Thus ACTH seems to be the only peptide that produces a completely "natural" grooming response compatible with the observations that novelty and stress situations both result in ACTH release.

ACTH-induced grooming can be altered pharmacologically. Pretreatment with the opiate antagonists, naloxone and naltrexone, prevents grooming, and low doses of morphine enhance grooming (Gispen and Wiegant 1976). Naloxone antagonizes ACTH-induced grooming in mice, as did naloxazone. This inhibition persisted until 96 hours postinjection, suggesting that resynthesis of opiate-binding sites was required for responsivity to return (Dunn et al. 1981). The type of opiate receptor involved has not been clear, leading most investigators to consider opiate receptor involvement as secondary rather than primary.

Dopaminergic antagonists are also effective in suppressing grooming response. Haloperidol decreased ACTH-induced grooming, while simultaneously increasing general locomotor activity; apomorphine increased ACTH grooming (Guild and Dunn 1982; Jackson et al. 1983). Low doses of metoclopramide, presumed to stimulate presynaptic dopaminergic receptors, potentiated ACTH-induced grooming, while higher doses, with postsynaptic action, prevented such grooming (Guild and Dunn 1982).

The role of the noradrenergic system is less clear, but a variety of investigations suggest roles for both norepinephrine and acetylcholine (Dunn, unpublished data; Dunn and Vigle 1985; Lassen 1977).

Additional studies localizing central nervous system (CNS) centers that mediate ACTH-induced grooming implicate the hippocampus and the periaqueductal gray matter. In contrast, lesions of the septal complex, medial and lateral preoptic areas, anterior hypothalamus, mammillary bodies, amygdala, posterior thalamus, and dorsal or ventral hippocampus have *no* effect (Gispen and Isaacson 1981; Wiegant et al. 1977). Local injections of ACTH into the substantia nigra elicited grooming (Wiegant et al. 1977), but less consistently (Ryan and Isaacson 1983).

Dunn (unpublished data) administered intraventricular ACTH following cold cream blockade of varying regions and found the anteroventral quadrant of the third ventricle near the oranum vasculosum of the lamina terminalis to be critical for the action of ACTH. Moreover, the short latency between ACTH administration and onset of grooming behavior suggested that the active site is quite close to the ventricular surface.

Studies of CNS glucose utilization have demonstrated changes in cerebral activity associated with grooming but have not pinpointed the direct site of ACTH action. ACTH-induced grooming was associated with decreased glucose uptake in the prefrontal and pyriform cortices, and was correlated with decreased glucose utilization in the olfactory bulbs and increased activity in the thalamus and cerebellum (Delanoy and Dunn 1978); (Dunn et al. 1980). Peripheral ACTH administration (which does not elicit grooming) produced no changes

(Delanoy and Dunn 1978). Naloxone (which antagonizes ACTH-induced grooming) attentuated the changes in glucose utilization (Dunn and Hurd 1982).

Adrian Dunn's extensive work with ACTH-induced rat-grooming behavior suggests that increased grooming in novel environments is due to secretion within the brain of ACTH, probably from the pituitary. Although grooming appears to be incongruous, it may actually serve as a neutral (nonthreatening but nonweak) signal, while the rat acclimates to a novel situation or decides whether to fight or flee. As with other fixed-action patterns, the grooming response can be overridden by stronger drive states such as hunger or thirst (Jolles et al. 1979).

In summary, the key external stimuli for grooming are novelty and conflict. If the drive state is receptive, these induce pituitary release of ACTH, which then acts most probably in the periventricular region as the internal key stimulus. In a receptive drive state, ACTH induces grooming behavior, a fixed-action pattern, which continues as long as the ACTH is active and the drive state is responsive.

The ACTH-induced rat-grooming behavior is intriguing in light of the phenomenology of OCD. Ritual washing could represent a fixed-action pattern released by an appropriate key stimulus and continuing unchecked until the stimulus waned or the drive state was no longer receptive. Two of our younger patients made such a comparison particularly compelling; they not only had elaborate washing rituals but also *licked* their hands in a ritualized, repetitive manner.

The importance of a receptive drive state and the ability of the key stimulus threshold to be raised by competing activity is also compatible with our patients' greater resistance to their compulsions when they are occupied (e.g., playing active games, carrying on a conversation, working).

The "key stimulus" in OCD must require integration, as patients do not ritualize in their sleep; either the key stimulus cannot be accepted during sleep or the drive state changes.

Nesting

Nesting is another highly ritualized behavior. Here, too, we find parallels with our patients' compulsive hoarding. The nesting fixed-action pattern consists of the location and collection of necessary building materials and the arrangement into the proper shape. Once the nest is built, it is fiercely protected. This fixed-action pattern is "innate," as it can be accurately performed by organisms raised in isolation, and it is "fixed," as the animals perform the entire sequence, once initiated, even if proper materials are unavailable. The nesting drive state is often hormonally influenced. For example, the pregnant mouse starts nest building after progesterone release. The key releasing stimulus can be internal (e.g., change in weather or the day/night cycle).

Obsessive-compulsive hoarders have patterns with some resemblance to lower species' nesting and hoarding. Our compulsive hoarders chose a particular "nesting/hoarding" area, often a bedroom, in which they draw together materials (e.g., bits of paper, string). They then protect this area from intrusion and contamination. Initially, the room must only be kept in a special order with everything in its own place.

The sanctity of the "nest" escalates until they are unable to disturb any of the room's contents or to even enter the room. One boy slept on the floor outside his room. Another slept on an air mattress in the basement furnace room for over 2 years rather than enter the bedroom. Other patients cannot allow anyone else entry to their room (particularly those who are suspected of being contaminated). A 16-year-old with AIDS contamination fears allowed only her mother into her room; her father's business travel could have "contaminated" him and her brother associated with rock musicians and therefore was contaminated by the "druggies."

The complexity of the nesting ritual makes it difficult to study. For invertebrates, such as the spider *Cupiennius salei*, nesting is restricted to building a cocoon for egg deposition. The spider builds a base plate, then a raised rim, and then deposits the eggs. After laying her eggs, she closes the opening. If disturbed after making the base plate and then returned to a different location, she starts from where she left off and constructs only the rim, lays the eggs in this bottomless shell, and covers the opening. In addition, an absence of spinning threads, which occurs when her glands dry up under the hot observation lights, does not preclude spinning activities. She will still make the predetermined 6,400 spinning movements (Eibl-Eibesfeldt 1970). The nesting behavior, like other fixed-action patterns once initiated, continues regardless of the appropriateness of the situation. Is this a model for situationally inappropriate yet perfectly executed compulsive rituals?

Vertebrates' nest-building fixed-action patterns are also innate, but the orienting patterns and the applications are often learned. Rats possess innate nest-building behavior patterns, but learn the sequencing of the component parts (Eibl-Eibesfeldt 1970). Canaries possess the component patterns for nest building but must learn the integration into a whole. Young ravens possess some specific nest-building skills, but must learn through their experimentation with twigs, ice, broken glass, tin cans, and other objects that twigs are the preferred nest material.

For African parrots (Genus *Acapornis*), the nesting impulse begins shortly after adults form pair bonds or after juvenile pairs attain adult plumage. A variety of building materials are carried between the ruffled-up feathers of their backs. Twigs and pieces of bark are cut, during which time the feathers are tucked close to the body. When a piece is obtained, the feathers fluff up and the bird tucks the material between them to carry it back to the nest. Males occasionally exhibit nesting behaviors, but this is thought to be mimicry of the female (Dilger 1965).

Releasers for nest-building behavior vary among species. Some, like parrots, carry nest-building materials throughout the year and throughout the reproductive cycle, only intensifying efforts immediately before and during the egg-laying phase. Cracks of light, splinters of wood, twigs, and fresh feces all prompt deposition of nesting material. The fresh feces seem to release nesting behavior because it is necessary for nest cleaning during the nesting stage. As the baby birds produce firmer, less messy stools, the deposition of new materials slows. In contrast, dove nest building is induced by progesterone release, which in turn is stimulated by the presence, or even just the sight of, a courting male; progesterone injection also induces nesting (Lehrman, et al. 1964).

House mice build a large nest four times the size of their sleeping nest shortly before giving birth, apparently under progesterone stimulation (Koller 1955). Postpartum, however, the nest-building is maintained by the presence of babies; if they are removed, nesting activity ceases.

Hormonal Control of Fixed-Action Patterns

The fixed-action pattern of nest building is clearly released by a hormonal key stimulus. Progesterone has been the best studied, but prolactin also can induce nesting (Nagasawa and Yanai 1972). Other key stimuli are external, such as day length cycle changes, presence of a courting male, and presence of young. The drive state required for responsivity to these key stimuli is also hormonally influenced. Prepubertal animals do not demonstrate nesting behavior under any circumstance, despite presence of multiple external key stimuli.

In humans, pubertal hormone changes could produce drive state alterations that release fixed-action patterns. Not only does OCD often start during puberty, postpartum OCD is also quite common. Rasmussen (personal communication) reported 20 representative cases, which showed an onset of symptoms 2 to 6 weeks postpartum as checking rituals that centered about the infant as well as obsessive thoughts that the newborn infant would be harmed. These obsessions were independent of depression. Five additional cases of postpartum OCD are currently under investigation at our clinic. One woman was first plagued by cleaning and counting rituals 2 weeks following the birth of her second child. Subsequently, these rituals waxed and waned in sequence with her menstrual cycle.

Pilot data from Spain and the National Institute of Mental Health (NIMH) also implicate hormonal modulation of OCD. Six patients with OCD experienced a remission in their symptoms following treatment with cyproterone acetate, a potent antiandrogen (Casas et al. 1986). In our pilot study, two clomipramine nonresponders showed improvement on testolactone (an antiestrogen) and spironolactone (an antiandrogen, particularly an antitestosterone compound). One adolescent male had slight lessening of his washing rituals and was able to sleep in his room for the first time in 2 years. The other, a prepubertal male, had a significant decrease in his obsessive thoughts, checking, and repeating rituals, and also could sleep in his own room for the first time in months.

It is common for compulsive rituals to change during adolescence; checking may convert to washing, counting to repeating, and so on (see Chapter 2). The role of hormonal shifts in initiating obsessive-compulsive symptoms deserves further investigation.

Hoarding

Like nesting, the hoarding rituals of obsessive-compulsive patients invite comparison with the fixed-action pattern of hoarding in animals. The hoarder fixes on a particular class of objects often to a bizarre degree. A 15-year-old girl collected a variety of trash, including used sanitary napkins, bits of paper, and empty apple juice cans. Partially chewed food would all be saved in small dishes or napkins in various places in the house. She had no evidence of thought disorder. Despite humiliation (being called a "bag lady" and teased for climbing into a garbage can) and her complete insight into the uselessness of these objects, she was unable to stop.

One young hoarder likened himself to a squirrel. Just as the squirrel carries nuts back to his nest, he told us, he carries things to his bed. He collected food wrappers and broken toys, storing them between mattress and box spring.

Winter food hoarding in animals has an obvious purpose. In common house mice *(Mus musculus)* no hoarding behavior is seen if the mice live with year-round ample food supplies, but in the field these mice collect 5 to 7 kg of seeds, which are stored in mounds beneath which the mice nest (Festetics 1961).

Rats' hoarding has been linked to caudate nucleus function (Borker and Gogate 1980). Laboratory rats hoard in response to environmental temperature and/or chronic food deprivation. After chronic deprivation, the rat adapts by collecting and hoarding all food during its availability and then consuming some after the provided food supply is removed. Following lesions of the caudate nucleus, both natural and induced hoarding behavior decreases. The hippocampus, septem, and anterior thalamus have also been implicated (Kolb 1974). Animals with medial frontal lesions still demonstrated some hoarding, and were able to increase hoarding appropriately in response to food deprivation, but hoarded less than control rats or rats with orbital frontal lesions. Lesions of the caudate-putamen and dorsomedial thalamic nucleus produced similar disturbances to medial frontal lesions (Kolb 1977). These rats also had impaired learning of spatial reversals and increased resistance to extinction. The similarity of effects of prefrontal, caudate, and dorsomedial thalamic lesions led Kolb to conclude that they were components of the same functional system. The defects observed in these lesioned rats are provocative, considering that children with OCD also exhibit spatial deficits on neuropsychological testing (Behar et al. 1984), and are consonant with increased orbito-frontal activity in OCD using positron emission tomography (PET) (see Chapters 5 and 19).

The Key Releasers

A search for "releasers" that could trigger compulsions should be a clinical research priority. We have hints that sensory stimuli can operate as releasers. Several of our patients avoid "key" situations to gain some freedom from ritual performance. For example, one girl rolled on the grass, touched and kissed the backyard trees, and waded in a muddy stream only if and when she saw the front door; entering the door prevented her outdoor ritual sequence.

Ethologists have long observed inappropriately released fixed-action repetitive patterns, such as the "mouse jump" one dog performed each time he approached the shed where he had first scared up a mouse. An old packhorse had to be unloaded and reloaded at a location where its owner had frequently camped. Unless this ritual was performed, the horse would not go on. Teleologically speaking, an "advantage" of such persistent habits is that "if it worked once, it may work again." The habit is difficult to extinguish, at least in part, because "deviation from it is accompanied by feelings of displeasure and fear" (Eibl-Eibesfeldt 1970, p. 224).

Konrad Lorenz (1963) kept his graylag geese in the house with him. One of these geese became accustomed to walking in a certain pattern on returning to the house:

> At first, she always walked past the bottom of the staircase toward a window in the hallway before returning to the steps, which she then ascended to get into the room on the upper floor. Gradually she shortened this detour, but persisted in initially orienting toward the window, without, however, going all the way to it. Instead she turned at a 90° angle once she was parallel to the stairs. Once, Lorenz forgot to let the goose into the house at the usual time. It was beginning to get dark and the goose ran, against her usual habit, directly toward the staircase as soon as the door opened and began to climb up. (p. 112)

Lorenz continued:

> Upon this something shattering happened: Arrived at the fifth step, she suddenly stopped, made a long neck, in geese a sign of fear, and spread her wings as for flight. Then she uttered a warning cry and very nearly took off. Now she hesitated a moment, turned around, ran hurriedly down the five steps and set forth resolutely, like someone on a very important mission, on her original path to the window and back. This time she mounted the steps according to her former custom from the left side. On the fifth step she stopped again, looked around, shook herself, and performed a greeting display behavior regularly seen in graylags when anxious tension has given place to relief. I hardly believed my eyes. To me there is no doubt about the interpretation of this occurrence: The habit had become a custom which the goose could not break without being stricken by fear. (p. 112)

Failure to perform the expected, released fixed-action pattern (compulsion) resulted in fear (ego-dystonic anxiety)!

Threshold-crossing rituals are particularly common in obsessive-compulsive patients. On arriving home in the family car, one male patient rolled the window down and up, opened and shut the door twice, got out of the car, walked to the mailbox and around the oak tree before entering the house. Are such rituals evolutionarily continuous with those of lower species?

Ritualized Movements

Insects, invertebrates, fish, birds, and mammals exhibit species-specific, predetermined mating rituals with visual, auditory, olfactory, or sensate cues from opposite sex as external releasers.

Hormonal motivation is necessary for the receptive drive state, and, as with other fixed-action patterns, the threshold for response to the presence of the key releasing stimuli increases in the presence of conflicting needs. The presence of a threatening aggressor can preclude courtship responses, as can hunger and other more powerful drives.

Courting rituals can be lengthy and complex, yet each male albatross performs the identical courtship dance. Some intraspecies variation occurs in isolated groups, suggesting a learned expression of the innate components. The dance sequence includes ritualized food begging, appeasement gestures, showing of nest, preening behavior, and others without interpretation (Eibl-Eibesfeldt 1970). Here again is the forced completion of an innate fixed-action pattern, once released.

Our ethological model complements our neurological model of OCD (see Chapter 19). Checking rituals of OCD may be a repetitive fixed-action pattern released inappropriately and lacking appropriate inhibition. We postulate that key releasing stimuli are not processed in a manner that extinguishes the checking fixed-action pattern. For example, the obsessive-compulsive patient who checks the light switch again and again, sees the switch is off and sees the light is dark. Despite accurate recall that they have checked, our patients have not "received" or integrated these stimuli centrally. The drive state has been conceived as dysfunctional in obsessive-compulsive patients who do not respond with an increased threshold until they have flipped the light switch on and off 100 times, or washed the germs from their contaminated hands 30 times. On another level, CNS processing, perhaps at the caudate, fails to get the extinguishing signal through.

Neural Models

Laboratory work by neuroethologists on the effects of selective ablations on these behavior patterns implicate the caudate nucleus, putamen, and the globus pallidus as mediating fixed-action patterns.

In addition to their role in "the automatic execution of learned motor plans" (Marsden 1982), the basal ganglia are also involved in the acquisition of motor skills (Heindel and Butters 1986). Which motor functions the basal ganglia dictate depends on information received by the striatum (caudate nucleus and putamen) from the cerebral cortex and midline thalamic nuclei and from the nigrostriatal dopaminergic system (Rolls et al. 1979). The basal ganglia filter these incoming signals in order to engender an appropriate efferent response (Schneider 1984). Based on focal ablations of individual extra-pyramidal structures, it appears that "the basal ganglia have all the aspects of a 'clearing house' that accumulates samples of all ongoing cortical projected activity and, on a competitive basis, can facilitate any one and suppress all others" (Denny-Brown and Yanagisawa 1976, p. 145).

The caudate nucleus is involved in the inhibition of sexual activity in male albino rats; caudate lesions resulted in increased mounts, genital grooming, and sniffing at female and decreased contact latency (Mulgaonker and Gogate 1980). Thus the caudate may function normally to increase the threshold of sexual response.

The caudate is also involved in recognition of patterns. Caudate neuron activity measurements during bar-press activity revealed that specific neurons respond to the sight of food, others to the bar-press activity itself, and still others to the combination of bar press and sighting of food (Nishino et al. 1981). In mice, caudate lesions decrease orienting responses to novel situations (Cigrang et al. 1986). Anther role of the caudate, therefore, appears to be sensory-motor integration, necessary for adaptation to environmental change.

Caudate dysfunction in primates produced by beta-carbachol injections disrupted both social communication and motor function (Vrijmoed-DeVries and Cools 1985).

The effect of caudate lesions on hoarding behavior and the effect of caudate ACTH injections on grooming behavior have been mentioned earlier. The caudate seems most involved in complex motor behaviors. Caudate nucleus lesions in cats caused serious disturbances in tasks requiring analysis and synthesis, with more severe impairment of higher integrative activity than of simple task differentiation (Adrianov et al. 1980). Simple conditioning and generalization were unaffected, whereas the ability to cope with complicated relations was lost. Van den Bercken and Cools (1982) showed that the

> caudate is responsible for establishing the relative priority of intra-individual and inter-individual constraints on the programming of behavior, thereby providing flexibility in the execution of ongoing behavior; the caudate is not primarily involved in motor control, nor in the control of particular categories of behavior. (p. 319)

In OCD, a growing body of information links the serotonergic system and the caudate and limbic system (cingulate gyrus). For patients with OCD, the serotonergic system may be malfunctioning (Zohar et al. 1987). Insufficient inhibitory input to the dopaminergic system would result in unchecked dopaminergic activity or stereotypies and hyperactivity. Brief spurts of such activity could result in repetitive thoughts and rituals. The inability to assess ego-dystonicity objectively in animals will complicate the establishment of an animal model to test this hypothesis, as it is the ego-dystonicity that separates OCD from the other stereotypic disorders.

Summary

In summary, a model of OCD is proposed in which there is inappropriate expression of a complex, ritualized fixed-action pattern. To further support such a model, key releasing stimuli must be identified. Are they internal (e.g., ACTH, serotonin, dopamine) or external (e.g., stress, visual or auditory images) or, most likely, some particular 'fit' of both? Research must identify a mechanism for altered drive state (e.g., why doesn't the drive state "click off"?). The role of hormonal changes is particularly suggestive and needs to be elucidated. Any model must account for the specificity of the symptoms, the response to pharmacologic and behavioral treatment, and developmental changes.

References

Adrianov OS, Molodkina LN, Mukhin EI, et al: Participation of caudate nucleus in different forms of voluntary activity in cats. Acta Neurobiol Exp (Warsz) 40:729–740, 1980

Behar D, Rapoport JL, Berg CJ, et al: Computerized tomography and neuropsychological test measures in adolescents with obsessive-compulsive disorder. Am J Psychiatry 141:363–369, 1984

Borker AS, Gogate MG: Hoarding in caudate lesioned rats. Indian J Exp Biol 18:690–692, 1980

Casas M, Alvarez E, Duro P, et al: Antiandrogenic treatment of obsessive compulsive neurosis. Acta Psychiatr Scand 73:221–222, 1986

Cigrang M, Vogel E, Misslin R: Reduction of neophobia in mice following lesions of the caudate-putamen. Physiol Behav 36:25–28, 1986

Delanoy RL, Dunn AJ: Mouse brain deoxyglucose uptake after footshock, ACTH analogs, alpha-MSH, corticosterone or lysine vasopressin. Pharmacol Biochem Behav 9:21–26, 1978

Denny-Brown D, Yanagisawa N: The role of the basal ganglia in the initiation of movement, in The Basal Ganglia. Edited by Yaar M. New York, Raven Press, 1976

Dilger WC: Excerpts from: the comparative etiology of the African parrot genus, *Acapornis*, in Readings in Animal Behavior. Edited by McGill TE. New York, Holt, Rinehart & Winston, 1965

Dorland's Medical Dictionary, illus, 25th ed. Philadelphia, WB Saunders Co, 1974

Dunn AJ, Hurd RW: Regional glucose metabolism in mouse brain following ACTH peptides & naloxone. Pharmacol Biochem Behav 17:37–41, 1982

Dunn AJ, Vigle G: Grooming behavior induced by ACTH involves cerebral cholinergic neurons and muscarinic receptors. Neuropharmacology 24:329–331, 1985

Dunn AJ, Green EJ, Isaacson RL: Intracerebral adrenocortiocotropic hormone mediates novelty-induced grooming in the rat. Science 203:281–283, 1979

Dunn AJ, Steelman S, Delanoy R: Intraventricular ACTH and vasopressin cause regionally specific changes in cerebral deoxyglucose uptake. J Neurosci Res 5:485–495, 1980

Dunn AJ, Childers SR, Kramarcy NR, et al: ACTH-induced grooming involves high-affinity opiate receptors. Behav Neural Biol 31:105–109, 1981

Eibl-Eibesfeldt I: Ethology: The Biology of Behavior. Translated by Klinghammer E. New York, Holt, Rinehart & Winston, 1970

Fentress JC: Development of grooming in mice with amputated forelimbs. Science 179:704–705, 1973

Festetics A: Ahren maushugel in Osterreich. Z Saugetierkde 26:1–14, 1961 [Cited in Eibl-Eibesfeldt 1970]

Gispen WH, Isaacson RL: ACTH-induced excessive grooming in the rat. Pharmacol Ther 12:209–240, 1981

Gispen WH, Wiegant VM: Opiate antagonists suppress $ACTH_{1-24}$-induced excessive grooming in the rat. Neurosci Lett 2:159–164, 1976

Guild AL, Dunn AJ: Dopamine involvement in ACTH-induced grooming behavior. Pharmacol Biochem Behav 17:31–36, 1982

Hainsworth FR: Saliva spreading activity and body temperature regulation in the rat. Am J Physiol 212:1288–1292, 1967

Heindel W, Butters N: Motor skill learning in Huntington's Disease (abstract). Abstracts, Society of Neurosciences 1986

Hess EH: Readings in animal behavior, in Ethology: An Approach Toward the Complete Analysis of Behavior. Edited by McGill T. New York, Holt, Rinehart & Winston, 1965

Ingle D, Crews D: Vertebrate neuroethology: definitions and paradigms. Annu Rev Neurosci 8:457–494, 1985

Jackson EA, Neumeyer J, Kelly P: Behavioral activity of some novel aporphines in rats with 6-hydroxydopamine lesions of caudate or nucleus accumbens. Eur J Pharmacol 87:15–23, 1983

Jolles J, Rompa-Barendez J, Gispen WH: ACTH-induced excessive grooming in the rat: the influence of environmental and motivational factors. Horm Behav 12:60–72, 1979

Kendon A, Ferber A: A description of some human greetings, in Comparative Ecology and Behavior of Primates. Edited by Michael RP, Crook JH. London, Academic Press, 1973

Kolb B: Prefrontal lesions alter eating and hoarding behavior in rats. Physiol Behav 12:507–511, 1974

Kolb B: Studies on the caudate putamen and the dorsomedial thalamic nucleus of the rat: implications for mammalian frontal lobe functions. Physiol Behav 18:237–244, 1977

Koller G: Hormonale und psychische steuerung beim Nestbau weisser Mause. Zoologischer Anzeiger Supplement 19:123–132, 1955

Lassen JB: Evidence for a noradrenergic mechanism in the grooming produced by (+)-amphetamine and 4, α-dimethyl-m-tyramine (h 77/77) in rats. Psychopharmacology 54:153–157, 1977

Lehrman OS, Brody PN, Wortis RP: The presence of the mate and nesting material as stimuli for the development of incubation behavior and for gonadotropin secretion of the ring dove (*Streptopelia risoria*). Endocrinology 68:507–516, 1964

Lorenz K: Uber den Begriff der Instinkthandlung. Folia Biol 17–50, 1937

Lorenz K: Das sogenannte Böse. Vienna, Borotha-Schoeler, 1963

Lorenz K: Studies in Animal and Human Behavior. Translated by Martin R. Cambridge, MA, Harvard University Press, 1970a

Lorenz K: Taxis and instinctive behavior pattern in egg-rolling by the greylag goose, in Studies in Animal and Human Behavior, Vol. 1, Translated by Martin R. Cambridge, MA, Harvard University Press, 1970b

Marsden CD: The mysterious motor function of the basal ganglia: The Robert Wartenberg Lecture. Neurology 32:514–539, 1982

Michael RP, Crook JH: Comparative ecology and behavior of primates. London, Academic Press, 1973

Mulgaonker VG, Gogate MG: Effect of lesion of caudate nucleus on sexual behavior of male rat (albino rat, Haffkine strain). Indian J Exp Biol 18:1342–1343, 1980

Nagasawa H, Yanai R: Changes in serum prolactin levels shortly before and after parturition in rats. Endocrinol Jpn 19:139, 1972

Nishino H, Ono T, Fukuda M, et al: Single unit activity in monkey caudate nucleus during operant bar pressing feeding behavior. Neurosci Lett 21:105–110, 1981

Richmond G, Sachs BD: Grooming in Norway rats: the development and adult expression of a complex motor pattern behavior. Behaviour 75:82–95, 1980

Rolls ET, Thorpe SJ, Maddison S, et al: Activity of neurones in the neostriatum and related structures in the alert animal, in The Neostriatum. Edited by Divac I, Oberg RGE. Oxford, Pergamon Press, 1979

Ryan JP, Isaacson RL: Intra-accumbens injections of ACTH induce excessive grooming in rats. Physiol Psychol 11:54–58, 1983

Schneider JS: Basal ganglia role in behavior: importance of sensory gating and its relevance to psychiatry. Biol Psychiatry 19:1693–1716, 1984

Spruijt BM, Gispen WH: ACTH and grooming behavior in the rat, in Hormones and Behavior in Higher Vertebrates. Edited by Balthazart J, Prove E, Gilles R. Berlin, Springer Verlag, 1983

Swenson RM, Randall WJ: Grooming behavior in cats with pontile lesions. J Comp Physiol Psychol 91:313–326, 1978

Van den Bercken JHL, Cools AR: Evidence for a role of the caudate nucleus in the sequential organization of behavior. Behav Brain Res 4:319–337, 1982

Vrijmoed-DeVries MC, Cools AR: Further evidence for the role of the caudate nucleus in programming motor and nonmotor behavior in Java monkeys. Exp Neurol 87:58–75, 1985

Wiegant VM, Cools AR, Gispen WH: ACTH-induced excessive grooming involves brain dopamine. Eur J Pharmacol 41:343–345, 1977

Wiepkema S: The social significance of self-grooming in rats. Netherlands Journal of Zoology 29:623, 1979

Zohar J, Mueller E, Insel T, et al: Serotonin receptor sensitivity in obsessive-compulsive disorder: comparison of patients and healthy controls. Arch Gen Psychiatry 44:946–951, 1987

Zwiers H, Aloyo VJ, Gispen W: Behavioral and neurochemical effects of the new opiod peptide dynorphin (1-13) comparison with other neuropeptides. Life Sci 28:2545–2551, 1981

Chapter 17

Childhood Rituals and Superstitions: Developmental and Cultural Perspective

Henrietta L. Leonard, M.D.

Men would never be superstitious if they could govern all their circumstances by set rules, or if they were always favoured by fortune; but being frequently driven into straits where rules are useless, and being often kept fluctuating pitiably between hope and fear by the uncertainty of fortune's greedily coveted favours, they are consequently, for the most part, very prone to credulity.

Spinoza, 1955
Tractatus Theologico-Politicus

It is often speculated that clinical obsessions and compulsions are extreme variants of normal development or cultural phenomena. Ritualistic play, repetitive behavior patterns of toddlers, common childhood games, and superstitions are hypothesized to be on some continuum with obsessive-compulsive disorder (OCD).

Implicit in such assumptions is that persons suffering from OCD would have had some exaggeration of these normal developmental phenomena, and that the superstitions and children's games themselves resemble obsessive-compulsive symptom patterns.

Despite reference to this notion in virtually any volume on OCD, there are almost no systematic studies of normal developmental patterns of rituals or of superstitions in childhood. The thesis of this review is that while rituals and superstitions are fairly common in our culture, most do not resemble the behavior patterns seen in OCD. Furthermore, preliminary data suggest that children and adolescents with OCD did not differ from their peers with respect to number or intensity of premorbid superstitions or childhood rituals. The scanty literature on childhood rituals and superstitions is reviewed, and these phenomena are rejected as models for this illness.

Childhood Rituals

At 2½ years of age, ritualistic behavior is evident in most children, but just how evident is surprisingly hard to find out. It is generally agreed that at this age, previously malleable infants will begin to expect routines and to have things done "just so." Transitions are difficult, and the familiar way is preferred. Mealtimes, bathing, and bedtimes are particularly likely to call forth these routines.

Anna Freud (1965) stressed the normalcy of childhood repetitive behaviors but provided no quantitative descriptions. Gesell et al. (1974) referred to the "ritualisms of the ritualist."

> There is the going-upstairs ritual, the brushing the teeth ritual, getting into bed, pulling down the shades, kissing and even a specially worded good night ritual. If the plug is pulled out the wrong way, the entire going to bed routine may be disturbed and a temper tantrum occurs. Even the shades must be pulled down to just the proper height. (p. 17)

When all is completed, the parent may be called back for another round on the premise that a detail has been forgotten, or that the youngster has a new bit of information to pass on, or a new question to ask. Most observers agree that a large component is anxiety about separation, but developmental issues mastery, cognitive control, and ordering must also play a role.

By age 3, children begin to give up much of their rituals, take less time, and become less rigid. By age 4, the rituals clearly diminish, and children are better able to deal with change.

Of course these stages represent only generalizations about widely varying phenomena. Nagera (1980) noted that marked increase in bedtime ceremonials and ritualistic behaviors can even be seen in the 4- to 6-year-old child, regarding this as, within limits, a normal developmental disturbance. Unfortunately, no quantification or follow-up is given for such a group. Children at this age (4 to 6 years) still have sleep disturbances, nightmares, and fears of the dark, monsters, ghosts, and so on, frequently leading to requests for another story, another glass of water, another hug or kiss. It is unusual if these rituals are not gone by 8 or 9 years of age (van Amerongen 1980).

As mentioned, virtually no systematic studies document the frequency and duration of childhood bedtime rituals. Albert et al. (1979) recorded bedtime rituals of 12 white upper-middle-class children from 3 to 8 years of age. All dialogue was recorded between the children and their parents from supper to sleep. Unfortunately, they did not descriptively detail individual variants or the components of the rituals.

The children's repeated request for "glasses of water" were seen as a social need for delaying bedtime. The frequency with which a child and parent called each other by name and displays of affection were increased. Albert et al. (1979) described the "rite of passage" as having parts of a macrolevel system transition (moving from sleep to awake states) and microlevel transition (moving from room to room).

Simonds and Parraga (1984) compared bedtime "behaviors" and sleep disturbance in 150 children and adolescents in a psychiatric clinic with those of 309 normal subjects. Although the study was flawed in that the clinic group had more males and a younger mean age than the control group, the psychiatric clinic population showed a significantly higher percentage of sleep problems. A reluctance to go to sleep was exhibited by 26 percent of the psychiatric patients as opposed to 8 percent of controls. Although limited, this is one of the few studies measuring the frequency of sleep-related ritual behaviors for clinical and nonclinical groups of children.

Luskin (1981) studied ritual greetings and leave taking in young children. She observed children entering and leaving school and pretending to talk on the phone, and found both situation and age determined differences in the use of greetings and leave-taking rituals. Rituals were more frequent on the telephone than in the classroom. No determinants were found. Correlations between social cognition and ritual use were few and inconsistent. Early ritualized play consists of solitary play such as playing with cards, dolls, and toys, and later develops into ritualized collective play where there are repetitive changes and behaviors.

At around 5 to 6 years of age, children's ritualization moves more into group play. Jump rope, jacks, and hopscotch are played with rules and elaborate rhymes (Rubin et al. 1983). At this and later stages, comparisons with obsessive-compulsive behavior are most often invoked.

From ages 6 to 11, games and rituals are apt to be governed by very specific rules, rare before age 4. Ritual prohibitions may dominate. Oremland (1973) described "the jinx game," a popular game of 7- to 11-year-old children consisting of stereotyped rituals. When a group of children are playing together and two of them happen to say the same word or phrase at the same time, one will say "jinx." Whichever child is able to say this first is in control, and the jinxed child must remain silent. The jinxed child is only freed when his or her name is called by the jinxer or another child. A variation of the jinx game is that the children saying the same thing must "fall into the ritual of hooking their little fingers together, making a silent wish . . . and remain mute until a third person speaks to one of them and so breaks the spell. If they forget and speak without this release, the wish is lost. All the other children are aware of their role in the rite and of their power to enforce silence until they choose to free the main participants. One assumption of the game is that the principals should not be liberated too quickly, and if anyone speaks too soon, this is felt as a gratuitous and offensive destruction of a magical moment to be greeted by the indignant and almost equally ritual cry of 'no fair!'" (Oremland, p. 422).

Around the age of 6, boys express their belief that girls have a kind of pernicious influence in ritual play. "Cooties" is frequently yelled out on a playground as someone is touched. Boys may vehemently avoid being touched by girls for fear of catching cooties (Adams 1973). Tag games are a variation on the theme. (Girls usually do not express such dramatic and pervasive fear of catching cooties from boys, but may manifest some fears of becoming dirty.) This contamination fear could be considered a mild variant of pathological obsessions.

Around age 7, children begin to take an interest in collecting objects and developing hobbies. Popular items are baseball cards, bottle caps, matchbooks, or the latest doll. Hoarding is relatively common in OCD, but the parallel is obvious. Moving into adolescence, kids become "obsessed" with an activity or an idol. They may spend hours and days playing "Dungeons and Dragons" or they may act out characters from *Star Wars*. They may dress like rock idols and play their songs in a seemingly incessant fashion. Here the analogy is particularly stretched as such intense preoccupations with culturally shared interests do not characterize obsessive-compulsive children.

Normal developmental "focused interests" are distinguished from pathological, "circumscribed interests" (Bender and Schilder 1940; Robinson and Vitale 1954). Bender and Schilder described "impulsions" of childhood, which were ego-syntonic preoccupations and actions that persist in the foreground of experience for months or years. These might be the precursors of obsessions and compulsions that at age 10 to 12 become an obsessional neurosis, but no follow-up data are given. Robinson and Vitale described a similar syndrome of "circumscribed interest patterns" in which interests are pursued with intensity and to the neglect of others. Three boys, ages 9 to 13 years, are presented who have "near obsessive interest" in chemistry, finance, transportation systems, maps, trolley routes, astronomy, electricity, railways, art, music, and mortgages. Such cases may be variants of Asberger's syndrome, although interestingly one of the boys barked and cleared his throat, suggesting the spectrum of Tourette's syndrome and OCD.

In summary, ritualized behavior occurs early in life and persists throughout childhood. Initially most evident as bedtime rituals and requiring things to be "just so," it later manifests as collective play, formalized games, collecting, and interests in music and sports. Whatever else its function, ritualizing has a role in socialization and in mastering anxiety. No clear evidence of continuity with obsessive-compulsive illness has been presented.

Superstitions

Besides, there are a hundred things one has to know, which we understand all about and you don't as yet. I mean passwords and signs, and saying which have power and effect, and plants you carry in your pocket, and verses you repeat, and dodges and tricks you practice; all simple enough when you know them, but they've got to be known if you're small, or you'll find yourself in trouble.

Rat to Mole in *The Wind in the Willows* (Grahame 1965, p. 53)

Webster's Dictionary defines superstition as: "a belief, conception, act or practice resulting from ignorance, unreasoning fear of the unknown or mysterious conception of causation."

Marmor defines superstitions as "beliefs or practices that appear to be without foundation in themselves and are inconsistent with the degree of enlightenment reached by the community in which they exist" (in Jahoda 1974, p. ix).

Dr. Wayland Hand (in Marmor 1956) compiled present superstitious beliefs and practices in this country, finding an enormous number, conservatively estimated at 80,000! For illustrative purposes, some common superstitions are listed in Table 1. For the most part, they deal with bringing good luck and protection from evil. The most common superstitions include knocking on wood, avoiding black cats and ladders, and spilling salt. Prominently absent are washing and grooming behaviors or concern with ritual purity.

Conceptual Models

Anxiety Reduction/Mastery Over Uncertainty

Freud noted the similarity between obsessions and social taboos, describing obsessional patients as having a "taboo sickness."

> The most obvious and striking point of agreement between the obsessional prohibitions of neurotics and taboos is that these prohibitions are equally lacking in motive and equally puzzling in their origin. Having made their appearance at some unspecified moment, they are forcibly maintained by an irresistible fear. No external threat of punishment is required, for there is an internal certainty, a moral conviction, that any violation will lead to intolerable disaster. (Freud 1950, p. 26)

There has been considerable psychoanalytic speculation about the basis for superstitions. Jung (1956) invoked superstitions as manifestations of a collective unconscious, a repository of either pathological fantasies or new but as yet unknown ideas. Fleiss (1944) suggested that "knocking on wood" symbolized the sexual act, with the magical ritual dispelling anxiety.

Fears of retaliation for boastful statements are ancient and universal: "By knocking on wood, the individual denies and undoes the aggressive boastful remark and magically propitiates the authority symbol (Marmor 1956, p. 122). In society, Marmor concluded, "knocking on wood represents an unconscious effort to achieve protection against envy and hostility from two potential sources, those representing parental or authority symbols and those representing sibling symbols" (p. 129).

Knocking on wood may have originated in times when men worshiped "good" spirits who lived in trees. To prevent the gods' punish-

Table 1.   Common superstitions in the United States

Events Bringing Bad Luck	Events Bringing Good Luck	Protective Superstition
Seeing black cats	Finding four-leaf clover	Spilling salt
Walking under ladders	Knocking on wood	Knocking on wood
Bad luck coming in threes	Keeping found penny	
Breaking a mirror	Wishing on a falling star	
The number 13	Keeping a rabbit's foot	
Opening an umbrella inside	Tossing coin in fountain	
Wishing good on important occasions	Seeing a horse show	
Receiving premature praise	Using a wishing well	
Stepping on pavement lines		

Note.   Adapted from Marmor 1956.

ment of man's boasting, one would magically touch the tree. In ancient Greece the oak was sacred to Zeus, in Scandinavia the ash tree to Thor, and in Egypt the sycamore to the goddess Hathor. It was thought that the winds would carry the boasting words of man to the leaves of the tree. Thus to touch the wood would be to be protected from the god's vengeance. After Jesus Christ's influence, a hunted person touching the wooden church door was "under the protection" of the church.

Conditioning/Learning Theories: Superstition as a Conditioned Response

> The chance knowledge of the marvelous effects of gifted springs is probably as ancient as any sound knowledge is to medicine whatever. No doubt it was mere casual luck at first that tried these springs and found them an answer. Somebody by accident was instantly cured. The chance which happily directed men in this one case, misdirected them in a thousand cases. Some expedition had answered when the resolution to undertake it was resolved on under an ancient tree, and accordingly that tree became lucky and sacred. Another expedition failed when a magpie crossed its path, and a magpie was said to be unlucky. A serpent crossed the path of another expedition, and it had a marvellous victory, and accordingly the serpent became a sign of great luck.... The worst of these superstitions is that they are easy to make and hard to destroy. A single run of luck has made the fortune of many a charm and many idols.
> Walter Bagehot, *Physics and Politics*
> (in Jahoda 1974, p. 71)

To behavioral scientists, "superstition" refers to the perception of an independent event as contingent on one's behavior. This behavioral paradigm is also referred to as adventitious, free, independent, or noncontingent reinforcement.

It was B.F. Skinner (1953) who first suggested that superstitions are based on an initial learned response. A child having had a bad experience with a dog may fear all dogs. "If there is only an accidental connection between the response and the appearance of a reinforcer, the behavior is superstitious" (p. 85). Although generalization to human learning has been questioned, some researchers have attempted studies on operant learning in people. An "ambiguity hypothesis" (the more ambiguous a notion is about a relationship between unrelated events, the more likely it is to be believed) was tentatively supported by an operant experimental paradigm in college students (Feingold 1978).

An operant model of human superstitious behavior (a repetitive response which is reinforced adventitiously) was explored in a study of college students who had to perform a three-choice learning task. Subjects observing the models imitated simulated superstitious behavior to a statistically significant degree (Dashefsky 1979).

Similarly, modeling clearly influences superstitious behavior. For example, Pole et al. (1974) hypothesized that a person would be more likely to walk under a ladder after having observed a model do so, predicting also that a model would only have an effect on ladder avoidance when the ladder was not in use (i.e., a superstitious situation). They watched 100 college students pass through the four situations (permutations of model, no model, empty ladder, worker on ladder). Both hypotheses were confirmed; 31 of 50 subjects walked under the ladder when seeing a model do so, as opposed to 17 of 50 who did not. The model increased the likelihood of walking under the ladder in the superstitious situation (where no worker was on ladder), supporting the learning hypothesis. In children, modeling increased key pressing in a noncontingent reinforcement situation, interpreted as social mediated acquisition of superstitious behavior (Hamm 1974).

Social psychologists focus on superstitions as a shift to an external "locus of control." Peterson (1978) speculated that a belief in "self-oriented" superstitions would correlate with "externality," and found a significant positive correlation between externality and superstition scores for a group of student teachers, suggesting that apparent relevance of the superstitions to the state of one's "luck" is a more important determiner of belief than is apparent internal control over superstitious contingency. "Perhaps the illogicality of the superstition is critical: externalizers, stressed as they are by fate's unpredictability, may be the only ones able to ignore the laws of physical causality enough to adhere to self-oriented superstitions" (p. 306).

In the laboratory, experimental "superstitions" can easily be induced in children. Zeiler (1972) studied "superstitious conditioning" in 12 children from age 4 to 5 using candy as a reinforcement in key pressing. In the absence of a response specification, responses that happen to precede reinforcement increase in probability, and the stimulus present when reinforcement occurs develops control over responding. He concluded that the essential process in operant behavior is the temporal contiguity among response and stimulus events. Higgins (1983) studied the development of superstitious operant behavior in 32 children between the ages of 3 and 5, who, despite the reinforcement being given intermittently, continued to respond for a long time. Others have confirmed that the free operant behavior of preschool children in a response-independent schedule of reinforcement is strongly determined by belief about causality even in the absence of any true relationship between response and reward (Wagner 1983).

Prevalence and Individual Differences

Plug (1976) compiled the most comprehensive (and one of the few) reviews of superstitions. Superstitions have been examined in relation to age, sex, education, instruction, intelligence, stress, and emotional adjustment.

Age. Although data on superstitions and age are poor, scanty, and inconclusive, qualitative changes in superstitious beliefs clearly take place with age. Opie and Opie (1959) reported several children's superstitions not found in adults. Plug (1976) pointed out that it is not "time as such" that is an independent variable in explaining changes in beliefs, but the events that have occurred during its passage.

Conklin (1919) asked 557 students, ages 16 to 25, to list superstitions they believed. There was a slight decrease with age in women from ages 16 to 25 ($p < .03$). Interestingly, one-half of the subjects retrospectively reported that from ages 12 to 16 were their most superstitious years. Similarly, Wagner (1928) found a significant decrease in superstitiousness in older subjects ($r = -.19$ between age and superstitions), but this could be attributed to older subjects feeling more uncomfortable disclosing their beliefs.

Maller and Lundeen (1933a) recorded acknowledged superstitions by junior (age 13) and senior (age 16) students, finding a slight decrease with age. Thouless and Brown (1964) found religious superstitions (petitionary prayer, crossing fingers, and using St. Christopher's medallions) decreased somewhat with age. In any case, the relation to age is not striking and others have not found a significant association (Lundeen and Caldwell 1930). Thus, while there may be some age-related decrease, this does not seem to be of major importance.

Sex. Plug (1976) reviewed studies comparing superstitiousness in men and in women. Of the 13 comparisons found, 7 revealed women more superstitious than men, 3 found a trend in that direction that did not reach significance, and 2 had no statistical analysis. Although some studies found that women were more superstitious ($p < .05$) (e.g., Blum and Blum 1974), instruments would need to be constructed to remove a sex bias (e.g., including business and sports superstitions) for a valid comparison. It may also be more socially acceptable for women to admit to superstitious beliefs. In any case, the effect is not striking; moreover, in childhood, males with OCD predominate.

Education. Educational level is confounded by many variables, including social status, age, intelligence, and experience. Lundeen and

Caldwell (1930) found that college students had heard of more superstitions, yet believed in fewer than high school students. Dudycha (1933) compared 853 college freshmen with 305 college seniors, finding seniors "more disbelieving," although the statistical analysis was not presented.

Pasachoff et al. (1970) administered a questionnaire about superstitions to 200 male Harvard students. Natural science students believed markedly less than other students in astrology, extrasensory perception, and flying saucers; there were no clear differences between students of the humanities and social sciences. Biological science majors tended to have higher superstitious belief scores than natural science peers. No correlation was found between years of university education and superstition. The interesting finding was that higher education and superstition frequently coexist. Within our culture at least, education does not show a dramatic relation to superstition. On the other hand, education about superstitions and superstitious behavior per se may have some effect (Emme 1940).

Intelligence.   Mixed results have been found in studying the association between intelligence and superstitiousness. Ter Keurst (1939) measured superstitiousness and intelligence in 663 secondary school children. The highly superstitious group had a significantly lower mean IQ score than the less superstitious group ($p < .001$). Killen et al. (1974) obtained similar findings. Other studies have not found such an association (Belanger 1944; Jahoda 1968; Maller and Lundeen 1933b; Powers 1931; Wagner 1928).

Urban versus rural setting.   There is a general consensus that superstitions are more common in rural areas. However, no study in this country has documented this.

Blum (1976) studied the difference in prevalence of superstitions between 69 urban and 64 rural men and women in Pennsylvania. The subjects completed a questionnaire about 12 common superstitions: walking under a ladder, the number 13, black cats, knocking on wood, four-leaf clovers, itching palm, opening an umbrella indoors, three on a match, keeping a found penny, wishing on a falling star, crossing fingers, and breaking a mirror. The level of superstitious beliefs was equivalent between the rural and urban locations, although differences were found in specific beliefs. Blum concluded that "within our over-all culture," subgroups, separated by distance and characterized by different conditions of population density and heterogeneity, evidence similar levels of beliefs.

Content of Childhood and Adolescent Superstitions

Whenever I walk in a London street,
I'm ever so careful to watch my feet;
And I keep in the squares,
And the masses of bears,
Who wait at the corners all ready to eat
The sillies who tread on the lines of the street,
Go back to their lairs,
And I say to them, "Bears,
Just look how I'm walking in all the squares!"
And the little bears growl to each other,
"He's mine,
As soon as he's silly and steps on a line."
And some of the bigger bears try to pretend
That they came round the corner to look for a friend;
And they try to pretend that nobody cares
Whether you walk on the lines or squares.
But only the sillies believe their talk;
It's ever so 'portant how you walk.
And it's ever so jolly to call out, "Bears,
Just watch me walking in all the squares!"

A.A. Milne 1952
Lines and Squares
(Milne 1952, pp. 14–15)

"Step on a crack, break your mother's back" is a familiar rhyme to city children who often avoid the cracks in the sidewalk. In hopscotch, you jump into the squares, avoiding all the lines lest you lose your turn. Milne wrote of this universal belief in danger that comes from stepping on a crack. The bear says "He's mine as soon as he's silly and steps on a line," and also stresses doing it right as "it's ever so 'portant how you walk."

There are no surveys of children's superstitions in the United States, although this belief is certainly common. Opie and Opie (1959), in collecting the lore of 5,000 schoolchildren throughout England, Scotland, Wales, and Ireland, found many rituals about avoiding cracks on the pavement or between stones. To step on a crack is unlucky: "you will get your sums wrong," "your hair will fall out," "you will fall downstairs next day," or "stand on a line and you'll marry a foreigner."

A way of telling whom one is going to marry is by hopping in and out of the squares on the pavement and if one stands on a black line then one is going to marry a foreigner, but if one should stand on a crack in the middle of the square, then one is going to marry of one's own country. If one stands with one foot on each, then one is going to marry a foreign person. (Opie and Opie 1959, p. 221)

Between the ages of 2 and 6, the child's cognition is characterized by magical thinking (Piaget 1969), with an assumption of omnipotence and omniscience. It is a good or evil world with unexpected certainties and no concepts of probabilities. There is "magic power" in thoughts, wishes, words, and actions (Wilder 1975). "Undoing" is normal in the thinking of 6- to 8-year-olds. Crossing one's fingers or legs to nullify a thought or to protect oneself from having told a lie is common, as is going back around a tree in the opposite direction to ward off an evil fate (Berman 1979). Opie and Opie (1959) collected examples of superstitions, labeling them as "half-beliefs" and eliciting them from the children by looking for "magic practices" or "ways of obtaining luck or averting ill luck." A wealth of beliefs and practices had been passed from generation to generation, derivatives that were remarkably similar in areas separated by many miles. Many of the rites are practiced "just for fun" because everyone does, whereas others are repeated because "there may be something in it." Others again are practiced because it is in the nature of children to be attracted by the mysterious: they indicate an innate awareness that there is more to the ordering of fate than appears on the surface. Most of these lores are about objects that bring good or bad luck, about reluctance to anticipate events, and about seeking safeguards. For example, after finding a "lucky" object, one must go through a prescribed action to bring the luck about. A 14-year-old girl believed: "When you pick up a button, say 'button, button, bring me luck or else I'll break you up.'"

If one finds a piece of coal, one should pick it up and spit on it, then throw it over the left shoulder and wish. Rituals about found coins include that it should be spat on, trod on, and then picked up or given away. The importance of wishing is felt at all ages as evidenced by wishing wells, wishes with rainbows, falling stars, and when blowing out birthday candles.

Many superstitions referred to good luck during times of stress such as exams. Students would bring a mascot, good luck charm, or lucky object to their tests. Faith is put in new pencils, which "have never written a mistake." Students cross their fingers and touch wood so that an answer is correct.

The most elaborate beliefs and sayings, however, were found about luck in games. Good luck chants and curse verse are common. Wearing socks inside out or mismatched, crossing one's fingers, and spitting on one's hands are pervasive practices. Common expressions before a sports trial include "here goes," "wish me luck," "thumbs up," "let's get it over," "one can only die once," or "I like dandelions on my grave."

Superstition and Ritual in Sports

Magical–religious practices of various kinds are found wherever one finds athletes. Religious–superstitious behaviors range from team prayers before games to personal idiosyncratic rituals. By far the best descriptive work on superstition and ritual has examined the high incidence and importance of sport superstitions. *The Journal of Sports Behavior* has numerous methodologically adequate studies. Interestingly, these behaviors are the most similar to clinical obsessive-compulsive rituals of any reviewed.

Stress and performance anxiety clearly increase their likelihood in otherwise rational individuals. It is generally agreed that a coach would be foolish to discourage such reassuring habits (Becker 1975).

Buhrmann and Zaugg (1983) studied the relationship between religion and superstition in sports. They administered a questionnaire that included items about church attendance, religious affiliation, and superstitious sports behaviors to 529 basketball players in junior and senior high school and college. The higher the frequency of church attendance, the greater the likelihood of superstitious beliefs and behaviors. Mormon basketball players had both the most frequent church attendance and a higher occurrence of superstitious practices than the other religions. Catholics were less superstitious than Mormons, but much more so than Protestants. They concluded that basketball players who attended church regularly were likely to have prayer-related thoughts and behaviors on the court.

A large percentage of superstitious behaviors are found in all the athletes (Buhrman et al. 1982). Commonplace activities, ritualized by the players, are listed in Table 2. There was no significant difference between the number of superstitions held nor the degree of superstitions between men and women although, not surprisingly, gender differences were found on specific items. Women were more likely to feel better prepared for a game if they were well dressed; men were more likely to feel prepared if they dressed sloppily.

Becker (1975) studied superstitious sports behavior in Yale athletes, attesting to their prevalence. Some behaviors somewhat resembled symptoms of OCD. For example:

- One lacrosse goalie has worn his favorite headband every game since high school and seldom washes it. One time after washing it, he severely injured his knee.

- A hockey player felt that "you never say the word 'shutout.'" Someone violated the rule and within 10 minutes their winning score of 4–0 lead was tied.
- A varsity runner states that "new shoes go fast," so he gets new spikes before each track meet.
- Borrowed or new clothes "can ruin an athlete's performance." One football player had a pair of lucky socks that were never washed.
- Another emphasizes that the *way* of getting dressed is crucial. He dresses the right side first "because it's the stronger side."
- Other superstitions are to prevent injury. One quarterback, who had to have his right shoulder bandaged after an injury, wears an elbow pad there permanently because it "protects the right side."
- A star tennis player preventively tapes his wrists exactly 5 inches above them. If taped differently, he fears something bad will happen.

Table 2. Sports superstition survey of 500 male and female basketball players

Superstitious Beliefs and Associated Behavior	Percentage Male ($N = 272$)	Percentage Female ($N = 257$)
Slap hand of scorer	93	95
Pep talks important for good performance	89	85
Team cheer	87	88
Stacking hands	87	91
Scoring first point	84	85
Unprepared if no pep talk	80	79
Make last basket in warm-up	80	85
Free throw—important to stand in identical spot	77	74
Music during warm-up	77	74
Cheerleading	77	54
Bounce ball same way before free throw	75	71
Need silence—seclusion before game	72	56
Bounce ball same number of times before free throw	66	64
Dressing well—feel better prepared	59	72
Snacks—energizers before contest (important for winning)	58	48
Pray for success before each game	57	61
Check appearance in mirror before games	53	68
Wear warm-up top same way	46	29
Coach encourages prayer—meditation	43	36

- The recent popular TV show *Cheers* featured a hockey player who had to have a club soda with lime, no ice, and a red straw the night prior to the game. He'd have to leave the napkin across the glass with the red straw across it. He'd have to walk back to his car in the exact same way for fear that his game would be ruined the next day.

In summary, superstitions or private rituals are prevalent and strongly ingrained in athletes. Presumably superstitious rituals give athletes some sense of control, thereby reducing anxiety.

As stressed by Neil (1982), players believing that their ability is fairly constant attribute the inconsistencies in their performance to some possibly connected piece of behavior, a charm, a piece of clothing, or something else. Superstitions appear to be a natural outcome of involvement in activities of an unpredictable and often dangerous

Table 2. *(continued)*

Superstitious Beliefs and Associated Behavior	Percentage Male ($N = 272$)	Percentage Female ($N = 257$)
Important for team to pray together	41	37
Gum chewing	38	68
Shifting weight before free throw	38	39
Coach is superstitious	39	41
Team has team player	33	36
Ritual before shooting free throw	32	42
Have lucky item of clothing	31	38
Team mascot helps cause	30	40
Afraid luck run out if no prayer	30	31
Toss ball between hands before shooting	28	23
Dressing sloppily—feel better prepared	25	17
Wears lucky charm on game days	22	29
Wearing luck charm so can't be seen	20	16
Coach takes lucky charm to game	20	20
Discarding lucky charm	19	12
When subbing in—take jacket to player	19	15
Wearing lucky charm so can be seen	15	12
Taping body—even if not injured	12	11
Tie double knot in laces	11	11
Wear socks inside out for luck	10	4
Good luck markings on shoes	5	8

Note. Reproduced with permission from Buhrmann et al. 1982.

nature. Through their use, athletes seem helped to maintain emotional balance under extreme pressure and some serve by contributing to team morale. Unlike obsessive-compulsive rituals that are deleterious and counterproductive, sports rituals were felt as helpful and noninterfering to these athletes.

Childhood Rituals and Superstitions and Childhood OCD: Are They Related?

To obtain systematic data, the number and strength of superstitions in 20 obsessive-compulsive children and 20 matched normal controls were compared. Superstitions were measured by a questionnaire about the most common superstitions believed by U.S. children. Children were also asked to recall if these were believed earlier (i.e., prior to the OCD).

Preliminary results from the superstition questionnaire confirm our clinical observation that obsessive-compulsive patients have occasional superstitions that followed their community pattern and did not differ from those of the control group. Even "superstitious" patients with OCD had no trouble in distinguishing superstitious behavior from their obsessive-compulsive behavior. Most important, obsessive-compulsive symptoms differ markedly from patterns of superstitions reviewed above and in clinical cases.

Checking, washing, and repeating rituals and obsessive thoughts of contamination and danger predominate in children (and adults) with OCD. Superstitions deal with brief "lucky" acts and objects.

Table 3 compares rituals and superstitions of normal children and children with OCD. The content, intensity, and distribution differ considerably. Obsessive-compulsive symptoms are elaborate, cumbersome, and somewhat bizarre. Note that the bedtime rituals and counting behaviors of normal childhood are seen in very young children. Retrospective data find no excess of bedtime rituals in obsessive-compulsive children compared to controls.

Childhood superstitions involve ladders, knocking on wood, and the number 13 and do not resemble obsessive-compulsive symptomatology. Sports rituals are different in that cleanliness and checking are virtually absent. Their intensity and idiosyncracies, however, *are* familiar, and suggest the importance of anxiety in initiating and maintaining these behaviors.

Summary

There are a few ways in which OCD rituals resemble developmentally normal childhood rituals. These include bedtime as a likely time for

Table 3. Patterns of ritual and superstition in normal and obsessive-compulsive children

Childhood Ritual or Superstition	Normal Development	Clinical Obsessive Compulsive Pattern
Bedtime rituals	Toddlers only	Elaborate, extensive, incapacitating, usually not related to going to bed per se
Stepping on crack	Young children commonly avoid	Rare as obsessive-compulsive symptom
Checking	Mild if at all	Extensive and incapacitating
Counting & lucky numbers	Normal developmental stage	Elaborate, pervasive, incapacitating but not common in OCD
Exactness/arranging	Brief stage, young age, often absent	Elaborate, incapacitating, fairly common
Touching	Minimal, seen in grade school games	In OCD can be elaborate, incapacitating
Collecting/hoarding	Usually collects things of significance and meaning, common in grade school	Hoards useless worn out objects, perhaps trash; not common
Bathing/hand washing	Preschool, not common in adolescence—usually mild preschool, not common	Major ritual of obsessive-compulsive children
Fear of contamination/germs	Brief, minimal features, if at all	Elaborate, incapacitating, most common obsession

rituals, not stepping on cracks, counting and having lucky and unlucky numbers, and wanting things in their right place. There are numerous and more important differences between developmental rituals, childhood superstitions, and childhood OCD. Normal developmental rituals are most intense in 4- to 8-year-olds, whereas OCD rituals persist far into adolescence. The hallmarks of OCD are washing, checking, hoarding, and repeating. The rituals of childhood stress rules about daily life with lucky numbers, avoiding cracks, and doing things right, incorporated into normal functioning. Rituals in normal children enhance their socializing process, help them master anxiety, and advance their development. In contrast, obsessive-compulsive rituals are incapacitating and painful, promoting social isolation and regressive behavior.

In the National Institute of Mental Health series, obsessive-compulsive children were not particularly superstitious (rated by structural interview) and had no exaggeration of normal developmental rituals. Thus the phenomena appear discontinuous on many levels, supporting a model of OCD that is discontinuous from normal development and relatively free from cultural influence. The data seem more compatible with a neuroethological approach, although undoubtedly there are cultural/environmental influences on expression.

References

Adams P: Obsessive Children. New York, Penguin Books, 1973

Albert S et al: Children's bedtime rituals as a prototype rite of safe passage. J Psychological Anthropology 2:85–105, 1979

Becker J: Superstition in sport. International Journal of Sport Psychology 6:148–152, 1975

Belanger AF: An empirical study of superstition and unfounded beliefs. Proceedings of the Iowa Academy of Science 51:355, 1944

Bender L, Schilder P: Impulsions: a specific disorder of the behavior of children. Arch Neurol Psychiatry 44:990–1008, 1940

Berman S: The psychodynamic aspects of behavior, in Basic Handbook of Child Psychiatry, Vol. 2. Edited by Noshpitz J. New York, Basic Books, 1979

Blum S: Some aspects of belief in prevailing superstitions. Psychol Reports 38:579–582, 1976

Blum SH, Blum LH: Do's and don'ts: an informal study of some prevailing superstitions. Psychol Reports 35:567–571, 1974

Buhrmann HG, Zaugg MK: Religion and superstition in the sport of basketball. The Journal of Sports Behavior 6:146–157, 1983

Buhrmann HG, Brown B, Zaugg MK: Superstitious beliefs and behavior: a comparison of male and female basketball players. The Journal of Sports Behavior 5:175–185, 1982

Conklin ES: Superstitious beliefs and practice among college students. Am J Psychol 30:83–102, 1919

Dashefsky PR: An operant investigation of the development of human superstitious behavior. Dissertation Abstracts 40:2358-B, 1979

Dudycha GJ: The superstitious beliefs of college students. Journal of Abnormal and Social Psychology 27:457–464, 1933

Emme EE: Modification and origin of superstition among 96 college students. J Psychol 10:279–291, 1940

Feingold BD: Superstition as a strategic research site for the investigation of belief: an extension of the operant superstition paradigm and an empirical inquiry into the role of hypothesis ambiguity in the development and maintenance of superstitious belief. Dissertation Abstracts 38:5059–5060, 1978

Fliess W: Knocking on wood: a note on the preoedipal nature of the magic effect. Psychoanal Q 13:327–340, 1944

Freud A: Normality and Pathology in Childhood: Assessments of Developments. New York, International Universities Press, 1965

Freud S: Totem and Taboo. London, Routledge & Kegan Paul, 1950

Gesell A, et al: Infant and Child in the Culture of Today. New York, Harper & Row, 1974

Grahame K: The Wind in the Willows. New York, Charles Scribner's Sons, 1965

Hamm P: An experimental investigation of socially mediated acquisition of superstitious behavior in children. Dissertation Abstracts 34:3532-B, 1974

Higgins ST: The social transmission of superstitions: operant behavior. Dissertation Abstracts 44:3561-B, 1983

Jahoda G: Scientific training and the persistence of traditional beliefs among West African university students. Nature 220:1356, 1968

Jahoda G: The Psychology of Superstition. New York, Jason Aronson, 1974

Jung CG: Collected Works, Vol. 5. London, Kegan Paul, 1956

Killen P, Wildman R, Wildman R: Superstitiousness and intelligence. Psychol Reports 34:1158, 1974

Lundeen GE, Caldwell OW: A study of unfounded beliefs among high school seniors. Journal of Educational Research 22:257–273, 1930

Luskin BR: The development of ritual greetings and leave takings in young children. Dissertation Abstracts International 41:2827-B, 1981

Maller JB, Lundeen GE: Sources of superstitious beliefs. Journal of Educational Research 26:321–343, 1933a

Maller JB, Lundeen GE: Superstition and emotional maladjustment. Journal of Educational Research 27:592–617, 1933b

Marmor J: Some observations on superstition in contemporary life. Am J Orthopsychiatry 13:119-30, 1956

Milne AA: When We Were Very Young. New York, EP Dutton & Co., 1952

Nagera H: The four-to-six year stage, in The Course of Life, Vol 1, Infancy and Early Childhood. Edited by Greenspan S, Pollock G. Washington, DC, Department of Health and Human Services, 1980

Neil GI: Demystifying sport superstition. International Review of Sport Sociology 17:99–124, 1982

Opie P, Opie I: The Lore and Language of School Children. London, Oxford University Press, 1959

Oremland JD: The Jinx Game. Psychoanal Study Child 28:419–431, 1973

Pasachoff JM, Cohen RJ, Pasachoff NW: Belief in the supernatural among Harvard and West African university students. Nature 227:971–972, 1970

Peterson C: Locus of control and belief in self-oriented superstitions. J Soc Psychol 105:305–306, 1978

Piaget J: The Child's Conception of the World. Totowa, NJ, Littlefield, Adams & Co, 1969

Plug C: The psychology of superstition: a review. Psychologia Africana 16:93–115, 1976

Pole J, Berenson N, Sass D, et al: Walking under a ladder: a field experiment on superstitious behavior. Personality and Social Psychology Bulletin 1:10–12, 1974

Powers EF: The influence of intelligence and personality traits upon false beliefs. J Soc Psychol 2:490–493, 1931

Robinson JF, Vitale LJ: Children with circumscribed interest patterns. Am J Orthopsychiatry 24:755–766, 1954

Rubin K, Fein G, Vandenberg B: Play, in Handbook of Child Psychology. Edited by Mussen P. New York, Wiley & Son, 1983

Simonds JE, Parraga H: Sleep behaviors and disorders in children and adolescents evaluated at psychiatric clinics. J Dev Behav Pediatr 5:6–10, 1984

Skinner BF: Science and Human Behavior. New York, Macmillan, 1953

Spinoza B: The Chief Works of Benedict de Spinoza. Translated from the Latin, introduction by Elwes RHM. New York, Dover Publications, 1955

Ter Keurst AJ: Comparative differences between superstitious and non-superstitious children. Journal of Experimental Education 7:261–267, 1939

Thouless RH, Brown LB: Petitionary prayer-belief in its appropriations and causal efficacy among adolescent girls, in From Religious Experience to a Religious Attitude. Edited by Goden A. Brussels, Lunnen Vitae Press, 1964 van Amerongen ST: Latency and prepubertal children, in Basic Handbook of Child Psychiatry, Vol. 3. Edited by Noshpitz J. New York, Basic Books, 1980

Wagner GA: The acquisition of superstitious behavior in children. Dissertation Abstracts 43:3762, 1983

Wagner ME: Superstitions and their social and psychological correlatives among college students. The Journal of the Educational Society 2:26-36, 1928

Wilder J: The lure of magic thinking. Am J Psychother 29:37–55, 1975

Zeiler M: Superstitious behavior in children: an experimental analysis. Adv Child Dev Behav 7:2–29, 1972

Chapter 18

Obsessive-Compulsive Disorder: The Religious Perspective

Larry Suess, D.O.
Martin S. Halpern

A vast literature untapped by psychiatry is that of the religious perspective on obsessive-compulsive disorder (OCD). This chapter examines both Catholic and Jewish sources in relation to this illness.

The Catholic Perspective

Definition

Within the Roman Catholic church, a version of OCD known as scrupulosity has been known for more than 400 years. From 1522 to 1523, Ignatius Loyola wrote *Spiritual Exercises to Conquer Self and Regulate One's Life and to Avoid Coming to a Determination Through any Inordinate Affection*, providing the Catholic Church a definition of scrupulosity through a description of his own obsessive behavior:

> After I have trodden upon a cross formed by two straws, or after I have thought, said or done some other thing, there comes to me from "without" a thought that I have sinned, and on the other hand it seems to me that I have not sinned; nevertheless I feel some uneasiness on the subject, inasmuch as I doubt and yet do not doubt. This is properly a scruple and temptation suggested by the enemy. (from Rickaby 1923, p. 164)

The term *scrupulosity* is derived from the Latin *scrupus*, whose diminutive form *scrupulus* means a small sharp stone. Conceptually, a minute weight could tip the scales of a sensitive balance, such as the scales of conscience (Palazziui 1962).

In 1615, the moral principles of scrupulous behavior were examined in Sanchez's *Praecepta Decalogi*. Another Spanish theologian, Gabriel Vazquez (1631) presented his arguments that scrupulosity was "judicium conscientiae erroneae" (an error in practical conscience). In 1660, the Anglican prelate Jeremy Taylor published the fascinating text *Doctor Dubitantium*, giving case materials to illustrate how religious scruples merge into obsessional disorder and then into nervous breakdown: "They repent when they have not sinned. [Scruple] is a trouble where the trouble is over, a doubt when doubts are resolved" (p. 36).

Catholic theologians further elaborated on the concept of scrupulosity. Saint Alphonus Liguori (1773) described scrupulosity as "a groundless fear of sinning that arises from erroneous ideas." Later definitions were similar; for example, "a disease, physical and moral, which produces a sort of derangement of conscience, and causes one to harbor vain fears of having offended God" (Tanquery 1923, p. 28), or "a groundless fear of having sinned grievously in an action which is perfectly lawful and praiseworthy" (Gearon 1927, p. 161).

O'Flaherty's (1966) summary is shown in Table 1, and is virtually the same as the DSM-III-R definition of OCD (American Psychiatric Association 1987).

The Church also carried out the first systematic survey of scrupulosity, predating any such efforts by psychiatrists in a sample of

Table 1. Comparison of scrupulosity with obsessive-compulsive disorder

Scrupulosity[a]	Obsessive-Compulsive Disorder[b]
Persistent concern with incident, thought, word, or deed.	Persistent intrusive idea, thought, or impulse.
Thoughts cause uneasiness and distress.	Ego dystonic (i.e., cause discomfort, uneasiness, and distress).
Person compelled and obsessional.	Obsessive thoughts and/or ritualized actions performed with subjective compulsion.
Occurs in person who is healthy, normal, and free of other pathological disorders.	Not due to another mental or physical disorder.

[a]O'Flaherty (1966)
[b]DSM-III-R (American Psychiatric Association 1987)

400 girls in a Catholic high school (Mullen 1927). Students were asked directly about their own awareness of their scrupulosity. Questions covered fears of committing some mortal sin unknown to oneself, praying excessively, and washing and cleaning habits. Seventeen were judged to be scrupulous (i.e., in some ways abnormal). Comments from the responders were strongly suggestive of OCD: "It seems to run in my family." "I always fear my analysis of an action is wrong. I fear that my judgment concerning a good or bad act is not correct." "When I was still younger, my mother was worried about my praying because I would say the prayers over and over and late into the night."

In *Scruples: Words of Consolation* (Gearon 1927), brief case histories are given:

> Z, the essence of good nature and charity, is ever pursued with the thought that she is always wishing harm. The more she examines her thought, the greater is her conviction of having a spiteful tendency. She prays fervently for those whom she think she hates, but the more she prays, the greater the hypocrite she feels. If she merely makes up her mind to do anything, she feels she has bound herself under the pain of mortal sin to do it.
>
> J, an employee in a boot shop, goes through veritable agony when selling a pair of boots. She examines the same pair again and again to see if there are any nails inside. She is haunted by dread that there may be a nail that will cause blood poisoning and then death. Thus she will be guilty of murder or, at least, manslaughter. The same person does not want to eat. She says she can't be tempted unless she exists. To take food helps her to exist, but this, she argues, will mean that she will make it possible for her to be tempted. Thus, to her mind, to eat is the occasion of sin. Therefore, she starves herself.
>
> L is continually wondering why water is wet, and why the leaves of trees are nearly always green. Moreover he has a dread of pouring water down the sink. If he pours it down, he begins to follow it in spirit through its various courses. He feels that when it reaches the river it may be frozen; children will skate in this ice; the ice may break; and he will be the cause of their being drowned. Seeing a notice in the street, he doubts whether he has read it right. He retraces his footsteps again, but the doubts only increase.

The National Institutes of Health (NIH) series has had a number of children and adults with religious preoccupations who would fit the definition of scrupulosity. Interviewing these cases, one feels forced into the role of confessor judge. It is easy to envision such patients as willing victims of a witch trial, and one is tempted to speculate how the flames of the Inquisition might have been fed by the occasional scrupulous case.

Etiology

Jean Charlier Gerson, Chancellor of the Sorbonne, in the early 1400s, outlined a systematic analysis of scrupulosity in his treatise *De Pusillanimitate* (Allers 1938). It was only after Loyola, however, that the Catholic Church found scrupulosity as an entity to be cherished. Eventually, during the 1960 ecumenical movement within the Catholic Church and in the Vatican II proclamations, parishioners with scrupulosity were referred to the psychiatrist (Larere 1964). Scrupulosity, however, was initially seen as a virtue to the church, although detrimental consequences to the individual were acknowledged.

For theologians prior to this century, a scruple involved a question of principle; they solved this question in accordance with their general doctrine about judgment of conscience. The 16th and 17th centuries' view was that scrupulosity arose from three causes: man (his nature and way of life), God, and the devil. Human nature allows a temperament disposed to fear. Other causes as relating to human nature are mania and melancholy—"aegritudo maniaca et melancholia." Because these "are diseases of the head, they engender disturbances of reason and memory" (Tesson 1964, p. 108).

It was reasoned that God was the probable cause of scruples. God withholds the enlightenment of mind that would enable one to see clearly what is right and what is wrong. God did not *cause* interior suffering, anxiety, and bad judgment of the afflicted person, but God *withholds* this enlightenment either in punishment for sin or for the purpose of promoting the victim's spiritual development through providing an occasion for the exercise of patience and humility and trust in God.

The alternate cause was Satan. The devil's object was to impede or destroy the victim's spiritual health, and this resulted in scrupulous behavior.

Scruples were said to arise from purely natural causes or supernatural intervention. Natural causes are physical and moral disease. Physical ailments that bring about scrupulosity are "a sort of depression" that tends to produce "the obsessing idea that one has sinned." The moral causes produce the same effect, such as the meticulous mind, a mind that loses itself amidst the most trifling details, that wants to reach absolute certitude in all things; a beclouded mind that represents God not as a just judge, but a merciless one; a mind that confuses feelings with consent in human acts (Tanquery 1923).

God uses obsession as a punishment for "inclinations of vainness" or as a trial to expiate past faults, to bring about a higher degree of sanctity. It's God's way of "fitting souls for contemplation." The devil, on the other hand, injects his activity "into the morbid predisposition of our nervous system in order to create a turmoil in our souls" (Tanquery 1923, p. 444).

Prummer's *Handbook of Moral Theology* (1949) also listed the causes of scrupulous conscience as natural or supernatural (i.e., God or the devil), but most frequently natural.

How could the clergy tell which is the correct etiology for a particular individual? Not easily. Saint Laurence Justian (quoted in Tesson 1964) proposed that scruples emanating from hell are "usually accompanied by a special darkening of the mind and by a notable bitterness of the heart, wherein they seek to engender distrust, lukewarmness, and the cooling of charity." On the other hand, "scruples deriving from human nature preserve a constant pattern, because they are consistent in their manifest effects. Experience shows naturally scrupulous people nearly always act in fear and perturbation of mind" (Tesson 1964, p. 109).

Treatment

The parallel between the Church's recommended treatment of scrupulosity and modern behavior therapy for OCD is humbling. Scruples must be attacked directly before they take deep root in the soul. The treatment for scruples was full and absolute obedience to an enlightened spiritual director. The spiritual director must, therefore, first attain the confidence of the sufferer of scrupulosity and wield his authority over the sufferer if he is to effect a cure. In order to gain confidence, one must not enter into discussion, but speak to them with authority, telling them categorically what they must do. To inspire this confidence, the spiritual director must merit it both by his confidence and his devotedness:

1. He will allow the penitent to speak first, limiting himself to a few remarks here and there to show that he has thoroughly understood. After that he will put a few questions to the penitent, to which the latter will answer yes or no, and thus the director will himself conduct the methodical examination of the penitent's conscience. Then he will add: I understand your case, you suffer in this or that manner. To see that he has been well understood is already a great comfort to the penitent, and at times suffices to win his confidence.
2. Devotedness must be joined to competence. The spiritual director must listen quietly to lengthy explanations of the penitent, at least in the beginning. He must be kind, taking an interest in that soul and expressing the desire and the hope of curing it. He must be gentle, refraining from taking a tone of severity or harshness, even when he is obliged to use the language of authority. Nothing wins confidence

more than this union between kindness and firmness." (Tanquery 1923, p. 447)

The alliance with the therapist and focus on changing the subject's behavior follow principles of a behaviorist text. The subject must have absolute obedience to the confessor and spiritual director: "Quod pro impossibile habeat posse scrupulosum curari confessorio non credentum ejus consiliis." (The cure of the scrupulous person must certainly be regarded as impossible if he does not trust his confessor and follow his counsel.) Once the penitent's confidence is obtained, the spiritual director exercises his authority and exacts obedience.

Tanquery (1923) further details treatment:

1. In giving this order the spiritual director must be direct, clear and precise, avoiding any equivocation, he must be positive, speaking categorically, never conditionally; for instance, he will not say: if this disturbs your peace, do not do it, rather he will say: do this, avoid that, spurn such temptation.
2. Generally no reasons must be given for the decisions especially at the beginning. Later on when the scrupulous penitent is capable of understanding them, and of feeling their weight, the director should briefly state these reasons in order to form his conscience little by little. But there must be no discussion of the decision itself. If there be any obstacles to prevent its immediate execution, they are to be taken into account, but the decision stands.
3. The spiritual director must not reverse his judgments. Before giving a decision he considers it fully, and gives no orders that cannot be insisted upon, but once an order has been given, it must not be revoked so long as there is no new fact requiring a change.
4. To ascertain if the order has been clearly understood, penitents should be asked to restate it, and then it but remains to have them carry it out. This is difficult, but they must be plainly told that they must report on it, and if they have failed to follow advice given, they will not be listened to until they have complied. There will be ample opportunity, therefore, to repeat the same injunction many times. This is done without losing patience but with increasing firmness, and in the end the scrupulous persons will yield obedience. (p. 448)

The spiritual director can also have the penitent put this principle in writing *in the form of an oath*, for example:

I am in conscience bound to take only evidence into account, that is to say, a certitude that excludes all doubt, a certitude as clear as the one that tells me that two and two makes four. I cannot, therefore, commit a sin either mortal or venial, unless I am absolutely certain that the action I am to perform is forbidden under pain of mortal or venial sin, and that fully aware of this fact, I will nevertheless do it just the same. I will, therefore, pay no attention whatsoever to probabilities, no matter how strong they may be, I will hold myself bound solely by clearcut and positive evidence. Barring such, there is no sin. (Tanquery 1923, p. 450)

In summary, much of our modern approach to OCD has been anticipated by church writings on scrupulosity. We are particularly impressed with the identification and treatment of young subjects. It is probable that some patients are still identified and treated entirely within the church.

While Catholic writings are the most extensive, obsessive-compulsive symptoms have occurred within other religions. In fact, Catholics were not overrepresented in the National Institute of Mental Health (NIMH) epidemiologic study (see Chapter 15). It may be, however, that a cultural emphasis on ritual directs symptoms toward religious expression.

The Jewish Perspective

The Biblical Approach to Vows and Its Development in Rabbinic Tradition

In Chapter 12, Daniel's story, we have the only known occasion in which Judaic religious law was formally invoked as a means of treatment of OCD. But because we have seen other children like Daniel, for whom Jewish ceremonies became part of their symptom pattern, this section contains the background that supplied the rationale for Daniel's treatment, and suggests that OCD has been a theological issue in Judaic tradition just as it has in Catholicism.

The Biblical period. In the Biblical Book of Numbers, the fourth of the first five books of the Hebrew Bible, there is a special section dealing with the sanctity of vows, and vows and promises are dealt with elsewhere in the Bible as well. Examples of vows a person might have assumed in Biblical times range from gift offerings to temple worship or the vow of the Nazirite to abstain from drinking wine and cutting one's hair. Others center around abstaining from normal relationships with fellow humans. An individual might also vow to avoid deriving satisfaction from certain pleasurable activities.

A vow was considered sacred, not to be taken lightly, and it was expected that the author of the vow would ordinarily fulfill it. In the post-Biblical period and onward, the mainstream of rabbinic tradition and Jewish theology greatly opposed the making of vows. From the New English Bible (1970): "If you forbear to vow, it shall be no sin in thee" (Deuteronomy 23:23); and "Be not rash with thy mouth.... Better is it that thou shouldest not vow, than that thou shouldest vow and not pay" (Ecclesiastes 5:1,4). From the Babylonian Talmud (1927): "Do not form the habit of making vows. He who makes a vow, even though he fulfill it, is called a wicked man" (Nedarim 22a:776).

During the Talmudic period, making vows was actually considered a sign of bad breeding and affected the honor of one's family. The making of vows was tolerated when it was made to rid oneself of bad habits, but the Jewish Law stresses that one should strive for the desired and without the aid of vows (Schulchan Aruch 1927).

However, since the ideal was not always achievable and people did make vows, rabbinical authorities were faced with a challenge as to how one can cope with vows that carried sanctity, but for various reasons could not be fulfilled. Such vows might, for example, clash with family obligations or interfere with interpersonal relationships. Such cases are alluded to in the Book of Numbers, where certain exceptions are stated that permitted the nullification of a vow by a wife or an unmarried daughter living in her father's house. In both cases the vow had to have been heard on the day it was made, otherwise it could not be retracted by father or husband.

Post-Biblical and Talmudic Legislation

In the post-Biblical period, especially in Talmudic legislation, a great deal of discussion centered around the ability to annul a vow that, due to circumstances beyond the control of the individual, could not be fulfilled. There were sages who took the position that a vow, once made, could never be withdrawn. In the Babylonian Talmud (1927), we find the statement: "The annulment of a vow is like an object fluttering in the air, and we have no source upon which to lean" (Tractate Hagigah 10a).

But many sages took the position that Jewish Law allows the possibility of annulment of vows. It was argued that a person might regret a vow and there should be a remedy for its retraction.

A good deal of discussion centers around a tragic story recorded in the Biblical Book of Judges (Tanakh 1985). Jeptha was a Warrior-Judge who led his people during a chaotic period in Jewish history. Just prior to an important battle, he evoked God to help him by promising to offer as a sacrifice the first living thing that came out to meet him when he returned victorious. What was Jeptha's horror to see his own child, his daughter, running out to meet him. The Bible is silent as to the actual fate of Jeptha's daughter. However, in the body of collective literature that seeks to interpret the Bible, called the "Midrash," there are references to the possibility for Jeptha to have annulled his vow by appearing before the recognized sage of his day and expressing regret for a thoughtless vow. One such reference takes the position that Jeptha refused to humble himself before the priest Pinhas, and Pinhas refused to initiate any procedure for him.

In would appear that those sages who favored the annulment of vows succeeded in establishing a methodology for the annulment of oaths that became a standard in Jewish Law and is still operative today.

A person who uttered a vow that cannot be fulfilled may appear before a sage or a quorum of three knowledgeable men, who would ask the individual: "If you had known the consequences of making this vow would you have done it?" If the person responded, "I would not have taken the vow," the sage or the quorum of three individuals would pronounce the person absolved of the oath. Such absolution would not apply if it involved damages or harm to an innocent victim of the vow. In such a case, proper restitution must first be made, be it an apology or some other remuneration.

A further remedy for the failure on the part of the community to fulfill vows is found in the sacred ceremony enacted each year prior to the beginning of the Jewish Holy Day "Yom Kippur"—the Day of Atonement. In the presence of the entire congregation, a special formula is recited, which is called "Kol Nidre"—All Vows—and which provides the means to begin by those who are to begin a 24-hour period of fasting in atonement for transgressions and for oaths which could not be fulfilled and/or which one regrets.

> All vows, bonds, promises, obligations, and oaths (to God) wherewith we have vowed, sworn and bound ourselves from this Day of Atonement unto the next Day of Atonement, may it come unto us for good; lo, of all these, we repent us in them. They shall be absolved, released, annulled, made void, and of none effect; they shall not be binding nor shall they have any power. Our vows (to God) shall not be vows; our bonds shall not be bonds; and our oaths shall not be oaths. (High Holy Day Prayer Book 1951, p. 207)

A lesser-known ceremony, but one that has been in vogue for many centuries and focuses more closely on individual vows, is referred to in Jewish tradition as "Hatarat Nedarim"—The Annulment of Vows. (See formula at end of article.)

The traditional time for this ceremony is just prior to "Rosh Ha-shanah"—the New Year. In this ceremony, three or more individuals band together and take turns constituting a quasi-ecclesiastical court. Each individual recites a formula whereby he or she renounces all oaths and promises. Reference in this formula is made to vows and various promises forgotten, as well as vows taken in a dreamlike state, and, of course, vows of which one is still aware.

The cathartic effect of this ceremony permits the individual to approach the High Holy Days free of nagging concern over vows taken or made that did not come to fruition.

Responsa Literature: T'Shuvot

Following the Talmudic period, Jewish Law was regulated to a great extent through the practice of questions directed to leading Jewish sages in all parts of the world. The responses (T'Shuvot) were often adopted as a standard practice.

Bar Ilan University in Israel has computerized many "Responsa" that for centuries had been available in manuscript form only. Through their project, precedents of unusual situations involving oaths that had been considered by Rabbinical authorities were obtained. It appears that from the Gaonic period (sixth century), there were attempts to find justification for the annulment of vows. The following is a brief selection from the Responsa Project (1987) to questions relating to vows:

A man vowed to abstain from use of the sea in the name of the Biblical Nazirite Samson, son of Manoah, husband of Delilah, who toppled the walls of Gaza. Rabbi Moses Ticktin (19th century) took the opinion that if the individual was now compelled by circumstances to undertake a sea voyage, his vow should be annulled despite the unusual formula invoked.

A man took an oath in a dream state in the presence of a number of people not to eat in the home of another person. Rabbi Solomon Ben Adret (1235–1310) ruled, based on Talmudic precedent, that in a situation of remorse, his vow should be annulled out of compassion for him. Furthermore, a vow in a dream is treated as a vow made while awake.

Rabbi Moses Isserles (1530–1572), in responding to instances of impossible vows or foolish vows, takes the position that they should be annulled. He records the case of a man who in a dream vows that if his son recovers from an illness he, the father, will not join in a festival dinner until his son reaches the age of 13. Rabbi Isserles terms this a virtually impossible vow that can bring on marital conflict. Furthermore, if he vows not to cut his son's hair until he reaches 13 years, it is the vow of a pious fool and a behavioral aberration.

Many Responsa justify the annulment of an oath on the basis that to do otherwise would be to create a stumbling block for the maker of the oath: "You shall not place a stumbling block before the blind." The annulment of such an oath becomes a "Mitzvah" (a good deed) and a meritorious act on behalf of an individual who is confronted with a variety of problems as the result of a vow.

Daniel's Treatment

Daniel (see Chapter 12) had resolved to punish himself by making some oath to abstain from a particularly pleasurable activity. In time he forgot the oath and, in order to maintain the sense of remorse, he made other oaths to compensate for those he had forgotten. Before long he had developed an entire system of negative oaths and promises that rendered him incapable of engaging in any pleasurable or productive activity.

My [Rabbi Halpern] initial contact with Daniel preceded any knowledge of the genesis of his disorder. He came to me from another synagogue seeking an understanding of the Jewish attitude toward oaths made to avoid pleasure. In our discussion, I tried to explain that Judaism did not look with favor on asceticism as a means of finding favor with God. Whenever possible, such an oath taken to abstain from pleasure should be discouraged. We did not discuss the annulment of oaths at that time.

Daniel's therapist later divulged, with the patient's permission, the nature of his disorder. Dr. Mansueto explained the religious ramification stemming from the patient's concern for his Jewish background, and he sought guidance in treating Daniel, possibly utilizing some religious mechanism within the framework of Jewish tradition.

I suggested that it might be possible to utilize the formula of "Hatarat Nedarim"—Annulment of Vows, inasmuch as it appeared to encompass many of the concerns that were afflicting his patient (Babylonian Talmud, Nedarim 1927).

The three of us met to discuss this procedure. It was necessary not only to explain the ceremony but, even more important, to establish in Daniel's mind a sense of the formula's efficacy and its validity in the sight of Jewish tradition. It should be recalled that where this procedure is used in a normal service during the High Holy Days, participants believe in its efficacy and a heightened spiritual upliftment results.

I emphasized that the use of the annulment procedure did not constitute a cure in itself, but was rather a means to an end. When used in conjunction with a positive therapeutic setting, and even repeated when necessary, it could help reverse the debilitating effects of the system of rules and vows with which Daniel had surrounded himself.

As already seen in Chapter 12, Daniel thought over the contemplated procedure and called a few days later to set a date for the actual ceremony. Two other rabbinical colleagues were contacted, and while maintaining confidentiality, I explained what we were planning to do.

The ritual was performed in the sanctuary of my congregation with only the patient, the two other rabbis, and the therapist present.

The patient had been given an opportunity to study the contents of the formula, and certain difficult terminologies were explained to him.

The ceremony of Hatarat Nedarim had a visible positive effect on Daniel. Daniel's therapist also saw an improvement. We met again some months later to clarify some aspects of the ceremony and of the Jewish attitude toward the attainment of pleasure and satisfaction.

It was emphasized that, far from being discouraged, the main stress of Judaism considers enjoyment a legitimate goal of life. We discussed statements by Jewish sages relating to joy as a vital ingredient in life. For example:

> Rabbi Aibo said: It is like a King who has filled his palace with enjoyments; if he has no visitors, what pleasure does he derive from them? Thus, when the Angels objected to the creation of man, God replied: "And of what use are all the good things I have created, unless men are there to enjoy them?"
>
> Midrash Rabbah, 1939, Vol 1, pp. 58–59

> Do not miss a day's enjoyment or forego your share of innocent pleasure.
>
> New English Bible
> Ecclesiasticus Apocrypha, 1970, 14:14, p. 135

> If you see anyone not taking food or drink when he should, refusing baths and oils, neglecting his clothes, sleeping on the ground, and fancying that he is thus practicing temperance, pity his self-deception and show him the true path of temperance.
>
> Philo
> De Decalogo, 1552

> Man will be called to account in the hereafter for each enjoyment he declined here without sufficient cause.
>
> Jerusalem Talmud, 1965

Summary

The oath always had and continues to have sanctity in Jewish tradition. One should fulfill sacred promises. But in cases where the fulfillment can be deleterious for the individual, the formula of annulment of oaths can be a beneficial aid. It is vital that the patient or client believe in the concept and formula. In its normal use for practicing Jews, the formula can be an important means of cleansing oneself of thoughts that impede the development of a healthy attitude toward life.

The effect of Hatarat Nedarim, by its very definition, is to cut away attachment to unfulfilled vows and promises that, like excess baggage, impede our progress in the journey through life.

Formula for Annulment of Vows

It is meritorious to annul vows on the day before Rosh Hashanah. The three "Judges" sit while the petitioner seeking annulment stands before them and states:

Listen, please, my masters, expert judges—every vow or oath or prohibition or restriction that I adopted by use of the term "konam" [Ed: vow of abstinence], or the term "cherem" [Ed: a ban or ostracism] that I vowed or swore while I was awake or in a dream; or that I swore by means of God's Holy Names that it is forbidden to erase or by means of the Name HASEM, Blessed is He; or any form of naziritism [Ed: abstinence from shaving or cutting one's hair], that I accepted upon myself, even the naziritism of Samson [which does not include a prohibition against contact with the dead]; or any prohibition, even a prohibition to derive enjoyment that I imposed upon myself or upon others by means of any expression of prohibition, whether by specifying the term "prohibition" or by use of the terms "konam" or "cherem" or any commitment—even to perform a mitzvah—that I accepted upon myself, whether the acceptance was in terms of a vow, a voluntary gift, an oath, naziritism, or by means of any other sort of expression, or whether it was made final through a handshake; any form of vow or voluntary gift, or any custom that constitutes a good deed to which I have accustomed myself; and any utterance that escaped my mouth or that I vowed in my heart to perform, any of the various optional good deeds, or good practices, or any good thing that I have performed three times without specifying that the practice does not have the force of a vow; whether the thing I did related to myself or to others, both regarding vows that are known to me and those that I have already forgotten regarding all of them, I regret retroactively and I ask and request of your eminences an annulment of them. [My reason is that] I am fearful that I will stumble and become entrapped, Heaven forbid, in the sin of vows, oaths, naziritism, cheremus, prohibitions, konams, and [violation of] agreements.

I do not regret, Heaven forbid, the performance of the good deeds I have done, rather I regret only having accepted them upon myself with an expression of a vow or oath or naziritism or prohibition or cherem or konam or agreement or acceptance of the heart, and I regret not having said, "Behold I do this without [adopting it in terms of] a vow, oath, naziritism, cherem, prohibition, konam, or acceptance of the heart."

Therefore, I request annulment for them all. I regret all of the aforementioned, whether they were matters relating to money, or whether they are matters relating to the body or whether they are matters relating to the soul. Regarding them all, I regret the terminology of vow, oath, naziritism, prohibition, cherem, konam and acceptance of the heart.

Now behold, according to the Law, one who regrets and seeks annulment must specify the vow, but please be informed, my masters, that it is impossible to specify them because they are many. Nor do I seek annulment of those vows that cannot be annulled; therefore may you consider as if I had specified them. (The Complete Art Scroll Machzor 1985, pp. 2–4)

References

Allers R: Confessor and alienist. American Ecclesiastical Review 119:410, 1938

American Psychiatric Association: Diagnostic and Statistical Manual of Mental Disorders, 3rd ed, revised (DSM-III-R). Washington, DC, American Psychiatric Association, 1987

Babylonian Talmud (Tractate Nedarim, Tractate Hagigah). The Widow & Brothers Romm, Vilna, Lithuania, 1927

Complete Art Scroll Machzor (High Holy Day Prayer Book: Vol. 1, Rosh Hashanah). Brooklyn, NY, Mesorah Publications, 1985

Gearon P: Scruples: Words of Consolation (3rd ed). Dublin & Cork, Talbot Press, 1927

High Holy Day Prayer Book, Silverman Ed. Hartford, United Synagogue of America Prayer Book Press, 1951

Jerusalem Talmud. Jerusalem, Talmudic Institute, 1965

Larere F: Pastoral behavior towards the scruples, in The Treatment of Scruples. Edited by Carroll MG. Illinois, Divine Word Publication, 1964, pp. 107–125

Liguori St. Alfonso: Theologia Moralis: Vol 1, Liber II, Tract 1, De Conscientia Scrupulorum. Vol. 3, Praxis Confessarii, Caput 7: Quomodo se gerere debeat cum scrupulosis. Bassano, Apud Remondini, 1773

Midrash Rabbah: Genesis. London, Soncino Press, 1939

Mullen J: Psychological Factors in the Pastoral Treatment of Scruples: Studies in Psychology and Psychiatry. Washington, DC, Catholic University of America Publishers, 1927

New English Bible, Ecclesiasticus Apocrypha. New York, Oxford Press, 1970

O'Flaherty VM: How to Cure Scruples. Milwaukee, The Bruce Publishing Co, 1966

Palazziui P (ed): Dictionary of Moral Theology. London, Burns & Oates, 1962

Philo of Alexandria, De Decalogo. Antwerpiae, Excudebat Verwithhaghen, 1553

Prummer DM (ed): Handbook of Moral Theology. New York, PJ Kennedy & Sons, 1949

Responsa Project (responsa cited by Rabbis Tictin, Ben Adret, Isserles, and Dembitzer). Bar Ilan University, Institute for Computers in Jewish Life, Chicago, 1987

Rickaby JJ: The Spiritual Exercises of St. Ignatius Loyola: Spanish and English, with a continuous commentary by JJ Rickaby. New York, Benziger Bros, 1923

Sanchez T: Opus Morale, in Percepta Decalogi. Lugdini, Anisson, 1615

Schulchan Aruch: The Code of Jewish Law. Translated by Golden H. New York, Star Hebrew Publishing Co, 1927

Tanakh: A New Translation of the Holy Scriptures. Philadelphia, Jewish Publication Society, 1985

Tanquery A: The Spiritual Life: A Treatise on Ascetical and Mystical Spirituality. Tournai, Belgium, Desclee & Co, 1923

Taylor J: Doctor Dubitantium, or the rule of conscience in all her general measures: serving as a great instrument for the determination of causes of conscience. London, J Flesher for R Royston, 1660

Tesson F: Doctrinal history, in The Treatment of Scruples. Edited by Carroll MG. Illinois, Divine Word Publication, 1964, pp. 11–87

Vazquez G: Commentariorum ad Disputatum in Primam Secundae Sancti Thomae. Lugdini, Jacobi Cardon, 1631

Chapter 19

Obsessive-Compulsive Disorder: Is It Basal Ganglia Dysfunction?

Steven P. Wise, Ph.D.
Judith L. Rapoport, M.D.

We present here a hypothesis that selective basal ganglia dysfunction underlies obsessive-compulsive disorder (OCD). At the basis of our hypothesis are neuroanatomical, neuropharmacological, and behavioral studies indicating a complex perceptual and cognitive role for the basal ganglia in addition to its more well-accepted motor functions. The hypothesis is also based on case reports suggesting increased obsessive-compulsive symptomatology in certain syndromes associated with basal ganglia disease, response to psychosurgery, and brain-imaging studies. As part of our hypothesis, we present a neural model in which the striatum acts to trigger behavior, and posit that permissive failure of such a system (i.e., the inappropriate triggering of genetically stored and learned behaviors) is the primary cause of OCD.

Basal Ganglia Disease and OCD

Tourette's Syndrome and Tics

In his original 1885 description of basal ganglia-associated syndrome that today bears his name, Gilles de la Tourette (1885) reported an association between recurrent motor and phonic tics and obsessive-compulsive behavior. He described a patient who suffered from tics and vocalizations, as well as tormenting, obsessive thoughts: "The more revolting these explosions are, the more tormented she becomes by the fear she will say them again; and this obsession forces these words into her mind and to the top of her tongue." The association between Tourette's syndrome and OCD had since been clarified and expanded. There is a strong genetic link between the multiple motor-verbal tics of Tourette's syndrome and OCD (Pauls et al. 1986). The disorders occur together in the same families, but not necessarily (although frequently) in the same individuals. In fact, from 15 to 80 percent of patients with Tourette's syndrome are described as having at least some abnormal obsessive-compulsive symptoms, a rate greatly in excess of the 2 percent lifetime prevalence of OCD in the general population (Karno et al., in press). Conversely, tics occur in childhood OCD far more frequently than would be expected by chance (Dr. S. Swedo, personal communication, 1988).

There is almost a century of recorded associations between simple motor tics and OCD. Osler, in his 1894 monograph *On Chorea and Choreiform Affections*, described a girl with "Tic of muscles of the face and neck; fixed ideas; arithromania":

> A.B., aged 13, was seen September 6, 1890. She is an only daughter in a family with marked neuropathic taint. The father died insane; the mother is a high-strung, nervous woman. The child is well grown, and well nourished, though rather stout for her age. She is very bright and intelligent, and perhaps has not had as much control as was good for her. For a year or more she has had occasional twitchings of the muscles of the face and neck, noticeable in the quick sudden elevations of the eyebrows, or in movements of the platysma muscles. They have not been severe, and for days it may not have been at all noticeable.

> A short time after the onset of the twitchings, it was noticed that she began gradually to have all sorts of queer notions and practices, many of which persisted for some weeks or months, and were then changed for others not less anomalous. Some of her vagaries are as follows, nearly all being modifications of the fixed idea known as arithromania: Before getting into bed at night she lifts each foot and taps nine times on the edge of the bed. After brushing her teeth she has to count to one hundred. For a year at least she has always entered the house by the back door, protesting that she never can enter by the front door again. Lest her mother should prevent her getting in by the back door, she for months carried the key herself. On reaching the door she knocks three times on the edge of the window near by, and three times on the door before unlocking it. She will not under any circumstances button her shoes. For a long time she would not pronounce the name of anyone, but would spell it, and if she wished for anything at the table she would spell the word, but not pronounce it. In drinking water she will take a mouthful, then put the tumbler down, turn it once or twice and repeat this act

every time she drinks. She would not brush her hair except at the extreme tips, and it is only under the strictest compulsion that she will allow the hair on the top of the head to be combed. Before putting on clean under-clothes she has to count so many numbers that there is a great difficulty in getting her to make the change, except under the strongest threats from her mother. (p. 82)

Postencephalitic Parkinson's Disease: A Dissociation of Will and Action

The best classic description of neurologically based OCD comes from Constantin von Economo, whose monograph of 1920 (translated to English in 1931) contains elegant clinical descriptions of postencephalitic disorders. In 1916 to 1917, an outbreak in Europe of viral encephalitis lethargica, as it was called, was followed, as previous smaller epidemics had been, by a somnolentlike state accompanied by parkinsonian features. In his study of hundreds of these patients, von Economo provided a comprehensive phenomenology, course, and neuropathology of the disorder. He reported that this infectious, neurotoxic lesion involved the basal ganglia and was associated with a sense of compulsion reminiscent of OCD in addition to motor changes. In discussing the psychological changes in these patients, von Economo argued against a role for the cerebral cortex in the generation of these uncontrollable movements and, instead, focused on subcortical centers, presumably including the basal ganglia:

> These patients do not say "I have a twitch in my hand," but rather as a rule "I have got to move my hand that way." The frequent subjectivization of these processes, experienced as compulsory by the patients is, I believe, one of their characteristic attributes. From this subjectivization we may deduce that in cases where the condition manifests itself, centres, probably in the diencephalon-mesencephalon, are affected whose motor function contributes intimately to the constitution of the "sensation of personality" and even to a greater extent than some parts of the cerebral cortex because, for instance, in Jacksonian fits affecting an arm as a result of a lesion of the anterior central convolution of the cerebrum itself, the patient says, "I have a twitch in my arm," that is, the movement does not become subjectivated, though it has its origin in the cerebral cortex. (p. 121)

Von Economo also noted a whole range of peculiar tics associated with these compulsions including blepharospasms, mimetic tics of clucking or hissing, torticollis, and tics of the upper and lower extremities, as well as fits of yelling and yawning. Von Economo concluded that "motor disturbances of encephalitics were reminiscent of compulsive movements and compulsive actions, with frequently ensuing utterances of speech and trends of thought of a compulsive character" (p. 120).

The problem of volitional disabilities continues to plague modern medicine as well as philosophy and reaches far beyond the particular disorders of obsessions and compulsions (Dunnet 1984). There are several disorders in which a dissociation of will and action are observed, as it was in von Economo's patients. But obsessive-compulsive patients are still, in a sense, "free" in that they "will *not* to will." This higher-order free will is a prominent and, in fact, defining feature of OCD: compulsive hand washers know that there are powerful reasons not to wash their hands (e.g., humiliation and waste of time), but simply do not act in accordance with those incentives and, at a simpler level, feel forced to carry out the rituals. Similarly, von Economo's (1931) postencephalitic patients describe "having to" act but not "wanting to":

> In spite of intact intelligence and the wish to execute a movement, in spite of the undisturbed possession of the imaginative faculty and the consequent existence of intention (e.g., to change an uncomfortable position) . . . [the] patient is unable to supply the impulse for the act of moving his otherwise sound limbs. (p. 162)

Although the possible linkage between postencephalitic and basal ganglia disease is intriguing, the lesions are by no means exclusively located in the basal ganglia; there tends to be a kaleidoscopic array of focal lesions and several brain regions. Indeed, von Economo stressed the involvement of the cerebral aqueduct, tegmentum, and gray matter ventral to the caudal third ventricle. Nevertheless, the basal ganglia are very much affected in the disease, which has a profound effect on the relation between volition and behavior.

Sydeham's Chorea

Sydenham's chorea, a disorder of children and adolescents, is characterized by sudden, aimless, irregular movements of the extremities frequently associated with emotional instability and muscle weakness. In children, the disorder occurs following rheumatic heart disease, as part of the complex of rheumatic fever. It is associated with high antibody titers to specific streptococcal antigens. These are usually high only for about 2 months following the infection, however, and the test is of limited value in chronic cases. Interestingly, the disorder, like OCD, is extremely rare in black populations. Postmortem studies in Sydenham's chorea have reported that perivascular cellular infiltration and neural degeneration is most pronounced in the striatum (Greenfield and Wolfsohn 1922). Further, Husby et al. (1976) reported that 50 percent of patients with postrheumatic chorea contain specific antibodies to caudate and putamen nucleus neurons, suggesting that the mechanism by which Sydenham's chorea is produced involves the immune system. Thus this disorder is of particular interest since it occurs exclusively in young people, may involve an autoimmunity toward basal ganglia, and has been linked with OCD.

Grimshaw (1964) reported an excess of Sydenham's chorea in the historic patients with OCD compared with a nonobsessional control group. Conversely, Freeman et al. (1965) described an increase in "neuroses," including OCD, in a group of 40 pediatric cases with Sydenham's chorea. In an ongoing survey of obsessive symptoms of 18 children with Sydenham's chorea, 3 of 18 cases examined to date show a clinical level of symptoms of OCD. Statistically, in the general adolescent population, a sample of 400 would be needed to yield two patients with OCD. This increase in automatic, compulsive, and stereotyped behaviors and thoughts occurred selectively in the patients with Syndenham's chorea and was not prominent in the comparison group of other patients from the same clinics who had rheumatic fever without Sydenham's chorea (Swedo et al. 1987).

Other Presumed Basal Ganglia Disorders and OCD

Several cases have been reported in which discrete lesions of the basal ganglia produced psychological changes that resemble obsessional illness. Laplane et al. (1984) reported a case of a 41-year-old man who suffered a rare but malignant neurotoxic reaction to a wasp sting. His initial drastic neurological disorder, coma followed by choreic movements and gait impairments, diminished over the next several months. But over the following 12 years, he had a rather apathetic, indifferent appearance and, in general, lacked motivation for life. The striking aspect of this case was that:

> two years after encephalopathy, he began to show stereotyped activities. The most frequent consisted in mental counting, for example up to twelve or a multiple of twelve, but sometimes it was a more complex calculation. Such mental activities sometimes were accompanied by gestures, such as finger pacing of the counts. To switch on and off a light for one hour or more was another of his most common compulsions. When asked about this behavior he answered that he had to count . . . that he could not stop . . . that it was stronger than him. . . . Once he was found on his knees pushing a stone with his hands: he gave the explanation that he must push the stone. (p. 377)

The computed tomography (CT) scan of this patient showed bilateral low-density lesions in the internal part of the lentiform nucleus (i.e., the globus pallidus). The case is of further interest in that after a variety of other drugs has been tried, clomipramine (250/mg/day) greatly improved, although did not cure, his behavior. This is one of the few demonstrations of clomipramine-linked improvement in obsessive-compulsive behavior following a known basal ganglia lesion.

Over the past decade, we and others have evaluated children with choreiform and athetoid movements that presented as OCD. Denckla (Chapter 7) summarized her neurological examinations of more than 50 children with OCD. Mild choreiform movements were prominent in this group, although other abnormal patterns were also found. These movements were less prominent in follow-up studies and, thus, seem an early characteristic of the disorder. Similarly, in our series of acute cases of childhood OCD, jerking peripheral movements are particularly prominent and resemble those seen in Sydenham's chorea.

This disturbance is fleeting, however, and disappears over the initial months of the disorder. One rather severe case will illustrate the several we have seen:

> A.B. had always been an "uptight" child, who worried at the start of each new school year, and for whom Hebrew school, with its preparation for the Bar Mitzvah, had been full of anxieties. His parents had consulted a psychologist because he was so worried over the ceremony, but reassurance and an easier studying schedule had seemed to solve this. But shortly after his 13th birthday, A. had told his parents of a new problem: He couldn't get "numbers" out of his head, and would say the number 4 and do things, touching, walking, jumping, counting, in 4s over and over again. Psychotherapy and a series of antianxiety and antidepressant medications were tried. At age 14, odd movements, a writhing of his body and arms, began, together with periods of muteness. He complained that he still could not stop numbers and words from going over and over, and that they were worse. The movements were unusual in pattern, puzzling the several neurologists who saw him. He would grimace, pursing his lips while making soft smacking sounds; his head would be to one side resting on his shoulder, and his body would writhe and jerk toward that same side. In between these bursts of writhing activity, he would sit mute, appearing to make a strained effort to respond when spoken to, but not producing any sound. During rare hours free from these symptoms, he complained about "the numbers." There appeared to be intellectual deterioration, but EED, LP, CT scans were normal.
>
> A diagnosis of atypical Tourette's syndrome was considered. There was slow but steady improvement on clomipramine, together with moderate doses of haloperidol. At 3-year follow-up, he is quite improved, and now attends regular school.

Brain-Imaging Studies

More direct data about a role of basal ganglia in OCD is provided by the study of Luxenberg et al. (in press), in which volumetric CT scan analyses were compared in 10 male patients with OCD (mean age, 20 years) and 10 matched normal controls. The only significant difference between the groups was a decreased volume of the caudate nuclei bilaterally in the patients with OCD ($p = .0002$); the lenticular nuclei and thalami did not differ from controls.

Baxter et al. (1987), using positron emission tomography (PET), found increased metabolic rates bilaterally in the caudate nuclei and the lateral orbito-frontal cortex in 14 obsessive-compulsive patients compared to 14 depressed patients and 14 normal controls. Interestingly, successful treatment with clomipramine did not lessen, and even increased, these differences. These important observations clearly need to be replicated and extended. For example, better quantification of the caudate volume and of associated limbic cortical regions could be achieved with magnetic resonance imaging (MRI) brain scans. Future work should include scans of familial patients with OCD as well as an examination of both state and trait markers and medical history (e.g., birth insults) in relation to these anatomical and metabolic measures.

Psychosurgery

Obsessive-compulsive disorder is one of the few psychiatric disorders for which psychosurgery may be indicated (Kettle and Marks 1986). We have reviewed 29 published reports of psychosurgical treatment in which OCD was one of the main disorders being treated. No studies were ideal; they varied widely in terms of their criteria for diagnosis, rating of illness, follow-up data, and reported improvement. The best documented studies are those following anterior capsulotomy, or cingulectomy, currently the preferred operation.

In capsulotomy, bilateral basal lesions in the anterior limb of the internal capsule are made. The lesions are thought to interrupt frontal cingulate projections, but the target zone for the lesion lies within the striatum, adjacent to the caudate nuclei. In cingulectomy, lesions are made in the anterior portion of the cingulate gyrus, interrupting tracks between cingulate gyrus and frontal lobes and several additional efferent projections of the anterior cingulate cortex. Further, Hassler (1981) reported that stereotaxic lesions in the mediodorsal and anterior nuclei of the thalamus, and their projection systems to the cortex, may diminish both Tourettic and obsessive-compulsive behaviors. It is noteworthy that these are the thalamic nuclei providing the main inputs to the cingulate and frontal cortex.

Although the psychosurgical results are far from conclusive, taken together with other evidence, these data are consistent with a model of OCD involving dysfunction of basal ganglia and frontal lobe–basal ganglia interactions.

Neuropharmacology

In the last decade, clomipramine, a drug with relatively selective action on the serotonergic system, appears to have selective benefit in ameliorating obsessive-compulsive symptoms. This striking clinical phenomenon has led to a "serotonergic hypothesis" of OCD (Flament et al. 1987; Insel et al. 1985). The 2- to 4-week delay before the drug is effective, the efficacy of other serotonergic agents, and the short-term worsening of symptoms following MCPP, a serotonergic agonist (Zohar et al. 1988), suggest that down-regulation of the serotonin system mediates the pharmacological efficacy of clomipramine in OCD.

Serotonin is not the aminergic neurotransmitter/neuromodulator most often thought of in relation to the basal ganglia, especially since the nigrostriatal dopamine system has been so intensively investigated. But recent studies have indicated higher concentration of serotonin receptors (5-HT-2) and serotonin itself in the basal ganglia than has previously been recognized (Pazos and Palacios 1985; Pazos et al. 1985; Steinbusch 1981; Stuart et al. 1986). In rats, concentration of serotonin was particularly high in the nucleus accumbens and ventral striatum, but was present throughout the striatum, including the caudate and putamen.

Hypothesis: Basal Ganglia Dysfunction as a Cause of OCD

There has been a prodigious accumulation of new information about the basal ganglia and its interactions with the cerebral cortex and other subcortical structures, most notably the thalamus (Alexander et al. 1986). The innerconnection among these structures can be viewed as forming "loops"; that is, "closed" polysynaptic circuits in which the cortex sends efferents to the basal ganglia, which, while not projecting back to the cortex directly, does so through the dorsal thalamus (Figure 1). An earlier concept of basal ganglia function restricted to motor control has proven too limited, and the initial proposals of one "motor loop" and another "complex loop" have also been found too simple. Nevertheless, the concept of a parallel array of "loops," including the striatum, pallidum, thalamus, and cerebral cortex, has found some

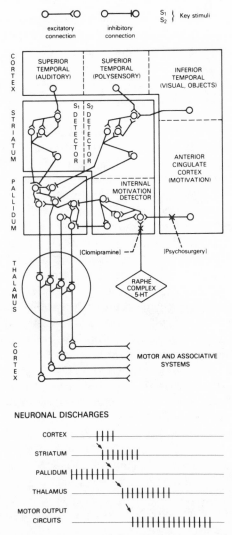

Figure 1. *(Top)* A neural model of obsessive-compulsive disorder. Circuits involved in transfer to the striatum of processed sensory information or information about an internal state are shown to emanate from the cerebral cortex. Two of a large number of stimulus detectors are illustrated in the striatum (the S_1 detector and the S_2 detector). The two detection circuits converge with an internal motivation detector onto one pallidal output cell group. This particular pallidal output is thought to project to the mediodorsal and ventroanterior thalamus, which in turn project to the orbito-frontal cortex. *(Bottom)* Timing of the discharges in structures sketched in the top part of the figure. Each vertical line indicates the time of an action potential discharging from the neural cell group in the structure indicated to the left. The arrows indicate proposed causal relations between the earliest changes in discharge rate of two structures.

general support in current anatomical thinking. It seems likely that some of the parallel loops may function primarily in a motor function, whereas others mediate numerous, complex perceptual and cognitive functions.

Basal Ganglia Anatomy

Before describing our model, it will be valuable to review some basic aspects of basal ganglia anatomy. In addition to the largest and most commonly cited striatal structures, the caudate and putamen, the striatum also includes the nucleus accumbens and parts of the olfactory tubercle. Similarly, in addition to the globus pallidus, the substantia nigra pars reticulata (SNr), parts of the olfactory tubercle, and aspects of the substantia innominata are also pallidal structures (Heimer and Wilson 1975; Heimer et al. 1987; Zahm et al. 1987).

The major input to basal ganglia is a glutamatergic, excitatory projection from the cerebral cortex to the striatum. Additional inputs to the striatum include the well-known dopaminergic input from the midbrain and a serotonergic input from the raphe complex in the brain stem. Within the basal ganglia, inhibitory, GABAergic neurons project from the striatum to the globus pallidus. The major output of the basal ganglia is a GABAergic, inhibitory projection from the globus pallidus to the thalamus, which in turn sends an excitatory input to the cortex. Thus a major pathway to, through, and out of the basal ganglia consists of a "four-neuron loop": (a) from cortex to striatum (excitatory), (b) from striatum to globus pallidus (inhibitory), (c) from globus pallidus to thalamus (inhibitory), and (d) from thalamus to cortex (excitatory). Of course, this simple scheme omits a number of important structures and pathways (including the thalamostriatal projection, the subthalamic nucleus and its connections, and many others). Further, one should not think of this circuit as consisting of four neurons, but rather as four groups of neurons following the basic pattern of the circuit.

The Model

Two ideas about basal ganglia function are central to our hypothesis. One is that the basal ganglia may be a repository of innate motor programs (Greenberg et al. 1979; MacLean 1978; Murphy et al. 1981). The other is that the basal ganglia function, in part, is a gating mechanism for sensory input (Caligiuri and Abbs 1987; Schneider 1984).

Figure 1 illustrates our hypothesis concerning the pathways and processes underlying the basal ganglia–OCD relationship. It is based on a simple model of an innate releasing mechanism in the basal ganglia: a detection mechanism for recognizing specific aspects of stimuli (key or sign stimuli) and a releasing mechanism for the species-typical behavioral response (sometimes known as a fixed-action pattern). Usually, detection of the key stimulus causes release (i.e., execution) of the appropriate behavior. But two sorts of behavior can occur in the absence of a key stimulus. Vacuum behaviors (Ingle and Crews 1985), for example, are often actions that would appropriately be directed toward a specific object but when the object is not present. A bird may snap at insects absent and go through the motions of preparing the nonexistent bugs for its meal (Lorenz 1981). Similarly, displacement behaviors are released when there are "conflicts between two strongly activated antagonistic drives" or "when the normal outlet for a certain motivation is blocked." Displacement activity is of particular relevance here since, as Lorenz has summarized:

> a vast majority of motor patterns appearing as displacement activities are common "everyday" activities . . . the so-called comfort activities of birds and mammals, such as scratching, preening, shaking, furnish the most common examples of displacement activities; when embarrassed, even humans tend to scratch behind the ear—and in other places. (p. 251)

Note that the term *displacement activity*, as used by ethologists, entirely differs from the term as used in dynamic psychiatry. Lorenz pointed out that the original German term would be translated as "sparking-over activities."

The crux of the model presented in Figure 1 involves the convergence of two sets of inputs onto the striatum, particularly the ventromedial aspect of the caudate nucleus and the nucleus accumbens: one from the anterior cingulate cortex and the orbito-frontal cortex and the other from cortical "association" areas thought to be involved in the recognition of objects and sounds (the superior and inferior temporal areas). We postulate that the striatum consists of cell groups acting as stimulus detectors. Some of these detectors can be thought of as innate pattern-recognition circuits; others may be completely or partially learned. We postulate further that in the same general part of the striatum is another type of cell assembly, which we term an "internal motivation detector." These striatal assemblies converge, in our model, to inhibit a pallidal cell assembly, postulated to be tonically discharging. Since the pallidal assembly, in turn, inhibits thalamic neurons, it can be seen that striatal inhibition of the pallidal circuits results in a disinhibition, or release, of the thalamic cell group (labeled "thalamus" in the bottom of Figure 1). In addition, it is postulated that the striatal serotonin system potentiates, by excitatory modulation, inputs to the striatum, including those from anterior cingulate cortex to the "internal motivation detector." This circuit corresponds to the "orbito-frontal loop" of Alexander et al. (1986) and includes the orbito-frontal cortex, the caudate nucleus (striatum), the globus pallidus and the SNr (pallidum), and the ventroanterior and mediodorsal thalamic nuclei.

The way in which we envision these circuits to perform is as follows: The sensory apparatus would relay the appropriate sensory information to the cortex and then to striatum. If the stimulus matches a stored representation in the striatum, then its cells would begin discharging, thus inhibiting the pallidal cells projecting to the thalamus. A simple example might involve the recognition of dirtiness. If sensory input to the striatum indicates that the hands are dirty, an innately programmed striatal cell group would recognize this input as dirtiness. That cell group would then discharge vigorously and stop the tonic discharging of the appropriate pallidal cell. Removal of the inhibitory inputs to the thalamus would release the thalamocortical circuits that lead to the normal behavioral response to dirty hands, hand washing.

The converging circuit, shown in Figure 1, originates from the anterior cingulate cortex and relays to the same pallidal cell group through a different set of striatal neurons. We envision that the circuit would provide a signal whenever the animal was to perform an act because of an exclusively internal motivation. There is some experimental evidence that the cingulate cortex could be important in this circuit, at least for learned movements. Brooks (1986) found that no electrical waves are recorded from the cingulate cortex when a monkey correctly performs a visually triggered limb movement. However, during the same behavior, emitted in the absence of the appropriate visual trigger stimulus, large cingulate cortex potentials are observed. Thus the cingulate cortex seems to be involved in generating behavior in the absence of an appropriate sensory signal, at least in this instance. If signals from cingulate cortex to striatum converge on the same pallidal cell group discussed above (the one responsible for producing the species-typical behavior), then activation of the cingulate cortex would serve to release the behavior without an appropriate sensory stimulus. In our example, hand washing is now triggered via this "internal motivation detector" in the absence of any sensory input signaling dirtiness. If, in OCD, hyperactivity in the cingulate cortex or in the striatum causes activation of this circuit in the absence of any motivation to perform the act, the behavior would be executed compulsively. A similar set of arguments could be made for the cognitive functions of the basal ganglia in relation to obsessional thoughts. Further, if the output of another circuit (not illustrated) were blocked or dysfunctional, build-up of basal ganglia activity with its extensive intrinsic collateral interactions might cause the "sparking over" to a displacement activity of the sort described by Lorenz (1981).

The Model and the Phenomenology of OCD

Several aspects of the OCD data are accounted for by this model, and it makes some testable predictions. First, the effects of psychosurgery are explained since destruction of the anterior cingulate cortex, its thalamic input, its efferent pathways to the caudate nucleus, or the caudate itself would eliminate the excitatory drive to the "internal motivation detector." Lesions of the mediodorsal or ventroanterior thalamus would eliminate the output of this cortico-striato-pallidal loop. Since the striatal cell groups involved in this circuit are viewed as releasing a vacuum behavior or displacement activity, destruction of this pathway should help prevent such release. The model also suggests that hyperexcitability of the anterior cingulate cortex or its striatal target cells may lie at the basis of OCD, and that OCD might be profitably considered a vacuum behavior or displacement activity in the sense that the latter term is used by ethologists. Thus, according to the model, a hyperactive striatal circuit (or of input to it) might periodically produce an output causing a movement pattern, such as grooming or obsessive thought.

The model also incorporates the neuropharmacology of OCD. Clomipramine could be viewed as blocking the potentiation by serotonin of striatal neurons by driving down the number of serotonin receptors. It is important to note that serotonin and its 5-HT-2 receptors are especially high in the caudate nucleus and nucleus accumbens (Pazos et al. 1985). One prediction made by the model is that local injection of serotonin and/or glutamate agonists into the ventromedial caudate nucleus or nucleus accumbens should promote vacuum behavior or other stereotypic motor acts. This idea is consistent with the finding of Zohar et al. (1988) that MCPP, a serotonin agonist, worsens OCD. Another prediction of the model is that glutamate and/or serotonin antagonists might inhibit the production of vacuum or stereotypic behavior, especially if locally injected in the appropriate region of the striatum.

Other observations outlined earlier are also consistent with the model. According to Alexander et al. (1986), only the so-called orbitofrontal loop receives converging inputs from the anterior cingulate cortex and from visual, auditory, and polysensory cortical fields. The specific involvement of this particular "loop" in OCD is indicated by the CT data showing shrinkage of caudate nuclei (but not the putamen) and by the PET data showing metabolic abnormalities in the orbito-frontal cortex and caudate nuclei. Further predictions of the model include the possibility that the thalamic relays of this "loop," the magnocellular division of the ventroanterior nucleus and the magnocellular mediodorsal nucleus, play an important role in OCD.

A question naturally arises as to the pathways by which this loop participates in producing the motor activity. Surprisingly little is known about the connectivity of the orbito-frontal cortex, but recent anatomical evidence from nonhuman primates suggests that it could relay information to the primary motor cortex through the ventral aspects of the premotor cortex (Barbas and Pandya 1987; Matelli et al. 1986).

Discussion

Several obvious difficulties are encountered by our hypothesis and model. Clinically, a great deal of information appears to be inconsistent with our "basal ganglia hypothesis" of OCD. Other neurological disorders of the basal ganglia, such as Huntington's disease and idiopathic parkinsonism, are associated with depression and psychotic symptoms, but not with OCD. In postencephalitic parkinsonian patients, as noted above, lesions outside the basal ganglia may be related to the obsessions. Moreover, a variety of brain insults such as head trauma, diabetes, and birth injury appear to be associated with OCD (Kettle and Marks 1986). It is possible that when these generalized disorders are associated with OCD, there is also basal ganglia damage, but we know of no evidence of such damage. However, differential sensitivity of the basal ganglia to anoxia, and to some neurotoxins, is well established (Laplane et al. 1984). Newer imaging techniques and/or autopsy data may eventually resolve these issues in favor of the "basal ganglia hypothesis," but for now they must be recognized as serious objections.

The present hypothesis also fails to account for three additional features of OCD: its time course, behavioral specificity (for one or two thoughts or actions at a time), and the efficacy of behavior therapy. As for time course, we can only speculate that degenerative changes in the basal ganglia or related part of the "orbito-frontal loop" might parallel the time course of the disease. But why such degeneration would lead to relatively long periods of symptom stability remains unaddressed by our model. Similarly, we have little to offer concerning the behavioral specificity of OCD beyond the invocation of highly localized brain abnormalities and the possibility that circuits producing one species-typical behavior, such as grooming, might overlap and share many of the same elements with that for another behavior, even cognitive functions like checking for contaminants. Regarding behavior modification, effectiveness of therapies based on behaviorist theory might appear to contradict our hypothesis, but the relationship between the cause of a disease and its treatment is not straightforward. A good example of this principle is seen in dyslexia. Although it is now thought that dyslexia is caused by disruption of species-specific learning (see e.g., Vallutino 1987), and that the disorder is not caused by malfunctional reinforcement history, this does not mean that special education is not an effective treatment. *Mutatis mutandum*; the same might be said of OCD.

In addition to being consistent with the phenomenology of OCD, the present hypothesis views the basal ganglia and OCD in a high, cognitive context, viewing it as did the French, as "folie de doute," the doubting disease. If one for the moment ignores the content of the obsessions and rituals (e.g., contamination, sex, violence), the other striking aspect of the disorder is the defect in knowing. Patients who are "checkers" or "washers" appear to be in a Berkleyan nightmare—tied to their immediate sensory systems, needing continuous reaffirmation that their hands are clean, the door is locked, and so on. The ruminators, on the other hand, are trying to "think their way out" using pure reason as the road to true knowledge. Ultimately, however, checkers and ruminators both are paralyzed skeptics who doubt their own senses and their own reasoning. The hypothesis presented here suggests a biological system underlying an "epistemological sense," in this case involving the rejection or acceptance of sensory input, ideas, explanations, and thoughts.

References

Alexander G, DeLong M, Strick P: Parallel organization of functionally segregated circuits linking basal ganglia and cortex. Annu Rev Neurosci 9:357–381, 1986

Barbas H, Pandya D: Architecture and frontal cortical connections of the premotor cortex (area 6) in the rhesus monkey. J Comp Neurol 256:211–228, 1987

Baxter L, Phelps M, Mazziotti J, et al: Local cerebral glucose metabolic rates of obsessive compulsive disorder compared to unipolar depression and normal controls. Arch Gen Psychiatry 44:211–218, 1987

Brooks V: Does the limbic system assist motor learning? A limbic comparator hypothesis. Brain Behav Evol 29:29–53, 1986

Caligiuri MP, Abbs JH: Response properties of the perioral reflex in Parkinson's disease. Exp Neurol 98:563–572, 1987

de la Tourette G: Etude sur une affection nerveuse caraterisee par de l'incoordination motrice accompagnee d'echolalie et de coprolie. Arch Neurol 9:19–42, 1885

Dunnett D: Elbow Room: The Varieties of Free Will Worth Wanting. Cambridge, MA, MIT Press, 1984

Flament M, Rapoport JL, Murphy D, et al: Biochemical changes during clomipramine treatment of childhood obsessive compulsive disorder. Arch Gen Psychiatry 44:219–225, 1987

Freeman J, Ann A, Collard J, et al: The emotional correlates of Sydenham's chorea. Pediatrics 35:42–49, 1965

Greenberg N, MacLean PD, Ferguson JL: Role of the paleostriatum in species-typical display behavior of the lizard. Brain Res 172:229–241, 1979

Greenfield G, Wolfsohn MJ: The pathology of Sydenham's chorea. Lancet 2:603–607, 1922

Grimshaw L: Obsessional disorder and neurological illness. J Neurol Neurosurg Psychiatry 27:229–231, 1964

Hassler R: The role of the thalamus and striatum in the causation of tics and compulsive vocalization. Presented at First International Tourette Syndrome Symposium, New York, 1981

Heimer L, Wilson R: The subcortical projections of allocortex: similarities in the neural associations of the hippocampus, the piriform cortex and the neocortex, in Golgi Centennial Symposium Proceedings. Edited by M. Santini. New York, Raven Press, 1975

Heimer L, Zaborszky L, Zahm D, et al: The ventral striatopallidothalamic projection: I: the striatopallidal link originating in the striatal parts of the olfactory tubercle. J Comp Neurol 255:571–591, 1987

Husby G, van de Rijn I, Zabriskie J, et al: Antibodies reacting with cytoplasm of subthalamic and caudate nuclei neurons in chorea and rheumatic fever. J Exp Med 144:1094–1110, 1976

Ingle D, Crews D: Vertebrate neurothology: definition and paradigms. Annu Rev Neurosci 8:457–495, 1985

Insel T, Mueller E, Alterman I: Obsessive compulsive disorder and serotonin: is there a connection? Biol Psychiatry 20:1174–1188, 1985

Karno M, Golding J, Sorensun S, et al: The epidemiology of obsessive compulsive disorder in five U.S. communities. Arch Gen Psychiatry (in press)

Kettle P, Marks I: Neurological factors in obsessive compulsive disorder. Br J Psychiatry 149:315–319, 1986

Laplane D, Baulac M, Widlocher D, et al: Pure psychic akinesia with bilateral lesions of basal ganglia. J Neurol Neurosurg Psychiatry 47:377–385, 1984

Lorenz KZ: The Foundations of Ethology. New York, Springer-Verlag, 1981

Luxenberg JS, Flament M, Swedo S, et al: Neuroanatomic abnormalities in obsessive-compulsive disorder detected in quantitative x-ray computed tomography. Am J Psychiatry (in press)

MacLean PD: Effects of lesions of globus pallidus on species-typical display behavior of squirrel monkeys. Brain Res 149:175–196, 1978

Matelli M, Camarda R, Glickstein M, et al: Afferent and efferent projections of the interior area 6 in the macaques monkey. J Comp Neurol 251:281–298, 1986

Murphy MR, MacLean PD, Hamilton SC: Species-typical behavior of hamsters deprived from birth of the neocortex. Science 213:459–461, 1981

Osler W: On Chorea and Choreiform Affections. Philadelphia, Blakiston & Sons, 1894

Pauls D, Towbin K, Leckman J, et al: Gilles de la Tourette syndrome and obsessive-compulsive disorder: evidence supporting a genetic relationship. Arch Gen Psychiatry 43:1180–1182, 1986

Pazos A, Palacios J: Quantitative autoradiographic mapping of serotonin receptors in rat brain: I: serotonin I receptors. Brain Res 346:205–230, 1985

Pazos A, Cortes R, Palacios J: Quantitative autoradiographic mapping of serotonin in rat brain: II: serotonin II receptors. Brain Res 356:231–249, 1985

Schneider JS: Basal ganglia role in behavior: importance of sensory gating and its relevance to psychiatry. Biol Psychiatry 19:1693–1709, 1984

Steinbusch H: Distribution of serotonin-immunoreactivity in the central nervous system of the rat. Neuroscience 6:557–618, 1981

Stuart A, Slater JM, Unwin HL, Crossman AR: A semiquantitative atlas of 5-hydroxytryptamine-1 receptors in the primate brain. Neuroscience 18:619–639, 1986

Swedo S, Rapoport J, Cheslow D, et al: Increased incidence of obsessive compulsive features in patients with Sydenham's Chorea. Poster presentation at 34th Annual Meeting of the American Academy of Child Psychiatry, Washington, DC, October 1987

Vallutino F: Dyslexia. Sci Am 256:34–41, 1987

von Economo C: Encephalitis Lethargica: its sequellae and treatment. London, Oxford University Press, 1931 [Translated from von Economo: Die enceptalitis lethargica Deuticke, Vienna 1917–1918. L'encephalik lethargica, Policlinica Rome, 1920]

Zahm DS, Zaborszky L, Alheid GF, et al: The ventral striatopallidothalamic projection: II: the ventral pallidothalamic link. J Comp Neurol 255:592–605, 1987

Zohar J, Mueller E, Insel T, et al: Serotonin receptor sensitivity in obsessive compulsive disorder: comparison of patients and healthy controls. Arch Gen Psychiatry 44:211–218, 1988

Section VII

Summary

Chapter 20

Summary

Judith L. Rapoport, M.D.

This book has had the ambitious goal of providing an up-to-date picture of clinical phenomenology, diagnosis, treatment, theory, and research relevant to childhood obsessive-compulsive disorder (OCD). Most of the data discussed here have been drawn from our own studies because the NIMH series comprises the largest cohort of such children ever to be studied systematically and prospectively. Reference to other studies has been made, however, where appropriate. The explosion of new clinical and research information only intensifies rather than settles the classic questions about OCD. We hope that the reader is left, as we are, with greater optimism about eventual understanding of this illness in view of these many new findings.

As the disease is far more frequent both in children and adults than had been previously thought, there will be a great increase in the recognition and treatment of OCD. These clinical data will be forthcoming with unprecedented speed, and the hypotheses put forth in this book and elsewhere will be tested over a few years rather than over a generation. Even now, however, a great deal has become clear.

The patient and family essays have been included because of the great lack of direct clinical experience and training with obsessive-compulsive children (or adults) in most psychiatrists' experience. It is obvious that more firsthand patient exposure is needed for adequate clinical training. In addition, there is a unique flavor of objectivity and shame in these writings that illustrates to us the painful progression of

347

uncontrollable habits or ruminations in otherwise rational and sensible individuals.

Then there is the remarkable similarity between the disorder as it presents in childhood and in adults. While psychological testing and checklists are useful and, indeed, we would not be without them, the diagnosis must still be made by clinical interview. Both adults and children show a preponderance of washing rituals. The preponderance of males is unmistakable and as yet unexplained. It may be that females with childhood onset manifest the disorder in different form. Trichotillomania may be a variant of OCD seen almost exclusively in girls. Are OCD and trichotillomania variants of instinctual grooming patterns run wild? Family and treatment studies are ongoing to address this issue.

The associated measures of neuropsychology, psycholinguistics, and neurology provide tantalizing evidence for subtle central nervous system dysfunction. These abnormalities appear more consistently in pediatric populations than they have in most adults series, perhaps because compensatory development has not yet taken place. As Dr. Cox et al. implied (Chapter 5), frontal lobe–caudate dysfunction may be reflected in the psychological test pattern. Does this mean that in OCD more "primitive" patterns are inappropriately activated by frontal lobe input?

Our own developmental data provide indirect support for OCD as an emergent illness relatively independent of both cultural and normal developmental factors. First there is little developmental continuity, either with respect to prevalence of superstitions or normal developmental routines of early childhood. In addition, parent description of development of patterns predating the disorder is usually normal. All this evidence for discontinuity mediates against the disorder as a variant of anxiety disorder.

There is amazingly little information on developmental norms for superstitions and for childhood rituals. It would be of great interest to study both the normal pattern as well as individual differences with respect to implications for development. We rely on our colleagues in child development and anthropology to work with us in this area.

The similarity of symptom patterns across widely different cultures and across ages also supports a biological basis for OCD. It is evident, however, that there is some culturally determined influence in the content of the obsessions. For example, preoccupation with AIDS has displayed itself prominently in our patients' presenting thoughts and rituals. Further cross-cultural studies of OCD are waiting to be undertaken.

Epidemiological research with adults has been extremely important for awakening interest in OCD. However, the NIMH Epidemiological Catchment Area study was so broad that OCD could only be covered in a relatively superficial fashion. An in-depth study of a large population to identify any associated stressors, subtypes of disorder, and associated features, as well as to examine the relationship to personality disorder, is badly needed.

Our own adolescent epidemiological and clinical samples both contained significant numbers of cases with anxiety disorders (see chapters on diagnosis and epidemiology). Here, too, there is considerable conceptual confusion. Although most agree that OCD has some comorbidity with anxiety disorders, still obsessive-compulsive patients generally are less anxious than patients with generalized-anxiety disorder and many are not anxious at all. Conceptual confusion is further generated by the findings in Sweden (and elsewhere) that psychosurgery is helpful for anxiety disorders, generalized anxiety disorder phobias, and OCD as well.

The relationship between OCD and compulsive personality remains completely unresolved. The data presented in this volume serve actually to confuse, rather than to resolve, the already uncertain relationship. We need to remember that the ICD-9 concept of ankastic personality is similar to our "subclinical disorder" or what we refer to as "obsessional features." There was a substantial group of such individuals, as important a subgroup as those meeting DSM-III (or DSM-III-R) criteria for compulsive personality disorder. DSM-III and DSM-III-R stress the ego-syntonic nature as well as the somewhat different behavioral descriptors for compulsive personality disorder.

With that in mind, it is already clear that compulsive personality (DSM-III) occurs with a small but significant percentage of our clinical obsessive-compulsive cases.

To make matters even more complex, follow-up studies (in progress) suggest that some cases of OCD may later present as compulsive personality disorder. Developmental studies will be crucial to see whether certain positive and adaptive traits may lead to a view of initial obsessive-compulsive symptom presentation as ego-syntonic, "accepted" and incorporated as a modus operandum.

The classic pattern of OCD in association with known brain disorders and lesions, the genetics of OCD per se (20 percent in first-degree relatives in our sample) and in relation to Tourette's syndrome, and the neurological and neuropsychological abnormalities within our patients all suggest a biological factor as etiologic. Furthermore, the specificity of clomipramine relative to other tricyclic antidepressants strongly invokes serotonergic dysfunction mediating this illness.

It remains mysterious how it is possible that complex behavior patterns such as washing, doubting, and checking, as well as "neutral" events such as images of tunes or neutral phrases are transmitted. Is there evolutionary significance to such transmission? What strategy is appropriate for further study?

The theoretical chapters on ethology and on a basal ganglia model have been included not because they are uniquely applicable to childhood OCD, but rather because childhood OCD has lent itself particularly well to the study of these models, and because pediatric cases are overrepresented in most neurologically based series. The remarkably similar and rigid patterns of these children's washing and checking would satisfy Konrad Lorenz that an instinctual pattern has been somehow "set loose!"

Treatment research in OCD has been particularly enthusiastic in the past decade. Despite these beginnings, the most important clinical questions remain. It is not known if there are certain children for whom behavioral treatment is not indicated. Should behavioral treatment be tried first for most cases? The intuitive answer would be yes for ritualizers and no for ruminators, but this has not been proven. Comparisons of behavioral and drug treatments have been carried out with adults in a very preliminary way, but parallel studies with unselected groups of adolescents have not been undertaken.

Finally, we do not know whether treatments will have any effect on long-term outcome. Our own prospective follow-up of children and adolescents maintained on drug and/or behavioral treatment is underway. Hopefully, there will be improvement in this new, more aggressively treated group over the generally poor follow-up seen in our pilot follow-up study (cited in Chapter 2).

Finally, the relation between obsessive-compulsive symptoms, individual preoccupations with cleanliness, and the communal symbolic rites of expiation and group safety invokes profound anthropological and philosophical issues. Understanding the interplay between such biologically induced patterns and cultural idiom will enrich us all.

Index